Edited by
Denise C. Murphy, DrPH, COHN

ERGONOMICS

AND

THE

DENTAL CARE WORKER

©1998 by the American Public Health Association

AMERICAN PUBLIC HEALTH ASSOCIATION
1015 Fifteenth Street, NW
Washington, DC 20005-2605

Mohammad N. Akhter, MD, MPH
Executive Director

Library of Congress card catalog number 98-072439.

ISBN: 0-87553-0233-0

2M 9/98

The use of trade names and commercial sources by authors in certain chapters of this compendium does not imply endorsement by either the APHA or the editorial board of this book.

Printed and bound in the United States of America
Typesetting: Patti Wolf, Wolf Publications, Inc.
Set in: Palatino and Helvetica
Cover Design: Steve Trapero Design
Printing: United Book Press, Inc.

Table of Contents

Foreword

The dental profession justifiably takes great pride in the accolades accorded it by the public and other health professionals with regard to the preventive orientation of its patient care and public health activities. It is, therefore, ironic that relatively little attention has been given, over the years, to the prevention of adverse health consequences among the practitioners of dentistry, dental hygiene, and associated occupations.

The mental and emotional stresses associated with clinical practice have been widely appreciated by the dental profession for many years. Less widely understood and of more recent interest is the level of disability caused by physical stress associated with the performance of clinical procedures, even when the mental and emotional demands are well within the adaptive capacity of the clinician.

Many years ago, common complaints of eye strain led to the development and use of supplemental lenses. Complaints about back strain led to the design of new chairs and the implementation of "sit-down dentistry." "Tired forearms" motivated development of mechanical condensers and ultrasonic scaling instruments. Ergonomic principles, limited by the knowledge base of the era, were used to make jobs fit workers, instead of making workers fit jobs. In the late 1960s, "four-handed dentistry" methods were developed in innovative clinics at dental schools, were evaluated and promoted by the U.S. Public Health Service, and by the mid-1970s were implemented in the majority of dental practices throughout the land. After many years of improved productivity, during which dental professionals were able to do more and more for their patients in shorter periods of time, other problems associated with modern treatment methods were recognized.

We are only now beginning to understand the prevalence and intensity of occupational health and safety problems in dentistry. Since most dentists are self-employed and their disability patterns are not recorded by the Bureau of Labor Statistics, the prevalence of musculoskeletal disorders and their contribution to disability in the dental profession have been underreported. Because of this underreporting, dentistry may not have received the attention and investment that it deserves from researchers, health agencies, and equipment manufacturers in the development of ergonomically designed instruments and work stations. However, the significance and consequences of the problem are clear. In their roles both as self-employed individuals and as employers (through disability and worker's compensation insurance) dentists ultimately bear a high share of the burden of compensating colleagues and auxiliaries who become disabled in the performance of clinical dental activities. Because of the high cost of dental education and the long period of time necessary to become an experienced dental practitioner, society pays a high price whenever dental professionals must curtail the performance of clinical activities as a result of the stress and strain of work-related health hazards.

The editor, Dr Denise Murphy, is to be commended for her foresight in recognizing the need for this book. She and the contributors to this volume have provided a great service to the dental profession and the public. The book is comprehensive, addressing a wide array of issues related to the promotion of modern ergonomic principles that would improve the safety, health, quality of work, and productivity of dental care workers. Its availability to the profession is an important step toward encouraging the exchange of ergonomic program experience and knowledge. Furthermore, this information will be useful to dental schools that are making efforts to emphasize the importance of good work practices to future dental clinicians, so that those clinicians may avoid disorders experienced by those who have preceded them.

This book describes and documents our knowledge of the state of the art and science of ergonomics in dentistry. It provides background in the principles of ergonomics and discusses specific problems with dental equipment and techniques commonly used by dental care workers. The volume also includes the perspective of the American Dental Association and describes the association's research and educational efforts. Other authors discuss promising efforts to improve clinical practice ergonomics by development of new approaches. Finally, the book offers practical tips of real "hands-on" information, including a working checklist for self-evaluation.

As this book is published, much controversy remains as to the merits of more aggressive promotion of ergonomic standards by the Occupational Safety and Health Administration. The alternative would be more independent establishment of voluntary guidelines by the dental profession, along with continuing education to improve awareness of hazards and of the means of avoiding those hazards. The debate is not resolved by this book. Ultimately, a combination of work site modification, including the development and use of more ergonomically sound instruments and equipment, and commitment by individuals to engage in healthier work habits and techniques will be most effective. However, this book will serve as a valuable primer for all dental care professionals, including students of each discipline, and will raise the level of knowledge about dental care ergonomics. From that more informed vantage point, we can begin to resolve the debate and move forward to address work factors, to reduce the risk of musculoskeletal disorders, and to build a healthier, more productive profession.

William R. Maas, D.D.S., M.P.H.
Chief Dental Officer
U.S. Public Health Service

Introduction

Denise C. Murphy, Editor

The need for a book in the field of dental ergonomics has developed over time. The early 1980s was the era of the "meat packing standard," a document developed by the Occupational Safety and Health Administration (OSHA) that focused on the ergonomic/biomechanical hazards associated with only this high-risk industry. However, this document was to serve as an early indicator of a future standard that would apply to multiple and varied sectors of the national workforce.

Numerous journal articles have documented the existence of ergonomic disorders among dental care workers. However, there is no one comprehensive document, and the level of awareness of this subject matter appears to be low among dental care workers. A short mail survey designed to ascertain this level of awareness was conducted in 1997. The results indicated a need for early education both among those preparing for and among those practicing in the field of dentistry.

The goal of this book is to provide the reader with a timely, interesting, user-friendly, comprehensive, and practical source of information about ergonomics and the dental care worker; it is intended to serve teachers as well as students and practitioners of dentistry including those in doctor of dental surgery, dental hygienist, and dental assistant programs. Various aspects of ergonomics and various viewpoints are included to allow a broad overview of the subject. The authors have many different disciplinary backgrounds—they are dentists, dental hygienists, architects, ergonomists, occupational therapists, physicians, academicians, occupational health and safety specialists, and public health experts. All authors have had personal experience with the subject matter.

In addition to an introduction to the field of ergonomics and chapters that address the various work-related biomechanical problems experienced by workers, other chapters stress prevention and control. Some chapters introduce the reader to the scope and impact of work-related disorders, and other chapters offer multiple strategies for prevention—always a much less costly alternative to treatment. Tools to assist readers in applying information to their own workplaces include definitions of ergonomic terminology, a list of resources, and a checklist to be used as benchmarks for individual practices.

There is now indication that OSHA will initiate a federal standard related to ergonomics in this decade. If that occurs, employers in all at-risk occupations, including dental care, will be required by law to assume specific responsibilities (following the format of the Bloodborne Pathogens Standard of 1991) to protect themselves and their employees. The costs associated with biomechanical work-related disorders in dentistry are large in terms of reduced productivity, worker compensation, lost work-days, and, most importantly, human suffering. Regardless of whether federal legislation is promulgated to mandate workplace controls, we, as responsible health care professionals, have an obligation to advocate for prevention of these disorders and to take whatever steps are necessary to achieve this goal.

I would like to thank each of the collaborating authors, as well as Doctor Alice Horowitz, who served as my liaison with the American Public Health Association, which supported this effort. All of the authors have generously contributed their time and energy in producing this book because we all recognize the importance of this endeavor. It is our sincere hope that you, the reader, will both enjoy and benefit from reading this book.

Contributors

Michael M. Belenky, DDS, MPH, FACD, FPFA, Associate Professor, Department of Oral Health Care Delivery, Dental School, University of Maryland at Baltimore.

Margit L. Bleecker, MD, PhD, Center for Occupational and Environmental Neurology, Baltimore, Maryland.

Marcia A. Boyd, DDS, MA, Department of Oral Health Sciences, The University of British Columbia.

Ralph Bruder, Prof. Dr. Ing.,Department of Design and Arts Education, University of Essen, Germany.

Martin Cherniack, MD, MPH, Director, Ergonomics Technology Center of Connecticut; Professor, University of Connecticut School of Medicine.

Eve Cuny, CDA, RDA, Director of Environmental Health and Safety, University of the Pacific School of Dentistry.

Jonathan Dropkin, MS, PT, Ergonomics Coordinator, Mount Sinai/I.J. Selikoff Center for Environmental and Occupational Medicine.

Richard E. Fredekind, DMD, MA, Group Practice Administrator, University of the Pacific School of Dentistry.

Fred Gerr, MD, Associate Professor, Environmental and Occupational Health Department, School of Public Health, Emory University.

Robin Mary Gillespie, MPH, Ergonomics Specialist, Hunter College Center for Occupational and Environmental Health, NY.

Edward G. Grace, DDS, MA, FAGD, Associate Professor and Director, Facial Pain Clinic, Facial Pain Center, Dental School, University of Maryland at Baltimore.

Albert H. Guay, DMD, Associate Executive Director, Division of Dental Practice, American Dental Association.

Manny Halpern, MA, CPE, Ergonomics Coordinator, Occupational and Industrial Orthopedic Center (OIOC), New York University Medical Center Hospital for Joint Diseases.

Alan Hedge, PhD, Professor, Department of Design and Environmental Analysis, College of Human Ecology, Cornell University.

Robin Herbert, MD, Medical Codirector, Mount Sinai/I.J. Selikoff Center for Environmental and Occupational Medicine, Associate Professor, Mount Sinai, Department of Community and Preventative Medicine.

Evie Jesin, RDH, BSc, Allied Health Department, George Brown College of Applied Arts and Technology.

Eckardt Johanning, MD, MSc, Eastern New York Occupational and Environmental Center.

Sachiko Kawaguchi, Human Space USA, Inc.

Ellen A. Kolber, MS, MA, OTR, CHT, Diversified Ergonomics, NYC.

Stephen Levin, MD, Medical Director, Mount Sinai/I.J. Selikoff Center for Environmental and Occupational Medicine.

Gary M. Liss, MD, MS, Medical Consultant, Ontario Ministry of Labor, Toronto, Ontario, Canada.

Jean Mangharam, PT, MS, University of Cincinnati, School of Medicine, Department of Environmental Health, Division of Environmental and Industrial Hygiene.

Phyllis E. Marino, MD, Medical Director, Occupational Health Services, Chilton Memorial Hospital.

James D. McGlothlin, Senior Research Ergonomist/Industrial Hygienist, Division of Physical Sciences and Engineering, Engineering Control Technology Branch, National Institute for Occupational Safety and Health, NIOSH, Cincinnatti, Ohio.

Denise C. Murphy, DrPH, COHN, Occupational Health/Infection Control, New York University College of Dentistry.

Patricia J. Nunn, RDH, MS, Associate Professor and Chair, Dental Hygiene Department, College of Dentistry, University of Oklahoma.

Gary Orr, PE, CPE, Ergonomist, Occupational Safety and Health Administration, Washington, DC.

Lance M. Rucker, DDS, Director of Clinical Simulation, Faculty of Dentistry, The University of British Columbia.

John C. Wittenstrom, DDS, Private Practice, Minneapolis, MN, former Coordinator, Human Performance and Informatics Institute of North America.

Chapter 1

Introduction to Ergonomics

Alan Hedge

Abstract

This chapter presents an overview of the discipline of ergonomics and its relevance to dental work. Following a brief account of the history of ergonomics, the chapter describes six categories of topics that ergonomists typically study: user-technology interface design issues (physical and cognitive design), workplace design and layout, physical environment conditions, job design, selection and training, and organizational design and management. The concept of a human-technology system, which is fundamental to ergonomic design analysis, is presented, and examples are given of how this system can be applied to dental situations. The chapter also covers the use of task analysis to improve human-technology system design. Many ergonomic product designs revolve around the concept of 'neutral' posture, and the basic principles of 'neutral' posture are summarized. Finally, the chapter gives some guidance on how to judge the ergonomic design of a product.

Ergonomics—A Source of Confusion?

From being an unfamiliar term only a few years ago, "ergonomics" has become a buzzword in the 1990s. Ergonomics has come to mean many things to different people, and, perhaps not surprisingly, the term has become shrouded by confusion and bewilderment. This confusion stems, in part, from widespread descriptions of products as being "ergonomically" designed. An amazing array of products, from cars, computers, and office furniture, to cutlery, clocks, wheels, and even tortilla chips, are advertised as being ergonomically designed. Unfortunately, the term 'ergonomic' is rapidly becoming so overused that it is losing any value as a way of distinguishing between a well-designed product and its less well-designed alternatives. What company, for example, would now set out to buy or sell office chairs that are specifically described as "not ergonomically designed"? So the adjective "ergonomic"

1

often is of limited value in helping with purchasing decisions, unless the consumer also has a good grasp of what the discipline of "ergonomics" strives to achieve and some understanding of the basic concepts and principles that form the basis for ergonomic product design.

What few people realize, however, is that ergonomics is an applied-science discipline that was founded almost 50 years ago. Again, recent marketing use of the term has created confusion about the discipline of ergonomics. For some, "ergonomics" becomes synonymous with therapeutic interventions and other actions that can prevent musculoskeletal injuries, such as back injuries or occupational overuse injuries like carpal tunnel syndrome. In 1996 the Occupational Safety and Health Administration developed a draft "ergonomics standard," specifically aimed at reducing injury risks to workers, which conveyed this image of the discipline. From this regulatory perspective ergonomics is seen as reactive approach to occupational injuries that have already arisen, and it involves the application of a collection of methods for physical work activities. To meet the anticipated demand for ergonomic analysis of workplaces, many health professionals, such as physical therapists and industrial hygienists, have become "ergonomists" almost overnight. However, much to the chagrin of many ergonomists, the discipline of ergonomics is, in fact, much broader than this use of the word implies.

This chapter attempts to clarify the considerable confusion that surrounds the term "ergonomics." It describes how the discipline of ergonomics has developed, what types of work ergonomists do, what criteria define a product as being ergonomically designed, what principles underlie judgments about whether a workplace is or is not 'ergonomic' and, above all, why ergonomics is important to everyone as a *proactive* discipline. This information will serve as a foundation for other material that will be presented in this book.

Ergonomics—The Laws of Work

The discipline of ergonomics was formalized after the end of World War II. Human performance studies, mainly of pilots, sonar and radar operators, conducted by psychologists in Great Britain during and immediately following World War II, had demonstrated the importance of designing technologies that fit the dimensions and capabilities of the human body and that complement human physical and mental abilities. Oborne (1982) gives an excellent summary of the history of ergonomics.[1] On February 16, 1950, the word "ergonomics," from the Greek "ergon" (work) and "nomos" (natural laws—hence, "the laws of work"), was adopted to describe this new human performance–oriented engineering design discipline.* The Ergonomics Research Society (now called the Ergonomics Society) was formed in the United Kingdom in 1949 as the professional body for this newly established discipline. Around this time, similar work was being undertaken in the United States, but mainly by engineers who, because they were dealing with the role of human beings in increasingly complex technological systems, named this same discipline "human factors." In 1957, the US Human Factors Society was founded. In the early days, other terms were applied to the study of ergonomics, including "human engineering" and "engineering psychology." All of these terms shared a focus on how best to design systems in which people would use technology to the greatest effect. As the study of ergonomics became a worldwide endeavor, the International Ergonomics Society was formed in 1959 to coordinate international activities. Today, 28 member countries have their own professional ergonomics societies, with over 16,000 members worldwide. In 1992, the US society renamed itself the Human Factors and Ergonomics Society. This society now has over 5000 professional members, and 20 different technical groups. Essentially there is no difference between Human Factors and Ergonomics, and the term "ergonomics" probably has gained greater public recognition merely because it has been used as an advertising adjective to describe many products.

Modern ergonomics is a multidisciplinary applied science that involves studying ways of optimizing the design of people-technology systems, through knowledge of human

---

*The earliest use of the word "ergonomics" was by Professor Wojciech Jastrzebowski, a Polish researcher interested in work performance, in 1857.

physical and mental abilities, human performance limits, factors affecting human reliability and errors, anthropometrics (the science of anatomy), work physiology, biomechanics, work environment conditions, human behavior as individuals and in teams, industrial design and engineering, skills learning and training, and management and organizational behavior. Figure 1 names some of the disciplines that contribute to ergonomics.

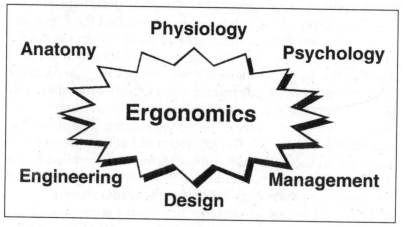

FIGURE 1.—Ergonomics is a multidisciplinary science.

The goal of ergonomics is to continually strive to develop new and better ways to optimize the performance of people using products (technology) to perform work more effectively in a given physical setting, by changing the design of the product, the job, the workplace layout, the work environment conditions, the organizational system, the training or some combination of these elements. Indeed, a good definition of ergonomics (human factors) is that this is a discipline that "discovers and applies information about human behavior, abilities, limitations, and other characteristics to the design of tools, machines, systems, tasks, jobs and environments for productive, safe, comfortable and effective human use" (Chapanis, 1985, cited in McCormick & Sanders, 1993).[2]

What Do Ergonomists Study?

Given the broad definition of the discipline of ergonomics, ergonomists must study a wide variety of aspects of workplaces, and ultimately, many specialize in specific areas. As Galer (1987)[3] points out, many topics are of interest to ergonomists, including at a minimum those shown in Figure 2.

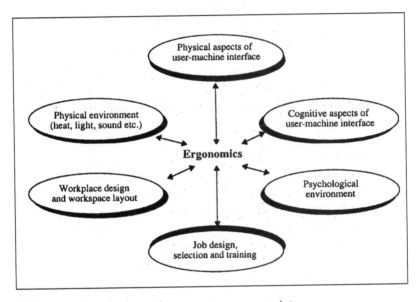

FIGURE 2.—Topic areas of interest to ergonomists.

User-Technology Interface Design: Physical Design

Understanding how people can most effectively interact with technology is fundamental to ergonomics. A basic requirement of any ergonomic design is that the physical dimensions of the technology must fit the anthropometric dimensions of the user or users. Anthropometry is the science of measuring the dimensions of the human body and its parts, and tables of anthropometric data can be used to determine appropriate product dimensions for different sets of users. Anthropometric dimensions are usually expressed as percentiles, and most ergonomic designs attempt to satisfy a range of users, usually from a 5th percentile woman to a 95th percentile man, for a given dimension. For example, a height-adjustable office chair may adjust from the seated leg height of a 5th percentile woman to that of a 95th percentile man. If a design can be adjusted to accommodate this range, then it should prove satisfactory for 90% of users (i.e., $95 - 5 = 90$). However, this means that even an ergonomically designed product perhaps will still not satisfy the requirements of 1 in 10 people (those women at less than the 5th percentile and those men above the 95th percentile represent 10% of all users). Depending on the type of product being designed, ergonomists use either static anthropometric dimensions for the appropriate body parts, such as a person's seated height or arm length, or dynamic anthropometric dimensions, such as the person's reach distance, or both. For example, in designing a dentist's chair the designer must look at how the chair should be contoured to accommodate a wide range of users (patients), and then over what range this chair can be height adjusted by the dentist, as well as where other equipment needs to be placed so that this can conveniently be reached by the dentist while he or she is examining a patient in the chair at that height.

Usually ergonomists try to influence product designs so that the greatest range of users can be accommodated. (For example, in designing the adjustments for a car seat, the designer wants to accommodate the greatest number of potential drivers.) Sometimes, when the user population is well defined or is even selected for a body dimension, the products are sized just for those users (e.g., the seat for a race car driver is contoured just for that driver and would be uncomfortable for another person). Thus, ergonomists apply anthropometric data to help with a continuum of design from custom-designed products to universal designs aimed at a general user population.

In addition to defining the size of a product or product component, ergonomists also help to define other attributes, such as its shape, color, and texture, along with the force that is required to operate the product and the direction of movement of any controls used to operate the product. These choices are usually also based on human-performance considerations. For example, the size of a product might be based on the body part that will operate the product, such as the hand or foot;

the shape of the product might be based on the type of grasp that is desirable, such as a power grip; and the color might be based on user expectations, such as green for "go" or red for "danger."

User-Technology Interface Design: Cognitive Design

As well as being able to physically operate technology, ergonomists also give careful consideration to people's expectations about how equipment works, and to any information displays associated with the equipment, such as warning signs, labels, and instructional materials. Arrangements of knobs (controls) and burners (information displays) on a stove frequently show the problems that can occur when designers fail to take account of people's expectations about which control operates which burner and, for rotary controls, which direction the control needs to be turned to raise the heat. A walk through a local appliances store will quickly confirm that designs vary greatly among models and manufacturers. Video-cassette recorders (VCRs) also often typify cognitive design problems. It has been suggested that most people never learn to correctly program their VCRs, and the plethora of small, strangely labeled buttons on most VCR remote controls confuses many users.

Ergonomists look at technology from the standpoint of what both naive users and trained users expect, what information needs to be presented to the users how best to present that information, what information users, need to learn, and how best to train them. When the layout and operation of controls and displays follow our expectations, the association is said to be compatible, and numerous research studies have confirmed that reaction times are fastest and error rates are lowest with compatible arrangements. For example, the widespread use of the graphical user interface (GUI) on modern personal computers has made these complicated devices easier to use.

Workplace Design and Workspace Layout

The way in which any work space is arranged can substantially affect a worker's health and how well work is done.

Ergonomists use several techniques to optimize the layout of a workplace and its workspaces along the following principles:
- *convenience* (the equipment used for those tasks performed most frequently is located most conveniently to the worker)
- *location* (equipment is located so that workers can access it without moving into a deviated posture such as bending down, leaning over, or twisting around), and
- *frequency* (those tasks most frequently performed in conjunction are located most closely together).

Resulting layouts ensure that workers maintain the best posture and use the least effort to perform the work. In this way work output can be sustained without the worker experiencing undue levels of fatigue. Physical and mental fatigue slow overall work performance, reduce work quality, and increase the chance of mistakes.

Physical Environment Conditions at Work

In the early years of ergonomics research, considerable effort was devoted to studying environmental hazards in factory and mining workplaces, such as heat or cold stress, noise stress, and inadequate lighting. Such industrial workplaces are still of interest to many ergonomists. However, a majority of today's labor force work in less physically challenging settings, and more recently, attention has focused on the same aspects of the white-collar workplace, especially issues of lighting for computerized offices; thermal comfort; indoor air quality; noise and disturbances; vibration (a particular problem in mobile workplaces such as cars, planes, and trains); and electromagnetic fields. Ergonomists also study extreme environments such as space, deep-sea habitats, desert habitats, and arctic or Antarctic habitats. The Human Factors and Ergonomics Society has a technical group devoted to environmental-design issues. The same environmental factors are also studied by other disciplines, such as industrial hygiene, but there is a difference in focus; industrial hygiene focuses on whether specific environmental conditions affect human health and safety, whereas ergonomics also studies how conditions affect human performance, comfort, and satisfaction, often at exposures that are less than those necessary to produce health effects.

Job Design, Selection, and Training

Virtually all jobs have to be designed—that is, the tasks that comprise the job have to be organized into some sequence. Tasks also have to be organized so that work is interspersed with rest pauses, to allow recovery from any fatigue, and working days have to be organized into patterns such as nine-to-five schedules or shift work. Ergonomists look at different ways of organizing work activities so that work output can be maximized without compromising job performance. Ergonomists use *task analysis* methods to analyze jobs so that the task sequences can be optimized and the skills necessary to perform each task can be defined. Typically, any job can be defined in terms of the following requirements:

- *physical skills requirements* (strength, size, reach, clearance, endurance, speed, and physical skills, etc.
- *cognitive skills requirements* (intellectual ability, problem solving, memory, language, math, etc.)
- *social skills requirements* (conversational skills, interview skills, interpersonal skills, empathy, personality type, leadership potential, etc.).

This *skills analysis* information can then be used as a basis for *job selection* decisions involving choices of different personnel for a job. Task and skills analysis information can also be used to define *training* needs, and it also helps with decisions about the type and content of training that is most likely to be most effective for the work under consideration.

Sometimes ergonomists work on the development of *simulations*, in which people are trained with a facsimile of a real situation. This may be necessary for some types of work for which the actual environment is not readily accessible. (For example, terrestrial training of astronauts to undertake repairs in space requires simulating the weightless conditions they will experience by using a large water tank.) Also, with recent developments in virtual reality capabilities, ergonomists are interested in the development of "virtual training" methods, whereby, for example, professionals, such as doctors or dentists, might be able to practice diagnostic and surgical skills using simulated patients.

Organizational Design and Management

Whether flying a commercial airplane, operating a modern fighting tank, running a dental practice, or managing a hospital, most types of workers engage in some degree of team effort. Ergonomists recognize that all of the factors discussed above influence how effectively any team can work. They also recognize that how a team is organized, how people are motivated, and how an organization is managed also affect the amount of work output and the quality of work performance. Often, changing the structure of an organization creates opportunities to save on costs and streamline how work can be done. The impact of new technologies, such as computers, forces us to rethink what work can best be done by people, what work can best be done by technology, how that work can best be done, and who can best do it. Inevitably, changes in technology bring opportunities for some people to enhance their skills, while for others there may be a deskilling of their work, or even a loss of jobs altogether. *Systems* ergonomists study how such organizational changes can best be coordinated, implemented, and managed. Because this approach to ergonomics tackles work issues at a larger scale, it is often referred to as *macroergonomics*.

Human-Technology Systems

When an ergonomist studies a work situation, he or she needs a framework that can encompass all of the topic areas described in the previous section. Usually, that framework is provided by the concept of a *human-technology system*. The concept of a human-technology system is fundamental to how ergonomists can systematically analyze and describe any situation in which a person is working with technology, whether that person is a pilot flying a plane, the driver of a car, or a dentist using a drill. The concept of a *system* dates back to the mid 1930s, when biologists realized that the human body is not only just a collection of organs, but also a self-sustaining set of interrelated components that function to create a purposeful "whole" entity, the organism. A basic definition of a system is "an entity that exists to carry out some purpose."[4] Thus conceptualized, a system is more than an assemblage of parts, and from an ergonomic viewpoint, a systems framework can be used to analyze and describe the functional performance of people and machines.

Early ergonomists quickly seized upon this idea of a purposeful system and realized that the performance of any technology, which can be anything from a single product as simple as a toothbrush to a complex product like the space shuttle, depends both on the design of that technology and on the capabilities of the people who operate it. The technology may be operated by a single person or many people, usually working in collaboration as a team. (For example, the members of the flight crew of a Boeing 747 have to work collaboratively to ensure the safe operation of this aircraft.) In other words, to optimize the performance of a system, one needs to consider how to design technologies that fit the capabilities of people, as well as how to train people to acquire the skills necessary to effectively operate the technology. For any human-technology system, ergonomists must also consider *allocation of function* between the person or people and the technology. This consideration is important because people are good at some things, such as decision making, recovering from errors, and creative problem solving, and technology is good at some things, such as accurate information retrieval, rapid data processing, strength, and endurance. To optimize the design of a human-technology system, the designer must appropriately allocate functions to the strengths of both the human and the machine components of the system.

Ergonomists have also recognized that for many technological systems, such as cars, videocassette recorders, computers, and even nuclear power plants, the scale of complexity of the technology of the system is not as relevant in determining overall system performance as is the design of the interface through which the user gains information from displays about the status of the technology and operates controls. Consequently, a good deal of ergonomic design work is devoted to optimizing the design of the control-display interface. A well-designed control-display interface produces faster learning, more accurate and faster performance with fewer errors and accidents, and better retention of skills and knowledge.

Figure 3 shows how one aspect of dental work, in this case filling a tooth, can be framed as a human-technology system. In this case, the performance of the dental team depends on the coordinated activities of two separate human-technology systems, the dentist and the dental assistant. In functional terms, the dentist is an information processor who must use displayed information from the dental drill (which includes visual, auditory, and tactile information, at a minimum); from the patient; from the assistant; and from any other relevant cues to determine what further manipulation of the controls (drill) is required to achieve the system objective (drilling out a cavity without inflicting pain). In this case, control may be complex and might involve multiple limbs (hand for the drill and foot for speed

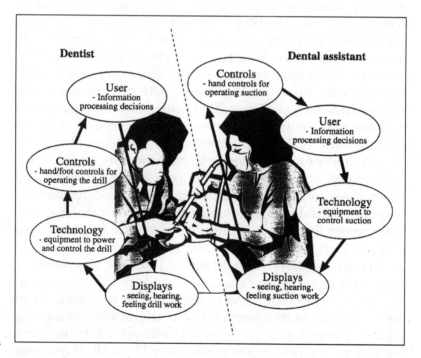

FIGURE 3.—Human-technology system analysis of a dental task.

control). Dexterity in manipulation of the drill depends on factors such as grip design, drill speed, tool vibration, hand posture, and glove design. For the dental assistant, the same analysis can be performed of the work involved in controlling suction to prevent the patient from choking and to maintain patient comfort. Here the displayed information is the sight and sound of the suction, any utterances from the patient or the dentist, and any other relevant cues. Obviously, the physical environment also must be adequate to support the operation of these systems. For example, dental work would be much more difficult in inadequate lighting or on a moving vehicle, such as a swaying ship.

Teaching a young child to use a toothbrush provides another simple example that illustrates the interdependence of components in a human-technology system. For the young child, the acts of inserting a tooth brush into the mouth and moving it up and down constitute unfamiliar skills. How well these actions are performed will, in part, depend on the design of the toothbrush. If the shaft of the toothbrush is too large or too small to correctly fit the child's hand, then the child will have difficulty effectively holding the toothbrush and consequently may fail to efficiently clean his or her teeth. If the head of the toothbrush is too large to allow it to reach the rear teeth or so small that it takes a long time to cover the surface of even a single tooth, then, again, the child will never acquire maximum proficiency with the toothbrush. In either situation, the system will perform suboptimally because of the physical design limitations of the control (in this case the toothbrush). However, even with a perfectly designed toothbrush the system may still fail because of suboptimal information *display* that limits the child's *information processing* ability. The child needs to know when he or she has brushed enough. Deficiencies in information may arise from a failure to correctly instruct the child on what to do (how to brush, how long to brush, etc.); incorrect gauging of the required quantity of toothpaste; or lack of feedback on adequate plaque removal (the use of dental dye tablets provides good visual feedback on the adequacy of brushing, but this information often is absent with normal brushing). Ergonomists looking to improve the overall performance of any human-technology system have to carefully consider the performance of each element of the system, and this requires the systematic analysis of what a worker does and how this is done using the methods of *task analysis*.

Task Analysis

To study someone working requires breaking down that person's job into a series of analyzable units called tasks. By definition, a task is a purposeful (i.e., goal-oriented) behavioral act that has a definite start and end. Thus, the time limits for any task can be observed. For most types of work, the jobs that are observed consist of a hierarchy of tasks in which sets of tasks consist of subtasks that in turn consist of smaller elements, such as individual movements. This approach to job analysis is known as *hierarchical task analysis*. The elements within any task can be physical, such as movements of parts of the body; verbal, such as uttering words; cognitive, such as thinking about a problem; or some combination of these, such as dictating into a tape recorder, which requires the coordination of hand and finger movements to operate the recorder with voice and thoughts. A task analysis of work usually helps to identify whether the tasks are organized in the most efficient way, what skills are required to perform the tasks, what equipment is required to perform the tasks, and whether the equipment is effectively designed. Task analysis also allows the ergonomist to identify the skills and knowledge that a worker needs and to determine what type of training, if any, is warranted.

In hierarchical task analysis, the elements of the analysis are usually shown diagramatically in a hierarchical tree or flow chart diagram. Task analysis is used by ergonomists to understand what a job entails, how the job might be improved, how any equipment might be improved, and how human errors can be reduced and human reliability can be enhanced.

To illustrate this process, consider the act of brushing one's teeth. The objective of brushing one's teeth is to clean the teeth to reduce the risks of oral disease. This daily task involves people interacting with technology. The controls are the toothbrush, the toothpaste dispenser, the faucet. The displays are the sight of the toothbrush and the toothpaste, any labeling and/or instructions on the toothpaste dispenser, and perhaps a mirror to provide visual feedback on goal attainment (are the teeth clean?). The activities involved in toothbrushing should occur in a coordinated manner and a logical sequence. The act of brushing teeth can be analyzed into a series of task components which in turn involve a series of musculoskeletal actions. Figure 4 shows a simple task analysis of the work of brushing teeth.

An ergonomist who wishes to improve the design of a toothbrush would try to improve overall system performance by addressing how each of the above tasks might be performed more effectively. Consequently, modern toothbrush designs include design elements such as the following:

- a broad, contoured-surface grip handle that helps the user to pick up, hold, and use the brush;
- a shaped, usually tapered, brush head that can reach to the rear of the teeth;
- a bent handle that allows the user to reach the brush into the corners of the mouth (recent designs also try to improve hand posture during brushing); and
- shaped bristles that allow easier cleaning of the tooth surface with the normal brushing motion.

Along with these design changes, toothpaste manufacturers have also responded by putting toothpaste into more stable, upright containers that allow the user to more easily dispense an appropriate quantity of toothpaste by pumping the toothpaste rather than squeezing a tube.

However, the ergonomist might also look to further improve system performance by trying to eliminate or combine tasks. So, for example, system performance could be improved by an automatic faucet (infrared automatic faucets are becoming increasingly commonplace), or by a toothbrush with a built-in toothpaste dispenser, or by exploration into other possible ways of cleaning teeth—by chewing gum, rinsing with a mouthwash, or eating certain foods, for example. Also, system objectives might be redefined to change the opportunities for system redesign. A broad set of objectives for toothbrushing might include

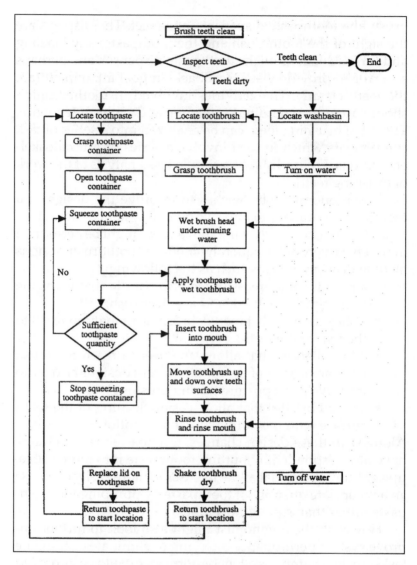

FIGURE 4.—Flowchart diagram of brushing teeth.

1. removal of residual food, plaque, and tartar from the surface of the teeth;
2. economical use of toothpaste;
3. efficient movements that maximize work (tooth area cleaned) relative to the energy expended;

4. pleasant experience that is desirable and therefore will be frequently repeated; and

5. engaging in a socially desirable behavior.

Whatever the outcome of the system analysis, the ergonomist strives to improve overall system performance in a systematic way. This example should illustrate that ergonomics involves much more than merely tinkering with design elements.

Design Application of Neutral Posture Principles

As we have seen thus far in this chapter, ergonomists strive to improve the design of the interface between people and technology that is being used to perform work. Technology changes at an increasingly rapid rate, but the dimensions and abilities of people change more slowly. This allows ergonomists to draw on information about human dimensions and human performance and apply this to design in a wide variety of situations. Whenever a design is analyzed and changed, the ergonomist pays particular attention to any postural implications that stem from the change to ensure that the new design will not increase and, preferably, will decrease the likelihood of any injury.

Sprain and strain injuries to the musculoskeletal system account for many occupational injuries among workers. Ergonomists generally agree that in many instances there appear to be three interrelated factors that are associated with an increased risk of injury while performing any task (Putz-Anderson, 1988)[5]:

1. *Force.* All movement requires some degree of force, but injury risks increase when a task requires high force from any muscle group or forceful overexertion. The amount of force that can be exerted also depends on posture. For example, when the hand is flexed or extended, or ulnarly or radially deviated, the power grip force is only about 65% of what can be generated when the hand is in a neutral posture. Force is also affected by the design of the technology that is being used. For example, it requires more force to pinch-grip a slender-

diameter pen than a pen with a larger diameter. Thus, performing the same work requires more effort when the hands
are deviated than when they are in a neutral posture (see Figure 5).

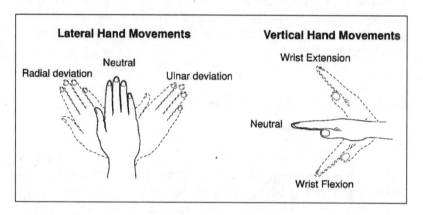

FIGURE 5.—Deviated and neutral hand positions.

2. *Repetition.* Repetition is the great multiplier! Repeated
performance of a task can increase the risks of injury, especially when the task requires a high amount of force or is being performed in a deviated posture. High levels of repetition
without appropriate pauses or breaks for the adequate recovery of fatigue or repair of tissue microtrauma are thought to
underlie the development of a variety of cumulative trauma
disorders (CTDs). Thus, an apparently low-force task such as
typing or playing the piano can become a more significant
injury risk when it requires a high number of finger movements every hour, every day, every week. For example, a typist frequently makes in excess of 12,000 finger movements per
hour, 8 hours per day, 5 days per week, which means that he
or she makes approximately half a million finger movements
per week. Studies of the key layout of most keyboards
(QWERTY layout) show that a typist can move the fingers in
excess of 15 miles per day.

3. *Posture.* There is a neutral zone of movement for every
articulating joint in the body. For each joint, the range of motion is defined by movements that do not require high muscular force or cause undue discomfort. For example, Figure 5
shows the neutral postures of motion for the hands. Injury risks

increase whenever work requires a person to perform tasks with body segments outside of their neutral range in a deviated posture. For example, research shows that the intracarpal pressure of the wrist, thought to be a significant factor in the etiology of carpal tunnel syndrome, rises as the hand deviates from a neutral posture into dorsiflexion (wrist extension) or palmar flexion, and ulnar or radial deviation.[6] Similarly, neutral postures can be defined for other body segments, such the upper arms and shoulders, which should not be abducted away from the body, overextended, or hunched while doing work. Also, neutral postures can be defined for standing and seated work. In a neutral standing posture, the trunk is not flexed forward or extended backwards, nor is it laterally bent or twisted. In a neutral sitting posture, the trunk is reclined back between 100° and 110° (where 90° is vertical); the buttocks, thighs, and legs are evenly supported; the popliteal arch behind the knees is open for free blood and fluid circulation; and the lumbar region of the spine is supported. Empirical studies show that pressure in the lumbar discs of the spine and electrical activity in the low back muscles are minimal when a person is sitting in this posture (see Figure 6). Lueder and Noro (1994)[7] provide an excellent compendium of recent studies on ergonomic sitting.

FIGURE 6.—Neutral sitting posture.

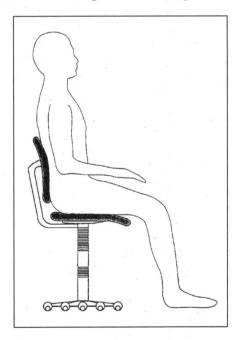

Personal observation of dental work suggests that dental staff may spend a substantial part of their work day in deviated postures. Figure 7 presents an example of a typical dental task to illustrate the postural deviations that can occur.

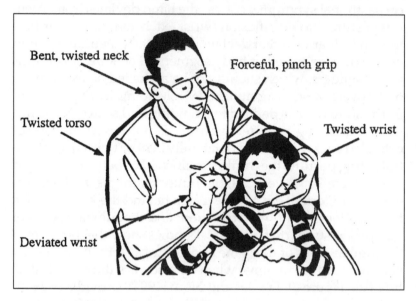

Bent, twisted neck

Forceful, pinch grip

Twisted torso

Twisted wrist

Deviated wrist

FIGURE 7.—Deviated upper-body positions during a dental task.

The central role played by poor posture in the etiology of musculoskeletal injuries allows ergonomists to use a variety of postural targeting methods to observe a worker's posture and to estimate injury risks on the basis of observation data. Postural targeting methods can also be used to assess the adequacy of the design of many products by observing how they affect posture, and to estimate the likelihood of success for any interventions.

The cumulative nature of most musculoskeletal injuries results in a progression of symptoms from initial sensations of musculoskeletal discomfort; through aches, pains, and other sensations (such as numbness and tingling); to the onset of an injury proper—a cumulative trauma injury (see Figure 8). Fortunately, this progression allows ergonomists to poll workers to determine the prevalence of discomfort and then estimate the size and seriousness of the injury risks. If interventions can be made that diminish the prevalence of discomfort.

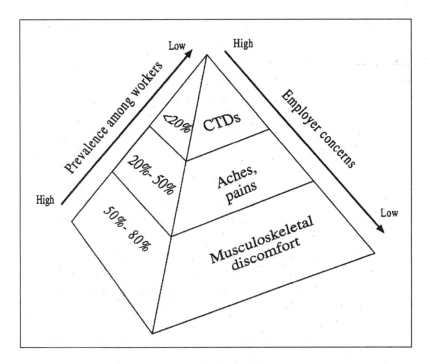

FIGURE 8.—Prevalence of musculoskeletal concerns among workers.

then these also will reduce the prevalence of any subsequent musculoskeletal injuries among workers.

Thus, the goal of many ergonomic interventions is to promote healthful working postures among workers when they use tools and perform tasks.

How to Judge the Ergonomic Design of a Product

Just because a label says that something is an ergonomic product does not mean that it is! The degree to which any product can be judged to be ergonomically designed depends on both the physical design of the product and how the product is supposed to be used. Many products that are marketed as being "ergonomically designed" give no instructions for how best to use the product. Rather than reducing injury risks and improving performance, incorrect use of such a product may result in more injuries and productivity decreases. Consequently, when considering the purchase of a product that is advertised as being "ergonomically designed," an informed user should ask the following questions:

1. Does the design of the product make intuitive sense given the goal of the design?
2. Does the product feel comfortable to use?
3. Does the product put the user into a more neutral posture?
4. Can the manufacturer/designer clearly articulate what the ergonomic objectives are for specific design elements? In other words, why is the product designed this way?
5. Does the manufacturer have any research evidence to demonstrate that their product works? How good is this evidence? Is it undertaken by reputable external bodies? What published evidence is there that the product works?
6. Can the manufacturer give contacts for others already using the product?
7. If you are still in doubt and if it is appropriate, is the manufacturer willing to let you have a 30-day trial period using the product?

If the answer to each of these questions is yes, then the chances are good that the product is ergonomically designed. If the answer to any one of the questions is no, then you should think carefully about whether the product meets your requirements. If you are still in doubt about the design of a product, you should seek advice from a professional ergonomist.

Conclusion

In the space of a single chapter it is impossible to cover all aspects of the diverse discipline of ergonomics. For an introductory discussion of many other areas of this discipline, such as human reliability, training, information design, and cognitive ergonomics, the reader is referred to additional texts.[2, 8] This chapter has introduced those aspects of the discipline that are most immediately relevant to dental work, specifically the importance of a systems approach, systematic task analysis, and principles of neutral posture for work and product design. These and other themes will be further explored in subsequent chapters.

REFERENCES

1. Oborne DJ. *Ergonomics at Work*. Chichester, England: John Wiley & Sons; 1982.
2. Sanders MS, McCormick EJ. *Human Factors in Engineering and Design*. 7th ed. New York: McGraw-Hill; 1993.
3. Galer I, ed. *Applied Ergonomics Handbook*. London: Butterworths; 1987.
4. Bailey R. *Human Performance Engineering: A Guide for Systems Design*. Englewood Cliffs, N.J.: Prentice-Hall; 1992.
5. Putz-Anderson V, ed. *Cumulative Trauma Disorders: A Manual for Musculoskeletal Diseases of the Upper Limbs*. Philadelphia: Taylor & Francis; 1988.
6. Bach JM, Rempel D. Carpel tunnel pressure while typing with the wrist at different postures. Marconi Research Conference, paper 17. Richmond, CA: University of California Ergonomics Program; April 13–16, 1997.
7. Lueder R, Noro K, eds. *Hard Facts about Soft Machines: The Ergonomics of Seating*. Philadelphia: Taylor & Francis; 1994.
8. Wilson JR, Corlett EN, eds. *Evaluation of Human Work: A Practical Ergonomics Methodology*. 2nd ed. Philadelphia: Taylor & Francis; 1995.

Chapter 2

Ergonomics and Dentistry:

A Literature Review

Jean Mangharam and James D. McGlothan

Abstract

This chapter provides a brief summary of selected literature on ergonomics and dentistry. It is organized into three main parts: musculoskeletal disorders and risk factors; psychosocial disorders and risk factors; and availability and effectiveness of current ergonomic interventions. The objective is to highlight selected works rather than to provide an exhaustive treatise of the literature in this area. Table 1 breaks the literature down by author, study design, sample size, instruments used (such as questionnaires), measures (from instruments used), and results and conclusions. Table 2 shows that dentists are more than twice as likely as dental assistants and dental hygienists are more than three times as likely to have repetitive musculoskeletal injuries and illnesses. Psychosocial-related musculoskeletal disorders appear to be connected with time pressures that may not allow dental personnel to fully recover between patients or tasks. These pressures may be driven by changes in the health care system that require extreme efficiency for a practice to be profitable. Finally, the availability of ergonomic interventions is limited because most solutions are reported anecdotally rather than studied systematically for effectiveness. However, recent advances in dental workplace layout, instruments, and operatory furniture show promise. Systematic, quantitative, epidemiologic evaluations of ergonomically designed dental furniture and instruments, as well as informative literature about good work practices and work postures in dentistry are needed to provide guidance in combating potentially career-ending musculoskeletal disorders such as carpal tunnel syndrome.

Introduction

The purpose of this chapter is to present a review of literature about ergonomics in dentistry. Ergonomics today requires the consideration and integration of both physical and psychosocial issues. Previous literature on ergonomics in dentistry may

25

be classified into three major categories: musculoskeletal disorders and associated risk factors, psychosocial disorders and associated risk factors, and the availability and effectiveness of current ergonomic interventions. Table 1 summarizes the literature under the classifications listed above.

Musculoskeletal Disorders and Risk Factors

Prevalence

Work-related musculoskeletal disorders in the service industry are common today, and their occurrence continues to proliferate globally. Statistics from 1995 (the latest available data at this writing) showed that "sprains" and "strains" accounted for 49.7% of all occupational injuries in service industries in the United States. Out of all musculoskeletal injuries, 2.1% were related to the neck, 31.4% were of the upper limbs, and 31.4% were of the back.[1]

Similarly, the prevalence of musculoskeletal injuries in the dental profession is high, showing significant differences among dentists, dental hygienists, and dental assistants. Table 2 lists the injury rates for the 1994 employed population (not including the self-employed) from the Bureau of Labor Statistics (BLS).

A number of studies have estimated the prevalence of work-related musculoskeletal disorders in dental work.[2–18] Most of the studies are cross-sectional, providing prevalence rates; because they lack comparisons with control groups they are unable to demonstrate true cause and effect. Many of these studies have not used statistical measures such as odds ratios, incidence rates, or risk ratios to analyze their results.

The most recent studies of the prevalence and incidence of work-related musculoskeletal disorders are briefly summarized below under the three major classifications of epidemiological studies: cross-sectional, case-control, and cohort studies.

CROSS-SECTIONAL

Auguston and Morken[2] administered a questionnaire to employees in the Public Dental Services of Hordaland County

Table 1.—A summary of Literature for Ergnomics in Dentistry

Musculoskeletal Disorders					
Authors	Study Design	Sample	Instruments Used	Measures	Results and Conclusions
Burke et al, 1997[6]	Retrospective analysis	393 dentists with premature retirement because of illness between 1981 and 1992	Records from one organization operating in the private medical sickness industry in the UK.	Causes of premature retirement	Premature retirements were due to musculoskeletal disorders (29.5%), cardiovascular disease (21.2%) and neurotic symptoms (16.5%). Eighty-two percent of cases examined were in the >50 years age group. Musculoskeletal disorders and stress related illnesses were the two most important groups of factors that influenced premature retirement.
Auguston and Morken, 1996[2]	Cross-sectional	329 employees in the public dental services of Hordaland (Norway)	Questionnaire	Musculoskeletal discomfort	Eighty-one percent experienced some sort of musculoskeletal discomfort in the last 12 months. Shoulder discomfort was experienced by 45%. Neck discomfort had been experienced by 47% and low back pain by 49%. Twenty-one percent hand/wrists and 20% upper back were reported. The dental personnel's experience of musculoskeletal discomfort did not differ from that found in the general Norwegian population. Neck discomfort increased with increasing age. Ergonomic equipment helped to alleviate discomfort in the shoulder. Perceived work load was positively associated with shoulder discomfort. Participation in sport activities showed negative association with discomfort in the lower back.

Table 1.—*Continued*

Authors	Study Design	Sample	Instruments Used	Measures	Results and Conclusions
Moen and Bjorvatn, 1996[8]	Cross-sectional	96 female dentists in a University (cases), 83 female dental auxiliaries and 25 female office workers	Questionnaire	Musculoskeletal symptoms	No significant differences in musculoskeletal symptoms between the female dentists and the other female employees were found. Female dentists reported more musculoskeletal symptoms than male. The study concluded that symptoms are not related to the work as dentists, but to female working conditions in general or to factors outside work. The dentists in this study treated patients only part of their working time and had varied types of work. The low occurrence of musculoskeletal symptoms may have been caused by less time spent in difficult positions and/or by the lack of stress factors such as time, economics, public attitudes, repetition, and professional isolation.
Jacobsen et al, 1996[9]	Case-control	489 male and 242 female dental laboratory technicians (cases) and 163 males and 160 females of other occupations (controls)	Questionnaire	Health complaints	Biannual prevalence comprising 68% of musculoskeletal complaints. Job-specific ergonomic and stress factors were responsible for musculoskeletal and neurological reactions. There were no age prevalence patterns. Female technicians consistently showed a larger prevalence of musculoskeletal complaints than their male counterparts. The prevalence of job-related health complaints was still higher among the technicians than in control groups. Only a few of the technicians had consulted medical personnel.

Table 1.—Continued

Authors	Study Design	Sample	Instruments Used	Measures	Results and Conclusions
Van Doorn, 1995[7]	a) Retrospective investigation b) intervention program	795 cases of self-employed dentists, veterinarians, physicians, and physical therapists.	Disability data from an insurance company in the Netherlands.	a) low back disability of 1987 and 1988 b) results after intervention program given in 1990	Among dentists over 44 years of age and veterinarians over 34 years of age had specific low back pain, nonspecific low back pain in combination with a deferred period of 14 days or more, low back problems before acceptance, and the presence of psychosocial problems at the start of the disability were significantly associated with the duration of low back disability. The same was not evident for physicians or physical therapists. After the introduction of an early intervention program the mean cumulative duration of low back disability decreased significantly. Standardized to 1990 (N=134), the number of claimants who reached a cumulative duration of 1 year was reduced by 56%. The early intervention program was cost-effective.
Kihara, 1995[23]	Cross-sectional	16 male dentists of an urban clinic in Japan	Questionnaire, time study of daily actions, electro-myography	Work-related complaints, daily action times	Most common posture was right-forward position. Neck and shoulder complaints were more than eyes, hands and arms and low back. The amplitude of electromyograms was increased by the extension of the muscles to lateral bending of 30 degrees and internal rotation of 15 degrees. It was concluded that body positions of daily dental practices cause an increase in work-related complaints.
Liss et al, 1995[12]	Cross-sectional	2,142 dental hygienists (DH) and 305 dental assistants (DA) (50% response rate)	Standardized Nordic Questionnaire	Musculo-skeletal symptoms	DHs compared to DAs (after adjusting for age) were 5.2 times (95% CI 0.9 - 32) more likely to have been told they had carpal tunnel syndrome, 3.7 times (95% CI 1.1 - 11.9) more likely to meet a carpal tunnel syndrome case definition. DHs more likely to have 2.5 times (95% CI 1.6 - 3.9) more hand/wrist, 2.8 times (95% CI 1.8 - 4.4) more shoulder and 1.8 times (95% CI 1.2 - 2.7) more neck problems than DAs. Less likely to complain of back problems.

Table 1.—*Continued*

Authors	Study Design	Sample	Instruments Used	Measures	Results and Conclusions
Jacobsen and Hensten-Petersen 1995[85]	Case-control	189 dental hygienists (cases) and 160 female and 163 male controls.	Questionnaire	General health problems	50% of industrial hygienists experienced occupationally related health problems. Most common health complaints were dermal reactions. Headache and dizziness were reported in about 25% of those surveyed. Headaches were associated with workload stress or musculoskeletal problems.
Milerad and Ericson, 1994[28]	Descriptive	12 healthy subjects	Electromyography	Electromyographic activities of six muscles during circular and eccentrically rotating track while holding a dental instrument with varying grip sizes and resistance against motion	The highest mean muscular activity was found in the dominant trapezius pars descends and supraspinatus/trapezius transversus muscles. Precision significantly affected the muscular load on extensor carpi radialis and infraspinatus muscles, while force had no impact on EMG activity in any of the muscles. Arm support during the task appeared to reduce the muscular load on the upper trapezius and supraspinatus.

Table 1.—*Continued*

Authors	Study Design	Sample	Instruments Used	Measures	Results and Conclusions
Stentz et al, 1994[39]	Cross-sectional	260 dental hygienists in the state of Nebraska (56.5% response rate)	Questionnaire	Subjective responses to questions on demography, working environment, workload, pain, discomfort, and numbness (altered sensation).	Sixty-one percent indicated that they experienced upper-extremity altered sensations related to physical stress. Pain, tingling, and numbness were most frequently reported. Sixteen percent had been previously diagnosed with an upper-extremity neuropathy. Ninety percent noticed altered sensations only after entering the profession.
Sinczuk-Walczak and Izycki, 1994[86]	Literature review	N/A	N/A	N/A	Aggregated data provide evidence that cervical and lumbosacral pains are the most common complaints as far as the locomotor system is concerned.
Pola-kowska, 1994[37]	Cross-sectional	31 dentists	Neurological examination, electroneuro-graphic and radiological examinations	Condition of peripheral nervous system, particularly cervical roots and peripheral nerves of the upper limb	All subjects complained of lumbar pain. In 80.6% of subjects, these pains indicated radicular neuralgia. Lesion of ulna nerve was found in 22.6% and lesion of median nerve in 35.5% of dentists examined.

Table 1.—*Continued*

Authors	Study Design	Sample	Instruments Used	Measures	Results and Conclusions
Visser and Straker, 1994[20]	Cross-sectional	28 qualified dental therapists and 26 qualified dental assistants	Written questionnaire, anthropometer and weight scale	Level of discomfort (visual analog scale on general body discomfort diagram), anthropometric measures and weights.	Discussed that since the 1960s, the introduction of the sitting posture, which was recommended to decrease lower-extremity problems, has not eliminated musculoskeletal injuries. Loads on soft-tissue structures of the lumbar spine and discs are increased in seating. Dental therapists and assistants experienced discomfort associated with their work, localized mainly in the back, neck, and shoulder areas. Dental assistants were shown to experience significantly lower levels of discomfort than dental therapists. Discomfort experienced by dental workers at work was also shown to significantly increase across the working day.
Stockstill et al, 1993[5]	Cross-sectional	1016 dentists in Nebraska	Survey	Musculoskeletal complaints	Twenty-nine percent of Nebraska dentists surveyed said they felt pain, followed by numbness and tingling. Frequency of symptoms was not associated significantly with age, years in practice, type of practice, or patient position. More frequent symptoms were associated with "crown and bridge" work. The prevalence suggests the possibility of an occupational concern.
Jacobsen and Peterson 1993[10]	Cross-sectional	101 women, 100 men employed in dental technology	Survey	Occupation-related health complaints	Fifty percent experienced job-related health complaints. Thirty-nine percent of the complaints were musculo-skeletal. In general the occupation-related health complaints were equally frequent among men and women. Self-reported occupational risk factors revealed that approximately one third of the musculoskeletal complaints were work related. Ergonomics and work-specific stress factors were important etiologic factors for the musculoskeletal reactions.

Table 1.—*Continued*

Authors	Study Design	Sample	Instruments Used	Measures	Results and Conclusions
Oberg and Oberg, 1993[11]	Cross-sectional	28 female dental hygienists, mean age of 40 years (most part-time workers)	Standard Nordic Questionnaire	Demographic data, presence and location of musculoskeletal complaints	Neck and shoulder complaints showed a clear predominance over other locations. Sixty-two percent of the subjects reported complaints of the neck and 81% reported complaints of one or both shoulders during the previous 12 months. The frequency of lower-extremity complaints was low. Most neck, shoulder, arm, and back complaints were considered work related by the dental hygienists themselves.
Izycki and Wagrowska-Koski, 1992[87]	Descriptive	Between 1984, and 1991, 188 dentists were referred for consultation with suspected occupational disease.	Assessed at the outpatient department of Occupational Diseases, Institute of Occupational Medicine, Poland	Musculoskeletal signs and symptoms were assessed for definite diagnosis.	In total, 122 (64.9%) of the cases referred were diagnosed with an occupational disease. Chronic inflammation of the humeral epicondyles (61.5%) and periarticular shoulder inflammation (25.4%) dominated the diagnoses. Low back disorders due to spondyloses or discopathies were rejected from the population because of high frequency in the general population and legal regulations that do not include them as an occupational disease in Poland.

Table 1.—*Continued*

Authors	Study Design	Sample	Instruments Used	Measures	Results and Conclusions
Rundcrantz 1991[86]	Cross-sectional	359 dentists	Questionnaire, ergonomic evaluation	Musculoskeletal complaints, ergonomic examination of 143 dentists' workplace	Seventy-two percent reported headache and pain and discomfort in the neck and shoulders. Female dentists had a higher prevalence of pain and discomfort. Younger dentists had pain and discomfort in the neck and shoulders as well as headaches, to a greater extent than older dentists. Male dentists, who positioned their patient carefully to gain a direct view suffered less from headache. Dentists who used the mirror reported less headache and pain and discomfort of the shoulders. Patient wedge cushions and intrinsic pauses in the work decreased the number of symptoms. Dentists having symptoms experienced unsatisfactory workload, were burdened by anxiety, and had poorer psychosomatic health and less confidence in the future. Regression analysis showed that personal harmony and age had the highest value for explaining the number of painful sites in the musculoskeletal system.
Kwahito et al, 1991[48]	Descriptive	5 instructors in the department of operative dentistry each preparing 5 cavities	Plastic-film-based stress-sensing element and a three-light emitted diode on the axis of a the bur	Measure finger stress and behavior of bur	Vibration emitted by the bur head is 500 000 rpm. The finger stress of forefingers had a tendency to be larger than the thumb. It appears that the middle finger controls the behavior of the hand-piece. The head end of the bur tended to incline into the buccal site.

Table 1.—*Continued*

Authors	Study Design	Sample	Instruments Used	Measures	Results and Conclusions
Rundcrantz et al, 1991a[14]	Cohort of 3 years	311 dentists (170 female) in 1987; 262 dentists (84%) reassessed in 1990.	Questionnaire	Information on pain experienced in the neck, shoulder, and low back areas and headache experienced during the past year and the past week and working postures.	Musculoskeletal pain symptoms increased in most body regions between 1987 and 1990 except low back. The incidence of musculoskeletal symptoms was greater in female dentists than in males. When stratified by age, the incidence of new cases of musculoskeletal problems was 0.2 case/person year for subjects 40 year old, 0.3 case/person years for subjects 40 to 49 years old, and 0.1 case/person year for subjects 50 to 65 years old. Attempts to relate working postures to development or resolution of symptoms between 1987 and 1990 surveys revealed no significant correlation. Ergonomic factors as indicated working postures have little predictive value for the recovery from or development of musculoskeletal problems.
Milerad et al, 1991[89]	Descriptive	12 dentists	Vocational electro-myography	Electro-myographic activity in different dental practice activities	Trapezius muscle showed similar activity between left and right. The right (dominant) extensor carpi radialis muscle had a significantly higher muscular load level than the left. The infraspinatus muscle had low activity levels on both sides.

Table 1.—*Continued*

Authors	Study Design	Sample	Instruments Used	Measures	Results and Conclusions
Lehto et al, 1991[3]	Cross-sectional	131 professionally active dentists	Questionnaire about health and general background; questionnaire on symptom checklist; Standard Clinical Examination; general fitness test (bicycle ergo-meter); hand grip force; radiographs of cervical spine and shoulder joint and lumbar spine (if over 40 years); psychological tests; and tempero-mandibular joint dysfunction test.	Multidisciplinary results-objective and subjective tests.	Forty-two percent had experienced pain and disability in the neck and shoulder in the preceding year (greater prevalence in salaried), and thirty-seven percent in the low back. Somatic symptoms or stress, perceiving dentistry as physically too heavy or mentally too straining, and a poorer general health status rating were all associated with greater than 1 year prevalence of neck-shoulder and lower back pain and disability and with poorer general physical fitness. The results provide evidence that physical exercise should be recommended to dentists and might also be applicable to subjects in other occupations with similar requirements.

Table 1.—Continued

Authors	Study Design	Sample	Instruments Used	Measures	Results and Conclusions
Lehto et al, 1990[40]	Case-control	136 dentists between ages 33 and 69 and 940 controls from general population of same age	X-rays of the hand	Prevalence of arthrosis in the hands and pinch power.	The prevalence of arthrosis was significantly higher in male than female dentists. Male dentists tended to have a higher and female dentists a similar prevalence of arthrosis as compared with the respective controls. The proportion of arthrotic distal interphalangeal joints (DIP) of all arthrotic joints of the hand was in both male and female dentists greater than that in controls, especially under the age of 50, suggesting earlier development in dentists. This might result from the extensive use of the precision grip in dentistry. Arthrosis of the DIP joint of the index finger was not associated with pinch power between the thumb and index finger, indicating good preservation of manual function in spite of increasing degeneration changes in hand joints with advancing age.
Milerad and Ekenvall 1990[4]	Case-control/ cross-sectional	99 dentists and 100 pharmacists	Telephone interview	Musculoskeletal symptoms	Forty-four percent of dentists and 26% pharmacists reported symptoms of the neck (RR = 2.1, 95% CI 1.4, 3.1). Symptoms of the shoulder were reported by 51% of the dentists and 23% pharmacists (RR = 2.2, 95% CI 1.5 , 3.3). Forearm symptoms were present almost exclusively in the dentists (12% versus 1%). Male dentists had increased prevalence of Raynaud@ phenomenon in the dominant hand, but the etiology was unclear. Numbness and paraesthesia were more common among the dentists than among pharmacists (RR= 4.2, 95% CI 2.3, 7.7). Symptoms of the dentists were probably related to their difficult work positions with arms abducted and elevated, cervical flexion and rotation, and repetitive precision-demanding hand grips.

Table 1.—*Continued*

Authors	Study Design	Sample	Instruments Used	Measures	Results and Conclusions
Ekenvall et al, 1990[49]	Case-control	26 dentists exposed to long-term, high-frequency vibration and 18 dentists with short-term exposure.	Survey	Differences between the dominant and non-dominant in the perception of vibration, temperature, heat and pain were compared between case and control groups.	Larger vibration thresholds were found in those with long-term exposure both for digit II (exposed to vibration) and digit V (unexposed). Temperature and pain thresholds were similar. The case group had neurological symptoms in the dominant hand more often than the controls. Vibration threshold (more advanced symptoms) differences were higher for the symptomatic dentists than for the symptom-free dentists. Since exposed and unexposed fingers were similarly affected, the neurological symptoms in the dominant hand of dentists with long-term exposure seem to have some other etiology than higher-frequency vibration.
Rundcrantz et al, 1990[13]	Cross-sectional	359 dentist (90.8% response rate)	Questionnaire	Musculoskeletal symptoms	Female dentists suffered more headaches (46% vs. 29%; $P < .001$), pain of the neck (61% vs. 46%; $P < .01$), and shoulder pain (62% vs. 43%; $P < 0.01$). Male dentists had pain and discomfort in neck, shoulders, and headaches to a greater extent in the younger sample. Younger female dentists had a significantly higher frequency of pain and discomfort in the neck and more headaches than older colleagues. If the patient was positioned carefully (direct view), significantly lower frequency of headaches was seen. Dentists who did not have discomfort in the upper locomotor system used the mirror (55% mostly used the mirror to facilitate a direct view).

Table 1.—*Continued*

Authors	Study Design	Sample	Instruments Used	Measures	Results and Conclusions
Persson and Brune, 1989[90]	Cross-sectional, descriptive		Survey, chemical air sampling, indoor air quality, observation.	Survey of health complaints and stress levels, exposure levels of methylmeth-acrylate, formal-dehyde and mercury vapor, dust exposure, ventilation system, observation of ergonomic status.	The potential hazards in the environment of the dental laboratory were related to ergonomics, chemicals (methylmethacrylate, formaldehyde, and mercury vapor), dust, noise, and light. Generally, headache was a common symptom among dental technicians and could be related to stress factors.
Hagberg and Hagberg, 1989[15]	Review	N/A	N/A	N/A	A review of literature was presented for posture; movement; and musculoskeletal load in dentistry, prevalence and risks of musculo-skeletal disorders, and prevention of musculo-skeletal disorders in dentistry.
Blewett and Hirsch, 1986[16]	Cross-sectional	168 dentists (out of 600)	Survey via professional newsletter	Demographic data, number of hours worked, type of seating, ratings of chair against certain criteria, musculoskeletal symptoms.	Eighty-eight percent reported pain, 54 reported no pain, and 24 were excluded from the study because they did not sit to work or the response did not have sufficient data.

Table 1.—*Continued*

Authors	Study Design	Sample	Instruments Used	Measures	Results and Conclusions
Shugars et al, 1984[18]	Cross-sectional	487 dentists of the South Carolina Dental Society (51% response)	Questionnaire	Prevalence and location of back pain, possible causative factors, (e.g., chair posture) and predisposing factors (e.g., age), years of practice, hours per week in practice, practice type, and percentage of time sitting.	Fifty-seven percent reported at least occasional general back pain. Twelve percent indicated they had sought professional treatment for back pain. Predisposing factors (26%) correlated more strongly with back pain than other factors. Good posture correlated negatively with back pain. Generally, dentists who sat 80 to 100 percent of the time reported more frequent low back pain.
Kajland et al, 1974[17]	Case-control	152 private and public health dentists 35-51 years old, majority of whom were females and 95 clerks (controls matched for age, sex and economic status).	Interview and questionnaire, kinocyclography motion analysis	Sociology background, professional environment, prevalence of medical conditions, equipment used, opinions on work positions, and observations of postures.	No significant differences were seen between dentists and comparisons with regard to reported absences from work because of sickness. Dentists suffered more musculoskeletal problems (shoulders and backs) than did comparisons. Those who reported musculoskeletal symptoms also reported lower work satisfaction or had a lower satisfaction index. Dentists with good working postures exhibited a lower frequency of absence because of illness.

Table 1.—*Continued*

Authors	Study Design	Sample	Instruments Used	Measures	Results and Conclusions
Powell and Smith, 1964[22]	Cross-sectional	49 dental operators	Visual and cinephotographic observations made during examinations, prosthetics, conservation and extraction operations.	Postures observed	For all operations, dentists spent most of their time either in a position of antero-posterior flexion, rotated counter-clockwise, or bent laterally to the right (in 70% of cases, all three at the same time). The cervical spine was involved to a greater degree. An outstanding problem is the provision of a satisfactory seat for the operator. The present dental stools tend to distort posture more than the equivalent standing attitudes, and to reduce mobility; some of this is due to the obstruction offered by the patient's chair.
Nystrom 1958[19]	N/A	N/A	N/A	N/A	Found that approximately 25% out of the 580 dentists surveyed reported backache and pains in the muscles and joints of the upper extremity. The clinical examination revealed that pains in the upper extremities were mainly located in the right hand and arm. Pains in muscles and ligaments were experienced, particularly from the flexors and extensors of the fingers, as well as from shoulders and neck. Joint symptoms were most pronounced in the index finger and thumb of the right hand.

Table 1.—*Continued*

Psychosocial					
Authors	Study Design	Sample	Instruments Used	Measures	Results and Conclusions
Reitemer, 1996[65]	Cross-sectional (over 72 workdays)	24 dentists	Heart rate periods, Nitsch self-assessment scale.	Workplace design (conventional versus ergonomic), light, noise, air movement, electro-cardiogram epidemiological data of occupational diseases (extracted from reports from various medical disciplines).	Analysis of the results revealed that dental work involves high psychic stress. Recommendations include the inclusion of dentists in occupational care, ergonomic design of working areas and their use, and coordinated advanced training in the field of dental work design. Dental extractions led to the highest working pulse in every proband, possibly being the procedure that causes the highest stress to the worker.
Newton and Gibbons, 1996[60]	Qualitative case comparisons	Two groups of dentists working under different systems of remuneration—NHS and independent capitation scheme	Questionnaire	Stress experienced	Both groups identified patient management, time pressures, and staff and practice management as sources of stress, although under the independent capitation scheme dentists felt that they were under less time pressure and faced considerably less paperwork. Results suggest that changing from a National Health System to an independent capitation scheme is of great benefit.

Table 1.—*Continued*

Authors	Study Design	Sample	Instruments Used	Measures	Results and Conclusions
Davidove, 1996[66]	Descriptive	Not specified	Ongoing discussions with dentists	Observation by Dr H. Adelson	Depression has a serious and adverse effect on the lives of many dentists today. Certain environmental demands, such as economy and constraints imposed by insurance companies, are accelerating and subjecting dentists to significant emotional pressures. Self-esteem may be compromised, and it has been recommended that self-criticism can help work as a prophylaxis against depression.
Joffe, 1996[67]	Descriptive	N/A	N/A	N/A	Written from a clinical psychologist's view point. Dentists have a number of common characteristics—hard-working and driven to achieve perfection at all costs. The critical inner voice can cause shame, anxiety, depression, exhaustion, and low self-esteem. It can lead to a compulsive lifestyle. Several studies suggest that the adult personality of dentists stem from patterns established in childhood and parental failure to provide adequate nurture. Dentists' cardiovascular systems have been shown to be stressed by difficult procedures. Burnout may result—a syndrome of physical and emotional fatigue.
Freeman et al, 1995[61]	Descriptive	N/A	N/A	N/A	Stressors that have been identified as being intrinsic to dentistry have included the heavy workload, the repetitive nature of the work, dealing with fears and anxieties of patients, and financial concerns. Time pressures have also been identified as stressors.

Table 1.—*Continued*

Authors	Study Design	Sample	Instruments Used	Measures	Results and Conclusions
Craven et al, 1995[62]	Cross-sectional	370 dental surgery assistants	Questionnaire	Psychological stress, job satisfaction, and organization	Results suggest that severe overall job stress and dissatisfaction were not prevalent but do present an important problem for the minority. The chief sources of stress were mainly time limitations, feeling undervalued, handling difficult patients, unclear job description, and annual salary review. Having a regular staff meeting, an annual salary review, and a clear job description were associated with significantly less job stress.
Osborne and Croucher, 1994[70]	Cross-sectional	340 dental practitioners	Questionnaire	Emotional exhaustion, depersonaliza- tion, personal accomplishment, demographic variables, frequency and type of practice.	Lower levels of emotional exhaustion were found in those working in practices containing four or more dentists and those working 3 days per week. Lower levels of depersonalization were found in married subjects and higher levels of personal accomplishment in those with postgraduate qualification.
Rundcrantz et al, 1991c[69]	Case-control	Case-96 dentists with cervico- brachial disorders and 47 controls are dentists without cervico-brachial disorders	Questionnaire	Psychosocial variables	Dentists with symptoms showed less satisfaction with work environment. Dentists with symptoms found (significant difference) work more unsatisfactory, were more burdened by anxiety, had poorer psychosomatic health, and less confidence in the future. Specialists were overall more satisfied (with or without symptoms). Specialists had more self-confidence and experienced less anxiety than general practitioners and head dentists.

Table 1.—*Continued*

Authors	Study Design	Sample	Instruments Used	Measures	Results and Conclusions
Katz, 1987[68]	Cross-sectional	291 members of the Texas Dental Association.	Survey	Predictor variables: hardiness (control, commitment, and challenge), dental attitude survey; situational predictors: outcome variables: dental stress (self-perception), career satisfaction, psychiatric symptoms.	Hardiness was found to be significantly related to lower levels of stress and psychiatric symptoms and higher levels of career satisfaction experienced. Dental attitude survey also was predictive of stress, symptoms, and career satisfaction. Income level and frequency of exercise were strongly related to dentists' career satisfaction. Specialization and number of weeks away from the office were significantly related to reduced stress.

Ergonomic Intervention

Authors	Study Design	Sample	Instruments Used	Measures	Results and Conclusions
Pollack 1996[72]	Descriptive	N/A	N/A	N/A	In dentistry, poor working habits, along with repetitive tasks such as scaling and root planning, contribute greatly to musculoskeletal disorders, stress claims, and lost productivity. The key objective for clinicians is to find a position that allows them to achieve optimum access, visibility, comfort, and control at all times.

Table 1.—*Continued*

Authors	Study Design	Sample	Instruments Used	Measures	Results and Conclusions
Powell et al, 1994[77]	2x2 intervention trial	176 dental hygienists	The distance between the two points with the hand in the modified pen grasp was subtracted from the distance between the two points in the relaxed position for each glove (converted into force)	Differences of forces exerted by ambidextrous and fitted gloves	Fitted gloves (f=0.792 N, SD=0.199) exerted significantly less force on the hand compared to ambidextrous gloves (f = 0.597N, SD=0.297) ;t=9.06, df = 175, P < .0001.
Oberg 1993[74]	Case-study	One Swedish dental hygienist	Time distributions study, posture targeting diagrams, biomechanical computations, serial photography and video recording	Critical factors causing work-related pain in the neck and shoulders	Fixed working postures, sparse movement patterns, limited work space, and long standing static load on the neck and shoulder muscles were shown. Horseshoe-shaped support for the patient chair and a special armrest for the operator chair were designed to provide an ergonomically desirable environment of decreased load.
Bruder and Rohmert, 1991[91]	Cross-sectional, descriptive	466 dentists	Questionnaire	Information on working conditions, individual characteristics and health problems	One of the major areas of concern and change was in the position of the dentist and the assistant in relation to the patient. Changes were suggested in the design of the chair for the patient.

Table 1.—*Continued*

Authors	Study Design	Sample	Instruments Used	Measures	Results and Conclusions
Rundcrantz et al., 1991b[27]	Case-control	96 dentists (64 males) who experienced neck and shoulder pain (cases) and 47 dentists (31 males) who did not report neck or shoulder problems	Observation/ Questionnaire	Musculoskeletal complaints from previous questionnaire, sitting work postures, use of mirror, clock-related working posture relative to patient, use of wedge cushion, active neck and shoulder mobility, and static endurance of the shoulder muscles	Approximately 26% of the asymptomatic dentists and 11% of the dentists with symptoms used a wedge cushion. No significant differences were found with mirror use. Cervico-brachial complaints in dentists cannot completely be explained by deficiencies in the neck and shoulder mobility or ergonomic factors.
Rundcrantz et al, 1991d[84]	Intervention study	Group A - dentists with occupational cervico-brachial disorders receiving physiotherapy treatment and psychosomatic approach and individual ergonomic instruction; Group B - as above, only receiving ergonomic instruction.	Ergonomic intervention, psychosomatic physiotherapy techniques, questionnaire	Pain and discomfort levels, experience of well-being, self-confidence, control over work, confidence in the future.	Both groups showed decrease in cervico-brachial disorders. In Group A significant decrease of pain and discomfort in the neck ($P < 0.05$) and a significant improvement was found concerning the experience of well-being ($P < 0.05$). The feeling of self-confidence had increased significantly in five weeks for Group A ($P < 0.05$).

Table 1.—*Continued*

Authors	Study Design	Sample	Instruments Used	Measures	Results and Conclusions
Jamar and Sevais, 1990[92]	Review	N/A	N/A	N/A	Recommendations of dentists' chairs and cupboards' designs and contents. Fixed furniture with fixed dentist's chairs are advised not ergonomic.
Grace et al, 1990[75]	Intervention	50 freshman dental student volunteers	Patient dental chair angle chosen by the subject	Volunteers were asked if they were comfor-table and the chair was subsequently adjusted in 5-degree intervals with the patient being questioned at each interval.	The initial sitting position of the patient affects the selected preferred inclination of the dental chair by the patient. If the patient is initially seated in a dental chair that has been present in the horizontal or supine position, this study suggests that the patient would not experience discomfort and therefore would have no objections to this position.
Micholt, 1990[93]	Review	N/A	N/A	N/A	Several studies indicate that there is still a large gap between the theoretical knowledge of work organization, working postures, and health risks on the one hand and its application in the dental practice on the other hand. Therefore it is useful again to take a closer look at the preventive measures that can contribute to less physical and psychological strain in the daily practice.
Eccles, 1976[71]	Descriptive/ Review	N/A	N/A	N/A	Discusses changes of posture and ergonomic intervention in dentistry over the years. Discusses the applications of ergonomics research to dentistry by using observation, timing operations, surveys, quantity of work measurements, physiological data, and other health hazards in dentistry. Areas of future research are urged for equipment design, building design, cost effectiveness, and human factors.

Table 1.—*Continued*

Authors	Study Design	Sample	Instruments Used	Measures	Results and Conclusions
Kwasman et al, 1975[78]	Intervention	Five interns and four dental assistants of the Eastman Dental Center (paired as dental teams). 150 actual dental treatment sessions in two dental treatment rooms of identical construction	Video recording	Observed frequency and duration of instrument transfer, critical incidents that interfered with instrument movements, and subjective responses of the dental team members.	The handpiece transfers were faster and more frequent in the 12 o'clock location where they were done by the assistant. The reverse was true for the transfers of the three-way syringe. The subjective responses indicated that the assistant working with the 12 o'clock instrument location had many more tasks and must be more highly trained.
Eccles and Davies, 1972[76]	Intervention	15 (10 male, 5 female) students of the Cardiff Dental School.	Posture of operator assessed by one examiner using a four-point scale for back tilt and back rotation, arm and shoulder movement, and right wrist and hand movements. The degree of undesirable movement was scored.	Postural score comparisons were made for operating positions (9 o'clock and 12 o'clock), handpiece position (5 o'clock and various positions), handpiece angle (vertical head up, horizontal, vertical head down), and tooth position (upper or lower)	In low-line dentistry, handpieces positioned in the mid-line above the patient are most convenient for operators working either at the 9 or 12 o'clock position and give fewer postural problems. For lower teeth the handpiece is best placed horizontally, and for upper teeth it is best placed with the head down.

Table 1.—*Continued*

Authors	Study Design	Sample	Instruments Used	Measures	Results and Conclusions
Eccles and Davies, 1971[83]	Intervention	32 male and 6 female dental students from the Cardiff Dental School	Patient stimulator to carry out a series of timed precision-movement tests	Accurate measure of time required to gain access to a number of cavities using a series of set operating positions	It was better to have the patient chair in the horizontal position than at 30 degrees since better posture could be achieved. In general it was better to have the patient's head facing forward and not rotated left or right. Though for some individual cavities, rotation may be desirable. The operator should work in the 9 o'clock or 12 o'clock position and not in the 3 o'clock position.
Kilpatrick, 1971[80]	Intervention	6 dentists and 8 assistants	Time studies (observation and stop watches)	Time differences between independent work, assistant utilization, workplace layout variances, and preparation prior to various dental procedures	Factors affecting efficiency were psychological factors (preference for working alone, patient temperament), use of the assistant (level of assistants' training), case involvement (complexity level of procedure), and physical factors (workplace layout).
Eccles, 1970[58]	Case-control, descriptive	10 male dentists carrying out treatment on 50 patients in total (5 patients to each dentist)	Two-channel galvanic skin response (GSR) apparatus measuring skin conductance. Electrodes placed on the palmar surfaces of the wrists.	Using the principle that skin conductance increases with arousal (as a measure of stress).	There was no real evidence that stress occurred in dentists that could be directly attributed to reactions of their patients and in only a few cases did dentists believe themselves to be affected by patients.

Table 1.—*Continued*

Authors	Study Design	Sample	Instruments Used	Measures	Results and Conclusions
Eccles, 1969[57]	Case-control, Descriptive	10 male dentists between ages 23 and 40	Electrocardiograph	Heart rate continuously monitored while patient reads a book, during conservative treatment carried out on a phantom head and during similar treatment carried out on a patient on four separate occasions each.	There was a significantly fall in heart rate from the first to the fourth trial indicating a reaction and subsequent adaptation to the experimental environment. There was a highly significant difference between the heart rate of different dentists and between the heart rates while patient reads book and while dentist carried out treatment. The difference in heart rate between treating a patient and a phantom head was just significant ($P < 0.05$), but not enough to warrant the firm conclusion that the dentist's heart rate was influenced by working on a living patient.
Fox and Jones, 1967[79]	Descriptive	N/A	N/A	N/A	Common working postures of dentists were presented. The dental chair role and design were discussed in terms of design parameters (working heights, access to patient, comfort of the patient, articulation, the operator's stool). The need for postural education was emphasized.

Table 1.—*Continued*

Authors	Study Design	Sample	Instruments Used	Measures	Results and Conclusions
Eccles and Powell, 1967[55]	Cross-sectional	231 (88.5% response) in the1965 Dentists Register in the counties of Carmarthen, Glamorgan, and Monmouth, Wales.	Questionnaire	Personal, morbidity, attitudes about work, surgery equipment and organization.	For most part they found their work fatiguing and considered the pace high. Nearly all made use of chairside assistance and more than half worked standing up. Dentists' satisfaction was obtained principally from relationships with patients and from achievements. The main source of dissatisfaction was from work restrictions and the pace of work. The dentists believed that their work was fatiguing because of long hours and severe pace, stress, and inadequate working environment. Poor posture was believed to be a contributory cause. Younger dentists and older dentists were the least dissatisfied.
Green and Brown, 1963[24]	Descriptive	11 subjects covering 3628 frames of film (one frame per second), and 163 tracings were made directly from selected frames. The frames were chosen on the basis of visibility of the dentist.	Memo-motion pictures	Observations of various postures adopted by the dentist.	More subjects stood than sat and only one dentist divided time between sitting and standing. Ten out of the 11 dentists assumed the 11 o'clock position with the subject in a head extension position. Cervical flexion (head down) position was assumed most often during work (69% of time). In most of the illustrations the dentist has a flexed cervical spine and rounded shoulders, the elbow is elevated, and the left hand is flexed at the wrist. A variety of stools were used (extent of adjustability unknown). For each of these observed postures, recommendations to improve posture were made. Education about good body mechanics was encouraged.

Table 2.—Estimates of Injury Rates from the Bureau of Labor Statistics[1] for the Employed Population (Does Not Include Self-Employed)

	Dentists		Dental Hygienists		Dental Assistants	
	Rates	Total count	Rates	Total count	Rates	Total count
Population employed in 1994 (excluding self-employed)	67 000		92 000		182 000	
Sprains and Strains	Not available for 1994	Not available for 1994	8 per 10 000	67	12 per 10 000	214
Repetitive trauma	22 per 10 000	149	30 per 10 000	270	8 per 10 000	135

in Norway. The purpose of the questionnaire was to measure the prevalence of musculoskeletal symptoms in various parts of the body. They found that out of the 329 satisfactory responses (76%), 81% had experienced musculoskeletal discomfort in the last 12 months, and among these, shoulder discomfort had been experienced by 45%, neck discomfort by 47%, and low back pain by 49%. Twenty-one percent reported hand and wrist symptoms, and 20% reported upper back symptoms.

CASE-CONTROL

A case-control study carried out by Jacobsen et al,[9] which studied female dental laboratory technicians ($n = 242$), consistently showed a higher frequency of musculoskeletal complaints ($P < .005$) than 160 matched controls of other occupations. Male technicians, although they had a higher frequency of musculoskeletal complaints than their respective controls, did not show significant differences.

COHORT

Two studies[7, 14] used a cohort design to determine the incidence rate and risk ratio of work-related musculoskeletal disorders in the dental industry. Rundcrantz et al.[14] carried out a cohort study on 311 dentists in 1987, and 262 of them were followed up in 1990, in the Municipality of Malmo, Sweden. Results of a questionnaire showed that the incidence of new cases of work-related musculoskeletal disorders was greater among female dentists than male dentists. When stratified by age, the difference in reported symptoms (between the period of 1987 and 1990) among three age groups (< 40, 40–50, 50–65) was not significant. Van Doorn[7] used a combined case-control and retrospective method to study 795 self-employed dentists, veterinarians, physicians, and physical therapists. Compared with dentists, physical therapists (relative risk [RR] = 2.67; 95% CI 2.23, 3.19) and veterinarians (RR = 2.04; 95% CI 0.72, 2.43) had a significantly greater risk of lowback disability claims, while physicians had a significantly lower risk (RR = 0.87; 95% CI 0.72, 1.06) . For all four professions combined, the annual incidence rate of lowback disability per 1000 persons at risk, adjusted for profession, age and deferred period for claims increased from 3.5 per 1000 in 1977 to 7.4 per 1000 in 1989.

The body of literature that supports the association between dental work and work-related musculoskeletal disorders has steadily accumulated since the 1950s. Nystrom,[19] cited in Kajland et al,[17] carried out one of the earlier studies in the field. Approximately 25% of the 580 dentists surveyed reported backache and pains in the muscles and joints of the upper extremity. Clinical examinations revealed that most pain in the upper extremities was located in the right hand and arm. Such pains were experienced not only in the flexor and extensor muscles (tendons and ligaments of the fingers), but also in the shoulders and neck. Joint symptoms were most pronounced in the index finger and thumb of the right hand. This literature prompted researchers to study the associations of occupational risk factors, environmental factors outside of work, age, and gender with the various types of musculoskeletal disorders commonly seen in this occupation. More recently, methods of prevention and specific ergonomic interventions have been studied: these will be addressed later in this chapter.

The remainder of the chapter will detail the specific types of musculoskeletal injuries common to dental practice and the risk factors associated with the profession for three major categories: neck and shoulder; hand and wrists; and low back.

Neck and Shoulder Disorders

Neck and shoulder symptoms among dentists, dental hygienists, and dental assistants have been commonly reported according to several researchers.[3, 4, 8, 11–14, 17, 20]

TYPES OF NECK AND SHOULDER DISORDERS

Pain and discomfort are the major symptoms of neck and shoulder complaints. A case control study carried out by Milerad and Ekenvall found that a group of 99 dentists had a higher frequency of cervical symptoms than a group of 100 pharmacists (44% versus 26%; RR = 2.1; 95% CI 1.4, 3.1)[4]. Female dentists reported neck symptoms 1.4 times more often than male dentists (95% CI 1.0, 2.0). Among the female dentists, the frequency of symptoms increased with age (not observed in male dentists or in either gender among pharmacists). Dentists with neck symptoms also experienced shoulder and arm symptoms more often than pharmacists with neck symptoms (RR = 5.4; 95% CI 1.6, 17.9). The shoulder on the dominant side was affected as often as that on the nondominant side. The authors felt that the result might reflect the effects of a work position in which both arms were abducted.

RISK FACTORS FOR NECK AND SHOULDER DISORDERS

Epidemiological studies have been designed to determine if sufficient evidence implicates physical workplace factors in neck and shoulder musculoskeletal disorders.[21] There is supportive evidence for a causal relation between highly repetitive work and neck and shoulder musculoskeletal disorders. Repetitive neck movements and continuous arm and hand movements affecting the neck and shoulder demonstrate significant associations. According to the National Institute for Occupational Safety and Health (NIOSH) Executive Summary (p. xiii), there is also evidence for a causal relation between forceful exertion and the occurrence of neck musculoskeletal disorders in epidemiological literature. However, there was insufficient evidence for positive association between force and shoulder musculoskeletal disorders.

There is a strong relationship between neck musculoskeletal disorders and high levels of static contraction, prolonged static loads, and extreme working postures involving neck and shoulder muscles.[21] There is also evidence for a relationship between shoulder musculoskeletal disorders and repeated or sustained shoulder postures involving greater than 60 degrees of shoulder flexion or abduction. However, there was insufficient evidence to provide support for the relationship of vibration and neck or shoulder musculoskeletal disorders, according to this investigation.[21]

Dentists and dental assistants are required to adopt nonneutral postures for much of the workday. The postures adopted usually require prolonged static contraction of the trunk and scapulothoracic and scapulohumeral musculature, combined with repetitive contraction of muscles in the wrist, hand, and fingers during fine hand motor control work. Dental workers usually assume awkward postures for several reasons:

- to obtain optimal view of teeth within the patient's mouth, often while maintaining a seated posture;
- to provide a comfortable position for the patient;
- to coordinate their positions relative to assistants, with whom they often share limited space; and
- to maneuver complex equipment and reach for instruments.

The posture and biomechanics of dental workers have been analyzed by several authors. Operating procedures can be identified in relation to a 12 o'clock position (Nield and Houseman cited in Liss et al[12] (see Figure 6 in Chapter 11, "Human-Centered Ergonomics: Proprioceptive Pathway to Occupational Health and Peak Performance in Dental Practice").

Operating positions are usually identified in relation to a 12-hour clock face:

1. the 8 o'clock position, to the front of the patient;
2. the 9 o'clock position, at the side of the patient;
3. the 10 o'clock position;
4. the 11 o'clock position; or
5. the 12 o'clock position, in back of the patient.

Powell and Smith[22] carried out visual and cinephotographic observations during dental examinations, prosthetics, conservation, and extraction operations. For all operations, the dentists spent most of their time either in a position of anteroposterior flexion, or rotated counterclockwise and bent laterally to the right (all three positions at the same time in 70% of cases).

Kihara[23] performed a cross-sectional study of 16 male dentists. Results from a questionnaire, time study of daily actions, and electromyography showed that the most common posture was the combination of the flexed and right side–flexion position of the neck. Similarly, Green and Brown[24] observed that dentists adopted a head-down position (45 to 90 degrees cervical flexion) for 58% to 83% of the studied period. The load upon the cervical muscles in such workers has been described as being 15% of maximal voluntary contraction at 30 degrees cervical flexion,[25] and it has been shown that significant muscular fatigue can occur within 2 hours in this position.[26]

To support the inference that awkward postures can lead to musculoskeletal symptoms, Rundcrantz et al.[27] found that dentists with cervico-brachial disorders adopted a posture of cervical flexion or rotation or a combination of the two more frequently than dentists without symptoms ($P < .01$).

Milerad and Ericson[28] carried out electromyographic (EMG) studies to identify the active musculature of dentists during dental procedures. The highest mean muscular activity was found in the dominant trapezius pars descends and supraspinatus/trapezius transversus muscles. High-precision work requiring dexterity significantly affected the muscular load on the extensor carpi radialis and infraspinatus muscles, but force had no impact on EMG activity in any of the muscles. Arm support during the task appeared to reduce the muscular load on the upper trapezius and supraspinatus muscles.

Prolonged static contraction of the upper trapezius may lead to fatigue, contributing to the high frequency of pain and discomfort in the neck and shoulder region.[29] The load of shoulder flexion and abduction may also lead to fatigue or irritation of the supraspinatus muscle.[30] According to Hagberg and Hagberg[15] the static elevation of the shoulders may cause chronic myalgia in the descending part of the trapezius muscle, often referred to as "tension neck syndrome." Hagberg and Hagberg[15] also described how at 30 degrees of shoulder abduction, the perfusion of the supraspinatus muscle may decrease, since the intramuscular pressure increases. The static contraction of a muscle in an abducted position may also cause impairment of the blood flow to the muscle. Decreased blood flow in the suprapinatus muscle may cause degeneration of the tendon and rotator cuff tendonitis.[15]

Although epidemiological studies reviewed by the National Institute for Occupational Safety and Health[21] showed a positive relationship between repetition and shoulder and neck symptoms, no specific studies in dentistry have examined the effects of repetitive movement on neck or shoulder problems. Most studies of repetition of movement have studied the more distal aspects of the upper limb.

As with repetition, no studies could be found that questioned the effects of forceful exertion in dentistry on the neck and shoulder problems.

Literature on neck and shoulder disorders has provided evidence that the prevalence of the disorders is high and that several risk factors are associated with dental work. Prolonged static neck flexion and shoulder abduction or flexion, lack of upper-extremity support, and inadequate work breaks seem to be major risk factors for neck and shoulder symptoms. A factor that has not been discussed is psychological stress and how it may increase tension in the neck and upper extremity musculature, possibly leading to overall musculoskeletal strain of this body region. The issue of stress is discussed in more detail in the section on psychosocial issues.

Wrist and Hand Disorders

Types of wrist and hand disorders

In addition to neck and shoulder problems, dental work has been associated with hand and wrist problems such as carpal tunnel syndrome and Raynaud's phenomenon (white finger).

Carpal tunnel syndrome is simply defined as symptomatic compression of the median nerve within the carpal tunnel.[31] The carpal tunnel is a space between the transverse carpal ligament on the palmar aspect of the wrist and the carpal bones on the dorsal aspect of the wrist. Through this tunnel pass the median nerve, the finger flexor tendons, and blood vessels. Swelling of the tendon sheaths, for example, can reduce the size of the tunnel, compressing its other contents.[32] Symptoms of carpal tunnel compression are reproduced by any activity causing prolonged increased (passive or active) pressure in the carpal canal. The condition appears to be primarily a compression neuropathy although some cases may involve an element of traction (symptoms reproduced by stretch). Acute neuropraxia occurs at greater than 30 mm mercury of compression upon the median nerve. The acute compression causes local interruption of function of the nodes of Ranvier (nodes on peripheral nerves between myelin-producing Schwann cells— their primary function is to increase nerve conduction rate). Chronic nerve compression leads to segmental demyelination and Wallerian degeneration (late stages). Chronic ischemia due to blood vessel compression is another factor that can lead to demyelination.[33]

Liss et al.[12] used a standardized questionnaire to measure the prevalence of musculoskeletal complaints in 2142 dental hygienists and 305 dental assistants. They found that after they had adjusted for age, dental hygienists were 5.2 times (95% CI 0.9, 3.2) more likely to have been told that they had carpal tunnel syndrome and 3.7 times more likely to meet a case definition of carpal tunnel syndrome than were dental assistants. However, these diagnoses were not confirmed by objective tests.

A cross-sectional study by Osborn et al,[34] used a questionnaire to survey 444 Minnesota dental hygienists. The results showed that 7% had been previously diagnosed with carpal tunnel syndrome and that 63% of the sample reported one or more symptomes of carpal tunnel syndrome. Similarly, a previous survey of 2400 California dental hygienists reported that 6.4% had been diagnosed with carpal tunnel syndrome and that up to 32% had reported symptoms common to carpal tunnel syndrome.[35]

Conrad et al.[36] used vibrometry testing of 58 practicing Minnesota dental hygienists to show that 12% of the nonrandom sample had mild carpal tunnel syndrome. Objective tests carried out by Polakowska et al,[37] used electroneurography and showed that lesions of the median nerve were found in 35.5% and lesions of the ulnar nerve in 22.6% of 31 dentists. No control groups, however, were used for comparisons in this study.

The condition termed secondary Raynaud's phenomenon, also known as vibration-induced white finger and constitutional white finger, is characterized by blanching (often painful) of the fingers. Initial signs and symptoms usually include numbness, tingling, and cyanosis (bluish discoloration). Exposure to vibration is required for a significant number of years before blanching occurs. Secondary Raynaud's phenomenon has been associated with changes that occur in the local vascular and neurological system as a result of exposure to long-term vibration. In contrast to carpal tunnel syndrome, numbness and tingling of the hands are not limited to the median nerve distribution. Temperature has more of an effect on the symptoms resulting from vascular involvement. Dose-effect guidelines and action levels have been proposed by several professional bodies, giving rise to International Standards, British Standards, and American National Standards. Various physical parameters, such as vibration magnitude, vibration frequencies, vibration directions, exposure durations, and grip forces, may play a role in the pathogenesis of secondary Raynaud's phenomenon, making it difficult to standardize guidelines for hand-tool vibration.[38]

Stentz et al,[39] carried out a cross-sectional study on 260 dental hygienists in Nebraska. Sixty-one percent indicated that they experienced altered sensations in the upper extremity related to physical stress. Pain, tingling, and numbness were the most frequently reported symptoms. Sixteen percent of the dental hygienists had been previously diagnosed with upper-extremity neuropathy, and 90% of those who complained of altered sensation stated that they only noticed the symptoms after entering the profession. In support of this finding, Milerad and Ekenvall[4] demonstrated in a case-control study that numbness and paresthesia were more common among dentists (99) than among pharmacists (100) (as described previously in this chapter). Because of the similar symptoms presented by carpal tunnel syndrome and Raynaud's (white finger) phenomena, these studies did not provide definite diagnoses of the conditions.

Looking at ailments related to the dental occupation, Lehto et al,[40] found that the distal interphalangeal joints had more degenerative changes in both male and female dentists than in controls. The difference was more predominant for those younger than 50 years of age, suggesting earlier development of joint degeneration in dentists.

RISK FACTORS FOR WRIST AND HAND DISORDERS

There is evidence of an association between carpal tunnel syndrome and highly repetitive work alone or in combination with other factors. Evidence also indicates an association between forceful work and carpal tunnel syndrome. There is insufficient evidence, however, for an association between carpal tunnel syndrome and extreme postures. There is evidence of a positive association between work involving hand/wrist vibration and carpal tunnel syndrome. Strong evidence indicates a positive relationship between high levels of hand-arm vibration and secondary Raynaud's phenomenon.[21]

The amount and type of repetitive movement performed during dental work has not been accurately quantified by previous studies. Liss et al,[12] however, highlighted that one of the predictors for high prevalence of carpal tunnel syndrome among dental hygienists was their longer clinical period of repetitive movements when work was done on parts of the mouth that were difficult to access.

It has been suggested that synovial tissue irritation results from repetitive movement. Repetitive movements within the enclosed sheath cause irritation and subsequently inflammation of the synovium lining, resulting in tenosynovitis. This may be the primary cause for increased pressure within the carpal tunnel. Treatment by removal of compression (carpal tunnel release surgery) has demonstrated partial subsequent relief from decreased constriction of the flexor tendons.[41]

A study by Neal et al,[42] found in fact that histopathological examination of the tenosynovium removed during surgery for carpal tunnel syndrome has shown a striking absence of inflammation. Barton et al,[43] feel that tenosynovitis is a distinct entity, in which the synovium around the tendon actually becomes inflamed. The term, according to Barton et al, is often

applied inappropriately to conditions that do not involve inflammation of the synovium

Skie et al,[44] reasoned that flexed wrist postures may reduce the volume of the carpal tunnel, thus increasing the
intracanal pressure and subsequently compressing the median
nerve. Szabo and Chidgey[45] showed that repetitive flexion and
extension of the wrist created pressures in the carpal tunnel,
that were more elevated in those who had reported symptoms than in normal subjects, and that the symptoms took
longer to dissipate. Laboratory studies support these findings,
demonstrating that carpal tunnel pressure is increased from
less than 5 mm mercury to more than 30 mm mercury during
wrist flexion and extension.[46]

Milerad and Ericson[28] found that precision work by dentists significantly affected the muscular load on extensor carpi
radialis and infraspinatus muscles, while force had no impact
on EMG activity in any of the muscles. In another study, it was
suggested that chronic disorders of the fingers resulting in arthritic joints may be caused by extensive use of the precision
grip in dentistry.[40] Increasing degenerative changes in the joint,
however, did not hinder manual function. Within dentistry, Liss
et al,[12] presented the predictors of wrist/hand disorders in the
past 12 months. The duration of work, the percentage of time
that the trunk was in a rotated position relative to the lower
body when operating, and instrument types were found to be
predictors of work-related musculoskeletal disorders. The impact of instrument type was less clear than that of other predictors because of possibly a greater mix of instruments and longer
clinical periods of repetitive movements when work was done
on patients with inaccessible calculus.

Because of the high precision required by much dental work,
the muscles used in sustaining such activity are at risk of becoming fatigued and causing discomfort. Stability maintained
through static muscle loading in the shoulder and elbow areas
for prolonged periods can lead to fatigue and discomfort.[20]
Grandjean[47] suggested that with prolonged contraction of upper
trapezius during upper extremity stabilization, adjacent blood
vessels and nerves may be compressed, making the upper extremity susceptible to temporary ischemia and neuropraxia.

Kwahito et al,[48] carried out finger stress measurements
during various "burr head" operations. It was found that

vibration emitted by the burr head was about 500,000 rpm and finger stress had a tendency to be greater than thumb stress, particularly for the middle finger, which controlled the behavior of the handpiece. Milerad and Ekenvall[4] found that male dentists had an increased prevalence of Raynaud's phenomenon in the dominant hand. Ekenvall et al,[49] found sensory-perceptions differences in the hands of dentists. In their research findings, they stated that "dentists with long term exposure had larger vibration threshold differences than those with short-term exposure, both for the digit II (exposed to high frequency vibration) and for digit V (unexposed), whereas the temperature and pain thresholds were similar." The former group had neurological symptoms in the dominant hand more often than the latter. Vibration threshold differences of exposed digit II and unexposed digit V were higher for the symptomatic dentists than for the symptom-free dentists. Since the exposed and unexposed fingers were similarly affected, the neurological symptoms in the dominant hand of dentists with long-term exposure seem to have some other etiology than high-frequency vibration.

Low Back Disorders

TYPES OF LOW BACK DISORDER

Low-back discomfort is a problem associated with dental work in numerous studies.[2, 3, 7, 10, 11, 17, 18, 20, 37]

Van Doorn[7] carried out a retrospective study of 795 cases of self-employed dentists, veterinarians, physicians, and physical therapists. His study showed that dentists over 44 years of age had significantly longer duration of low back disability if they had

1. specific low back pain,
2. nonspecific low back pain in combination with a deferred period of 14 days or more,
3. low back disorders before acceptance of the disorder, and
4. psychosocial problems at the start of the disability.

Polakowska et al,[37] carried out a study using electromyography and radiological examination of 31 dentists. All subjects complained of lumbar pain. In 80.6% of the subjects, the pains were associated with objective signs of radicular neuralgia.

RISK FACTORS FOR LOW BACK DISORDERS

The NIOSH literature review[21] showed evidence indicated a positive relationship between lowback disorder and heavy physical work, work-related lifting, forceful movements, and work-related awkward postures. There was strong evidence also for a positive relationship between whole body vibration and low back disorders. The only risk factor that pertains to dental work is work-related awkward posture.

Changes in operating methods in dentistry, which have occurred since the late 1950s, have altered the occupation from a standing to a sitting profession. Shugars et al, [18] found that good (neutral) posture correlated negatively with back pain and, generally, dentists who sat 80% to 100% of the day reported more frequent lower-back pain. Static work in the sitting posture requiring spinal flexion and rotation has been associated with increased risk of low back pain.[20, 50-52] According to Visser and Straker,[20] since the introduction of the sitting posture, lower-extremity problems of the worker have decreased, but musculoskeletal injuries of upper extremities and the low back have not been eliminated. Loads on soft-tissue structures of the lumbar spine and discs are increased by sitting. Additionally, extensor muscle activity in the lumbar spine area in the unsupported sitting posture is greater than in standing. Discomfort experienced by dental workers was shown to increase over the working day.

Psychosocial Disorders Related to Dentistry

Types of Psychosocial Disorders

Studies of psychosocial stress levels experienced by dentists are numerous.[53-55] Litchfield[53] commented that a high level of stress is associated with dentistry because it involves fine, meticulous surgery and little or no rest or diversion. The stresses experienced may be internally or externally provoked.[54]

Risk Factors for Psychosocial Disorders

Eccles and Powell[55] surveyed 358 male dentists in South Wales to determine the health of dentists, as defined by the World Health Organization: *"Health is a state of complete mental, physical and social well-being and not merely the absence of disease or disability."* The questionnaire found that 60% liked their work. Younger dentists (between 23 and 34 years of age) were more satisfied than older dentists, and the 45 to 54 age group was the most dissatisfied. These findings occurred possibly because the younger dentists worked shorter hours and had less responsibility (being assisted), while those over 65 years of age had adapted by reducing their work load. It seemed that the greatest sources of dissatisfaction lay in the external limitations (e.g., finance constraints, fearful patients, time pressures, length of working day, and health care system) imposed on the dentist and the pace at which the work was carried out.

According to Diakow and Cassidy[59] financial obligations of dentists may promote longer and harder working hours, placing more stress on the worker psychologically and physically. Basset[56] reasoned that dentists kept working despite physical discomfort because, like many others who are self-employed, dentists suffer direct loss of income if they are unable to work.

Basset[56] found that one psychosocial stress factor that may increase low back pain is the constant coping with fearful patients. Eccles[57] studied whether the presence or absence of a patient affects the degree of stress experienced by dentists carrying out conservation work. It was found that precision activities or activities requiring high levels of concentration, such as reading, giving injections, cavity preparation, and insertion of a lining, were associated with short, low-amplitude electrocardiogram waves, preceded by a cardio-decelerator reflex. According to the researchers, the short, low-amplitude waves may be significant of an increased respiratory rate. The researchers felt it could not be concluded from the study that dentists were influenced strongly by the presence of a living patient as compared with a mannequin head.

Eccles[58] used skin conductance to assess the level of arousal of dentists during practice. An elevated skin conductance is believed to be associated with increased arousal. It was shown that a rise in skin conductance before treatment events indicates some apprehension. Specific behaviors of patients, however, did not influence the skin conductance of dentists. Eccles reported that "it seems likely that dentists have learned to adapt successfully to reactions of their patients which might otherwise be stressful but that they sometimes show apprehension before certain phases of treatment, such as injection of local anesthetic and cavity preparation."

Time pressures have been found to be one of the major sources of extrinsic stress for the dentist.[60–62] Freeman et al,[61] reported that dentists had to schedule more work in less time to stay profitable. There was a perception among dentists, especially the National Health System (NHS) dentists, that they were constantly running late, and it was found that this perception itself was stressful.[60] In two studies that investigated potential dentist stresses, it was found that running behind schedule and constant time pressures ranked high. In the first study, Cecchini[63] found that dentists from the United Kingdom reported that running behind schedule and constant time pressures ranked third and fourth, respectively, among 20 other stresses reported in the survey. In the second study, Cooper et al,[64] reported that running behind schedule and constant time pressures ranked seventh and third, respectively, among the other 20 stresses.

Reitemeier[65] found that the length of the working day can affect the motivation and social qualities of a dentist. When working long hours, practitioners tend to decrease their manual contacts and efforts later in the day. Decline in sociability is evident in the younger dentists, while senior professionals tend to have significant decline in the ability to relax. For experienced workers, symptoms of general physical fatigue were significantly higher, but the trade-off was greater emotional stability at the end of the working day.

The organization of the health care system has been shown to influence the stress levels of the dentist. Newton and Gibbons of Guy's Hospital, London,[60] showed that changing from a National Health System to an independent capitation scheme is of great benefit. In the independent capitation scheme, dentists felt that they were under less time pressure and faced considerably less paperwork, although both groups still identified patient management, time pressures, and staff and practice management as sources of stress. Davidove[66] found that environmental demands, such as economy and constraints imposed by insurance companies, were accelerating and subjecting dentists to significant pressures. Although both systems are very different, it is evident that dentists in both countries face stress from the different health system changes imposed upon them.

Joffe[67] pointed out that there was a basic personality profile for dentists: hard-working, dedicated, altruistic, empathic, humble, well-balanced, and selfless. Many use their inner voice to criticize themselves in a negative manner, causing shame, anxiety, depression, exhaustion, and low self-esteem. Burnout may result from the combination of physical and emotional fatigue.

Katz[68] surveyed 291 members of the Texas Dental Association. From this survey, it was concluded that higher levels of control (belief that they have control over their life); commitment (ability to feel deeply involved or committed to the activities, people, or institutions in their lives); and challenge (anticipation of change as an exciting challenge) were found to be significantly related to lower levels of stress and psychiatric symptoms and higher levels of career satisfaction.

It was found that specialized dentists were overall more satisfied, having more self-confidence and less anxiety than general practitioners.[68–70]

Stress and Work-Related Musculoskeletal dDsorders

There has been speculation that work-related musculoskeletal disorders may be associated not only with the physical stresses imposed on the dental professional but also the psychological stresses.[20] Rundcrantz et al,[69] carried out a case control study of 96 dentists with cervico-brachial disorders and 47 dentists without cervico-brachial disorders (controls). Dentists with symptoms showed a significant tendency to be more dissatisfied at work and to be more burdened by anxiety, experiencing poorer psychosomatic health and feeling less confident in their future.

Lehto et al,[3] found that dentists who perceived dentistry as physically too heavy had a greater 1-year prevalence of neck, shoulder, and low back pain than those who perceived dentistry as physically light or optimal (odd ratio (OR) = 4.0 [CI 1.3, 12.2] for neck and shoulder pain; (OR = 5.4 [CI 1.7, 17.2] for low back pain). Dentists who perceived dentistry as mentally too straining had a greater 1-year prevalence of neck, shoulder, and low back pain than those who perceived dentistry as mentally too undemanding or optimal (OR = 2.5 [CI 0.9, 0.2] for neck and shoulder pain; (OR = 4.6 [CI 1.5, 14.2] for low back pain). Dentists who perceived their work as fast paced had a greater 1-year prevalence of neck, shoulder, and low back pain than those who did not perceive dentistry as fast paced (OR = 6.8 [CI 1.5, 30.1] for neck and shoulder pain; (OR = 3.4 [CI 0.8, 13.8] for low back pain).

To reduce stress, the dentist can make efforts initially by recognizing or unmasking it.[54] Exercising and taking a greater number of weeks away from the office,[68] employing healthy and useful self-criticism,[66] and paying attention to ergonomic design[65] have decreased stress in dental practice.

The Availability and Effectiveness of Current Ergonomic Intervention

Eccles[71] discussed the changes of ergonomics in dentistry. Modification of the patient dental chair did not occur until the 19th century. Mechanisms for elevating and tilting the chair slightly backwards so that it could be adapted to operators of different heights and operations in different parts of the mouth were the first modifications. The modern dentist works seated on a low stool, and the assistant, also seated, provides continuous chairside assistance: this is commonly called four-handed low-seated dentistry. Instruments and equipment are placed within close reach of the dentist and the assistant. The patterns of floor area design have evolved on an empirical basis for each functional area and for flow in occupants' movements.

Aims of Ergonomic Principles

According to Pollack[72] the aim of ergonomic intervention should be to achieve optimum access, visibility, comfort, and control at all times of treatment. Many ergonomists have urged an evaluation of the dental work space and process to improve not only health, but also productivity.

Equipment Design

Hardage et al,[73] used electromyography to study 20 dental students and faculty members to evaluate the effects of stool height and lumbar support. They found that lumbar support reduced muscle activity in the upper and lower spine and that the stool height had no significant influence on the muscle activity of the back. They suggested, however, that knee angles of 90 and 75 degrees were more desirable than 105 degrees as the back was more supported in this position.

Oberg[74] considered the working postures, sparse movement patterns, limited workspace, and long standing static load on the neck and shoulder musculature in designing a reference workplace to provide an ergonomically desirable dental practice environment for a single dental hygienist. A horseshoe-shaped support for the patient chair and a special armrest for the operator chair were designed to alleviate the static load on the neck and shoulders. The dental hygienist experienced fewer complaints in her shoulder region. These prototypes are now available commercially. No other study, however, was found to support this design.

Grace et al,[75] found that the position in which the patient is placed in when first seated in the dental chair significantly determines the patient's final chosen position for optimum comfort. Patients who are first placed in an upright position will choose a position that is closer to upright. Similarly, patients who are first placed in a supine position choose a final position that is close to supine. If the patient is initially seated in a dental chair that has been preset in the horizontal or supine position, the study suggests that the patient will not experience discomfort sitting up and therefore will have no objections to this position.

Eccles and Davies[76] found that in low-line dentistry, handpieces positioned in the mid-line above the patients are most convenient for operators working at the 9 and 12 o'clock positions, thus decreasing postural problems. However, mid-line position may not be accepted well by all patients. The position on the right side is not at all convenient for the surgery assistant, but may be less threatening to the patient. The best handpiece angle would seem to be somewhere between horizontal and head down. A hand piece placed head up, which is common practice in dental equipment, was less favored by dentists.

Accessories

Rundcrantz et al,[27] carried out an ergonomic analysis and locomotor function analysis on 96 dentists who experienced neck and shoulder pain and 47 dentists who did not report neck or shoulder problems. They found that approximately 26% of the asymptomatic dentists and 11% of the symptomatic dentists used a wedge cushion under the upper part of the back of the patient to get an optimal view ($P < .05$).

Rundcrantz et al,[13] found that if the dentist worked with a direct view, it was probably appropriate for the dentist to sit in the 9 o'clock position when working in the upper jaw to reduce stress in the neck. Dentists who sat in the 11 or 10 o'clock position ought to use the mirror to reduce the load to the neck. Dentists without pain who worked in this position used the mirror to a greater extent. However, no significant differences in neck stress were seen with the use of a mirror by or Rundcrantz et al,.[14]

Powell et al,[77] found that fitted gloves exerted significantly less force on the hand compared with ambidextrous gloves (i.e., one size fits all). The findings from this study and further research in this area may provide some guidance toward decreasing prolonged high-forced static gripping during dental practice.

Kwasman et al,[78] showed that rather than elect to retract the instrument back into the cabinet, some dentists or assistants had the option of placing the instrument on the holding pad on top of the cabinet while working. This practice made it easier to access the instrument when it was used often during a procedure. Although both the 8 and 12 o'clock positions showed that the dynamic instruments were stored in the cabinet more than on the holding pad, the holding pad was used three times more frequently in the 8 o'clock location, where the dentist transferred the handpiece, than in the 12 o'clock location, where the assistant transferred the handpiece.

Recovery Period

A study by Hellerstein (1959, cited in Fox and Jones,[79]) showed that dentists had a low calorie output during hours of practice, but that they nevertheless felt fatigued at the end of the workday. It appears that the dental operator averages 1.2 calories per minute during a working day (walking burns approximately 4 to 5 calories per minute). The fatigue that is felt by the dental professional may result from the static muscular contraction required in prolonged postures. Muscular imbalance may result from certain muscles remaining in prolonged contraction while the relaxed muscles remain in neutral or lengthened positions.

Rundcrantz et al,[27] found that significantly more dentists without pain and discomfort took advantage of the intermittent interruptions provided in their work (e.g., when the assistant was preparing the amalgam), using them for a rest or taking the chance to raise and lower their shoulders.

Workplace Layout

The arrangement of the equipment can affect efficiency and whether the operator works alone or with assistants.[80] According to Kilpatrick, dynamic instruments, such as turbines, multiplex syringe, and suction lines, should be accessible.[80] Medications, linings, cements, amalgam and plastic fillings, impression trays and materials, instruments, and other essentials should be arranged in such a way that the operating team does not have to leave the seated position at the chair to retrieve them.

Rundcrantz et al,[27] pointed out that in restricted working spaces, the dentist may have more difficulty when assisted by a nurse. The dentist's working position is influenced not only by the limited work but also by the dentist's position relative to the dental assistant when instruments are being handed over or when reach is required, in using dynamic equipment.

Green and Lynam,[81] used motion film analysis to carry out "work simplification" principles during dental operations. The analysis resulted in recommendations that considered the layout of the workspace. All of the equipment could be recessed in a cabinet such that pressure on various buttons would allow necessary pieces of equipment to glide out and the spotlight to be foot controlled. Green and Lyman stressed that objective time studies and motion analysis were necessary to work out ideal patient flow patterns; working arrangements for multiple workers in a room; and workspace layout for equipment (cabinets, trays, spotlight, hand instruments) and personnel.

Kwasman et al,[78] found that the high-speed handpiece transfers were faster and more frequent in the 12 o'clock location when carried out by an assistant. The dentist was able to make the transfer without moving his body or refocusing his eyes from the mouth to the unit. However, the passing of three-way syringes was less efficient in the 12 o'clock position by an assistant, compared with an 8 o'clock position without use of an assistant. In the transfer of the three-way syringe, additional time was required by the dentist and the dental assistant using the 12 o'clock position. Hand positions of the dentist and dental assistants needed to be changed from a pen to a palm grasp and vice versa. If the dentist was positioned in the 8 o'clock position, directly picking up the instrument with a palmar grasp increased efficiency.

Job Design

Kilpatrick[80] argued that if chairside assistants were trained and permitted, under supervision, to do more of the simple, time-consuming intraoral duties that are required of the dentist, more people could be served with quality dentistry. Subsequently, this would decrease the external (time-pressures) and internal (self-esteem, job satisfaction), stresses on dentists. The studies were designed to determine efficiency of patient service by a dentist working without a chairside assistant, with one assistant, and with two assistants. Significant amounts of time were saved by preplanning procedures and the use of assistants.

Factors that affected efficiency were psychological (dentist's comfort working with an assistant and patient's temperament controlled by conditioning education, proper anesthetic, and medication); use of a trained assistant; level of case complexity; and physical factors such as workplace layout.

Training

The working positions of dental professionals vary depending on where in the mouth the dentist is working and on which surface of the tooth procedures are required. Rundcrantz et al,[27] found that most (82%) dentists sat in the traditional way with a 90- degree hip angle when working on the 26d tooth (the distal surface of tooth 6 in the left upper jaw). Among dentists with seats that could be tilted, very few used this feature of the chair. Hence, training is required for the profession, as Bruder and Rohmert[91] also pointed out; they showed that ergonomic faults in positioning the patient lead to unfavorable postures for the dental professional.

A study by Davies and Eccles[82] showed that patients tend to prefer being in the 30-degree cervical flexion position while the operator prefers the patient to be in a nearly horizontal position of 15 degrees for clearer viewing without neck flexion. From this study, a list of requirements for the design of dental chairs was derived, pertaining to adjustability of the seat pan and back rest.

Eccles and Davies[83] carried out postural studies using a phantom head. Each operator was asked to carry out a cavity correction procedure on six standard teeth—both upper first molar teeth, both lower second molar teeth, and labial cervical cavities in the upper left canine and lower right canine. They recommended that the operator work in a 9 o'clock or 12 o'clock position relative to the patient and not in a 3 o'clock position. They also found that it was better to have the chair in the horizontal position than at 30 degrees to achieve a posture of less stress for the dentist, and that in general the patient's head should face forwards and not be rotated, except for certain tooth cavities.

Training on using as much support as possible for the upper limbs during precision work has been recommended.

Rundcrantz et al,[27] found that among dentists without pain and discomfort more worked with the left arm resting than those with pain. They noticed that dentists were able to decrease the load of the nondominant arm by resting it against the head of the patient, against the patient's chair, or against the instrument tray. Most dentists worked with the right arm abducted less than 40 degrees, resting their hand or wrist against the patient. Resting the dominant arm has to be intermittent and may be made dependent on the shoulder or thorax of the patient.

Exercise and Stress Reduction

Van Doorn[7] showed that an early intervention program (consisting of education on back care and body mechanics, early return to work, exercises to increase mobility and strength, and professional psychological advice) was cost-effective, significantly decreasing the mean cumulative duration of low back disability. Auguston and Morken[2] also showed that participation in sport activities was negatively associated with discomfort in the lower back.

Shugars et al,[18] conducted a survey of 1057 American Dental Association (ADA) members and showed that out of the 746 who reported musculoskeletal pain, 523 used exercise to alleviate pain with the result that 16% received complete relief and 16% received permanent relief. Two-hundred and thirty-four ADA members changed position relative to the patient; 9% received complete relief and 12% received permanent relief.

Rundcrantz et al,[84] carried out an intervention study on a group of dentists with occupational cervico-brachial disorders. Group A received physiotherapy, psychosomatic approach treatment, and ergonomic instruction. Group B only received ergonomic instruction. Both groups showed a decrease in cervico-brachial disorders. Group A showed significant improvement in pain and discomfort of the neck and increased self-confidence within a five-week period. The concentration required for the psychosomatic approach and the stretches and strengthening exercises provided by the physiotherapy program require dentists to take responsibility for the musculoskeletal conditions that they have acquired.

Lehto et al, [3] found that general physical fitness as measured by total work index was associated with a lower-stress symptoms score, lower score on somatic aspects of depression more favorable health status rating, and perception of dentistry as physically optimal or too light and as mentally optimal or without strain. Lehto et al, concluded that physical exercise can act as a prophylaxis against musculoskeletal illness and stress for dentists of a wide range of ages.

Conclusion

Ergonomics requires understanding of both the physical and the psychological aspects of the workplace. From the review of literature, it is evident that ergonomics plays a significant role in the health of dental professionals, but only after the dentist has recognized and integrated both physical and psychological systems. The musculoskeletal and stress-related disorders associated with dentistry seem to be interrelated. Literature about work-related musculoskeletal disorders and psychosocial disorders associated with dentistry is plentiful. However, ergonomic solutions for dental practitioners are under-reported in the literature. Furthermore, the few ergonomic solutions that have been provided have not been adequately evaluated or validated.

REFERENCES

1. Bureau of Labor Statistics. 1995. Statistics of injuries categorized by industry, ftp://stats.bls.goc/pub/special.requests/ocwc/osh/cftb0067.txt.
2. Auguston TE, Morken T. Musculoskeletal problems among dental health personnel. A survey of the public dental health services in Hordaland (Norwegien). *Tidsskrift for Den Norske Laegeforening*. 1996;116(23):2776–2780.
3. Lehto TU, Helenius HY, Alaranta HT. Musculoskeletal symptoms of dentists assessed by a multidisciplinary approach. *Community Dentistry and Oral Epidemiology*. 1991;19(1):38–44.
4. Milerad E, Ekenvall L. Symptoms of the neck and upper extremities in dentists. *Scandinavian Journal of Work, Environment and Health*. 1990;16(2):129–134.

5. Stockstill JW, Harn SD, Strickland D, Hruska R. Prevalence of upper extremity neuropthy in a clinical dentist population. *Journal of the American Dental Association*. 1993;124(8):67–72.
6. Burke FJ, Main JR, Freeman R. The practice of dentistry: an assessment of reasons for premature retirement. *British Dental Journal*. 1997;182(7):250–254.
7. Van Doorn JW. Low back disability among self-employed dentists, veterinarians, physicians and physical therapists in the Netherlands. A retrospective study over a 13-year period (N=1,119) and an early intervention program with 1 year follow-up (N=134). *Acta Orthopaedica Scandinavica. Supplementum*. 1995;263:1–64.
8. Moen BE, Bjorvatn K. Musculoskeletal symptoms among dentists in a dental school. *Occupational Medicine*. 1996;46(1):65–68.
9. Jacobsen N, Derand T, Hensten-Pettersen A. Profile of work-related health complaints among Swedish dental laboratory technicians. *Community Dentistry and Oral Epidemiology*. 1996; 24(2):138–144.
10. Jacobsen N, Peterson AH. Self-reported occupation-related health complaints among dental laboratory technicians. *Quintessence International*. 1993; 24(6):409–415.
11. Oberg T, Oberg U. Musculoskeletal complaints in dental hygiene: a survey study from Swedish county. *Journal of Dental Hygiene*. 1993;67(5):257–261.
12. Liss GM, Jesin E, Kusiak RA, White P. Musculoskeletal problems among Ontario dental hygienists. *American Journal of Industrial Medicine*. 1995;28(4):521–540.
13. Rundcrantz BL, Johnsson B, and Moritz U. Cervical pain and discomfort among dentists. *Swedish Dental Journal*. 1990;14(2):71–80.
14. Rundcrantz BL, Johnsson B, Moritz U. Pain and discomfort in the musculoskeletal system among dentists—a prospective study. *Swedish Dental Journal*. 1991a;15(5):219–228.
15. Hagberg M, Hagberg C. Risks and prevention of musculokeletal disorders among dentists. In: Brune DK, Edling C, eds. *Occupational Hazards in the Health Professions*. Boca Raton, Florida: CRC Press;1989:323–332.
16. Blewett V, Hirsch R. Seating for dentists: ergonomic requirements and assessment of available chairs. In: Morrison D, Hartley L, Kemp D, eds. *Trends in the Ergonomics of Work, Proceedings of the 23rd Annual Conference of the Ergonomics Society of Australia and New Zealand*. 1986:219–221.
17. Kajland A, Lindvall T, Nilsson T. Occupational medical aspects of the dental profession. *Work, Environment Health*. 1974:11(2);100–107.

18. Shugars DA, Williams D, Cline SJ, Fishburne C. Musculoskeletal back pain among dentists. *General Dentistry.* 1984;32:481–485.
19. Nystrom A. Yrkesbetingade sjukdomstillstand bland tandlakare. Sverig. *Tanlakarforbunds tidning.* 1958;21(1).
20. Visser JL, Straker LM. An investigation of discomfort experienced by dental therapists and assistants at work. *Australian Dental Journal.* 1994;39(1):39–44.
21. NIOSH [Second Printing, 1997.] *Musculoskeletal Disorders and Workplace Factors: A Critical Review of Epidemiologic Evidence for Work-Related Musculoskeletal Disorders of the Neck, Upper Extremity, and Low Back.* Cincinnati, OH: US Department of Health and Human Services, Public Health Service, Centers for Disease Control and Prevention, National Institute for Occupational Safety and Health. DHHS (NIOSH) Publication No. 97–141.
22. Powell M, Smith JW. Occupational stress in dentistry: the postural component. *Ergonomics, Supplement, Proceedings of the Second International Congress on Ergonomics.* Dortmund, West Germany: International Congress of Ergonomics;1964:337–340.
23. Kihara T. Dental care works and work-related complaints of dentists. *Kurume Medical Journal.* 1995;42(4):251–257.
24. Green EJ, Brown ME. An aid to the elimination of tension and fatigue: body mechanics applied to the practice of dentistry. *Journal of the American Dental Association.* 1963;67:679.
25. Chaffin DB, Andersson GBJ. *Occupational Biomechanics.* New York: John Wiley and Sons; 1984.
26. Chaffin DB. Localized muscle fatigue—definition and measurement. *Journal of Occupational Medicine.* 1973;15:346.
27. Rundcrantz BL, Johnsson B, Moritz U. Occupational cervicobrachial disorders among dentists—analysis of ergonomics and locomotor functions. *Swedish Dental Journal.* 1991b;15(3):105–115.
28. Milerad E, Ericson MO. Effects of precision and force demands, grip diameter and arm support during manual work. *Ergonomics.* 1994;37(2):255–264.
29. Jonsson B, Rugan P. Besvar fran rorelseorganen bland tandhygienister. Arbetatarskyddstyrelsen. *Undersokningsrapport.* 1982.
30. Hagberg M. Electromyographic signs of shoulder muscular fatigue in two elevated arm positions. *American Journal of Physical Medicine.* 1981;60:111–121
31. Nathan PA. Cumulative trauma disorders of the upper extremity: II. *American Association for Hand Surgeons Conference Proceedings.* August 1995, Cincinnati, OH.
32. Williams R, Westmorland M. Occupational cumulative trauma disorders of the extremity. *The American Journal of Occupational Therapy.* 1994;48(5):411–420.

33. Armadio PC. Cumulative trauma disorders of the upper extremity: II. *American Association for Hand Surgeons Conference Proceedings*, August 1995, Cincinnati, OH.
34. Osborn JB, Newell KJ, Rudney JD, Stoltenberg JL. Carpal tunnel syndrome among Minnesota dental hygienists. *Journal of Dental Hygienists*. 1990;Feb:79–85.
35. McDonald G, Robertson MM, Erikson JA. Carpal tunnel syndrome among California dental hygienists. *Dental Hygiene*. 1988;July/Aug:322–327.
36. Conrad JC, Osborn JB, Conrad KJ, Jetzer TC. Peripheral nerve dysfunction in practicing dental hygienists. *Journal of Dental Hygiene*. 1990;Oct:382–320.
37. Polakowska B, Gluszcz-Zielinska A. Neurological assessment of health status in dentists [Polish]. *Medycyna Pracy*. 1994; 45(3):221–225.
38. Griffin MJ. Occupational human vibration. In: Bhattacharya A, McGlothlin JD, eds. *Occupational Ergonomics*. New York: Marcel Dekker;1996:605–626.
39. Stentz TL, Riley MW, Harn SD, Sposato RC, Stockstill JM, Harn JA. Upper extremity altered sensations in dental hygienists. *International Journal of Industrial Ergonomics*. 1994;13(2):107–112.
40. Lehto TU, Ronnemaa TE, Aalto TV, Helenius HY. Roentgenological arthrosis of the hand in dentists with reference to manual function. *Community Dentistry and Oral Epidemiology*. 1990; 18(1):37–41.
41. Beckenbaugh RD. Cumulative trauma disorders of the upper extremity: ii. In: *American Association for Hand Surgeons Conference Proceedings*. August 1995; Cincinnati, Ohio.
42. Neal NC, McManners J, Stirling GA. Pathology of the flexor tendon sheath in spontaneous carpal tunnel syndrome. *Journal of Hand Surgery (Br.)*. 1987;12B:229–232.
43. Barton NJ, Hooper G, Noble J, Steel WM. Occupational causes of disorders in the upper limb. *British Medical Journal*. 1992; 304:309–311.
44. Skie M, Zeiss J, Ebraheim NA, Jackson WT. Carpal tunnel changes and median nerve compression during wrist flexion and extension seen by magnetic resonance imaging. *Journal of Hand Surgery (Am)*. 1990;15A(6):939.
45. Szabo RM, Chidgey LK. Stress carpal tunnel pressures in patients with carpal tunnel syndrome and normal patients. *Journal of Hand Surgery (Am)*. 1989;14A:624–627.
46. Gelberman RH, Herginroeder PT, Hargens AR, Lundborg GN, Akeson WH. The carpal tunnel syndrome: a study of carpal tunnel pressures. *Journal of Bone and Joint Surgery*. 1981; 63A(3): 380–383

47. Grandjean E. *Fitting the Task to the Man*. London: Taylor and Francis; 1981.
48. Kwahito T, Onchi Y, Inowe M, Fujii B. Three dimensional finger control on cavity preparation especially on hand-piece control and finger stress. In: Queinnec Y, Daniellou F, eds. *Designing for Everyone, Proceedings of the 11ᵗʰ Congress of the International Ergonomic Association*. London: Taylor and Francis;1991:170–172.
49. Ekenvall L, Nilsson BY, Flaconer C. Sensory perception in the hands of dentists. *Scandinavian Journal of Work, Environment and Health*. 1990;16(5):334–339.
50. Bergquist-Ullman M, Larsson U. Acute low back pain in industry. A controlled prospective study with special reference to therapy and confounding factors. *Acta Ortopaedica Scandinavia (Supplement 170)*. 1977:1–117.
51. Brown JR. Factors contributing to the development of low back pain in industrial workers. *American Industrial Hygiene Association Journal*. 1975;36:26–31.
52. Damkot DK, Pope MH, Lord J, Frymoyer JW. The relationship between work history, work environment and low back pain in men. *Spine*. 1984;9:395–399.
53. Litchfield NB. Stress-related problems of dentists. *International Journal of Psychosomatics*. 1989;36(1–4):41–44.
54. Domeyer N. Stress as a synonym for marriage. *Florida Dental Journal*. 1988;59(1):27–28.
55. Eccles JD, Powell M. The health of dentists: a survey on South Wales 1965/1966. *British Dental Journal*. 1967;123:379–387.
56. Basset S. Back problems among dentists. *Journal of Canadian Dental Association*. 1983;49:251–256.
57. Eccles JD. The heart rate of dentists at work. *British Dental Journal*. 1969;126:216–220.
58. Eccles JD. Skin conductance changes in dentists and patients during conservation treatment. *Dental Practitioner and Dental Record*. 1970;21:43–48.
59. Diakow PRP, Cassidy J. Back pain in dentists. *Journal of Manipulative Physiological Therapy*. 1984;7:85–88.
60. Newton JT, Gibbons DE. Stress in dental practice: a qualitative comparison of dentists working within the NHS and those working within an independent capitation scheme. *British Dental J*. 1996;180(9):329–334.
61. Freeman R, Main JR, Burke FJ. Occupational stress and dentistry: theory and practice part II assessment and control. *British Dental Journal*. 1995;178(6):218–222.
62. Craven RC, Blinkhom AS, Roberts CA. Survey of job satisfaction among DSAs in the North-West of England. *British Dental Journal*. 1995;178(3):101–104.

63. Cecchini JG. Differences of anxiety and dental stresses between dental students and dentists. *International Journal of Psychosomatics.* 1985;32:6–11.

64. Cooper CL, Watts J, Kelly M. Job satisfaction, mental health and job stressors among general dental practitioners in the UK. *British Dental Journal.* 1987;162:77–81.

65. Reitemeier B. Psychophysiological and epidemiological investigations on the dentist. *Reviews on Environmental Health.* 1996;11(1–2):57–63.

66. Davidove DM. Dentistry, self-esteem and criticism. *New York State Dental Journal.* 1996;62(4):43–45.

67. Joffe H. Dentistry on the couch. *Australian Dental Journal.* 1996;41(3):206–210.

68. Katz CA. Are you a hardy dentist? The relationship between personality and stress. *Journal of Dental Practice Administration.* 1987;4(3):100–107.

69. Rundcrantz BL, Johnsson B, Moritz U, Roxendal G. Occupational cervico-brachial disorders among dentists. Psychosocial work environment, personal harmony and life-satisfaction. *Scandinavian Journal of Rehabilitation Medicine.* 1991c;19(3):174–180.

70. Osborne D, Croucher R. Levels of burnout in general dental practitioners in the south-east of England. *British Dental Journal.* 1994;177(10):372–277.

71. Eccles JD. Dental practice—a field for ergonomics research. *Applied Ergonomics.* 1976;7(3):151–155.

72. Pollack R. Dental office ergonomics: how to reduce stress factors and increase efficiency. *Journal de l'Association Dentaire Canadienne.* 1996;62(6):508–510.

73. Hardage JL, Gildersleeve JR, Rugh JD. Clinical work posture for the dentist: an electromyographic study. *Journal of the American Dental Association.* 1983;107:937.

74. Oberg T. Ergonomic evaluation and construction of a reference workplace in dental hygiene: a case study. *Journal of Dental Hygiene.* 1993;67(5):262–267.

75. Grace EG, Schoen DH, Cohen LA. Chair inclination and patient comfort. *Behavioral Science.* 1990;7(2):76–78.

76. Eccles JD, Davies MH. Hand piece positions in low-line dentistry. *The Dental Practitioner.* 1972;22:308–310.

77. Powell BJ, Winkley GP, Brown JO, Etersque S. Evaluating the fit of ambidextrous and fitted gloves. *Journal of the American Dental Association.* 1994;125(9):1235–1242.

78. Kwasman R, Handelman SL, McIntyre B, Barret G. Comparison of the effects of two hand-piece locations on dental team performance. *Journal of the American Dental Association.* 1975; 91:1203–1209.

79. Fox JG, Jones JM. Occupational stress in dental practice. *British Dental Journal.* 1967;123(10):465–473.
80. Kilpatrick HC. Production increases due to chairside assistance. *Journal of American Dental Association.* 1971;82:1367–1971.
81. Green ES, Lyman WA. Work simplification: an application to dentistry. *Journal of the American Dental Association.* 1958;57:242–252.
82. Davies MH, Eccles JD. Attitudes of dental patients to conservation treatment in different chair positions. *Journal of Dentistry.* 1978;6:294.
83. Eccles JD, Davies MH. A study of operating positions in conservative dentistry. *Dental Practitioner.* 1971;21:221.
84. Rundcrantz BL, Johnsson B, Moritz U, Roxendal G. Cervico-brachial disorders in dentists. A comparison between two kinds of physiotherapeutic interventions. *Scandinavian Journal of Rehabilitation Medicine.* 1991d;23(1):11–17.
85. Jacobsen N, Hensten-Petersen A. Occupational health problems among dental hygienists. *Community Dentistry and Oral Epidemiology.* 1995;23(3):177–181.
86. Sinczuk-Walczak H, Izycki J. Back pain syndromes in dentists. Diagnosis and differential diagnosis [Polish]. *Medycyna Pracy.* 1994;45 (1):71–74.
87. Izycki J, Wagrowska-Koski E. Musculoskeletal system diseases in dentists—an analysis of consultation cases referred to outpatient department of occupational disease [Polish]. *Medycyna Pracy.* 1992;43(6):525–529.
88. Rundcrantz BL. Pain and discomfort in the musculoskeletal system among dentists. *Swedish Dental Journal—Supplement.* 1991;76:1–102.
89. Milerad E, Ericson MO, Nisell R, Kilbom A. An electromyographic study of dental work. *Ergonomics.* 1991;34(7):953–962.
90. Persson B, Brune D. Dental laboratories. In: Brune DK. Edling C, eds. *Occupational Hazards in the Health Professions.* Boca Raton, Florida: CRC Press;1989:333–345.
91. Bruder R, Rohmert W. Ergonomic research of dentists—an example of a co-operation between industrial and university research departments. In: Queinnec Y, Daniellou F, eds. *Designing for Everyone, Proceedings of the 11th Congress of the International Ergonomic Association.* London: Taylor and Francis;1991:1159–1161.
92. Jamar P, Servais J. Choosing one's furniture, one's dental chair in a more ergonomic style [French]. *Revue Belge de Medecine Dentaire.* 1990;45(2):9–16.
93. Micholt F. Ergonomics and health risks for the dentists: overview [French]. *Revue Belge de Medecine Dentaire.* 1990;45(2):17–33.

Chapter 3

Job and Task Analysis

Manny Halpern

Abstract

A task or job analysis can be defined as a process by which we collect information about how work is done. This information is then translated into a format that will represent the job, or some aspects of it, for the purpose of design and evaluation. The analysis considers where work is done and what, when, how, why, and by whom an activity is performed. The chapter describes methods of ergonomic analysis suitable for dental care. The analysis assesses task demands that put the care provider at risk for developing musculoskeletal disorders. Recent guidelines recommend that the process start with hazard surveillance, which uses screening tools such as checklists to identify activities that require further evaluation. The methods described address the in-depth analysis done by professionals trained in ergonomics. The chapter suggests using a suite of methods to cover in moderate detail specific hazards that were identified in the initial screening.

Introduction

Many ergonomic research or intervention programs require a description of what and how things are done on the job. In programs that aim to prevent occupational musculoskeletal disorders, the analysis typically occurs when an existing job has been identified as involving a potential risk. An analysis of what is happening on the job may be initiated through a regular screening following a complaint about work conditions, as a result of a medical report on an individual case, or as a result of a review of injury records. Alternatively, a hazard assessment may be initiated as part of a comprehensive ergonomics program.

The information derived from such an analysis has the potential to

1. reduce the stressors acting on the musculoskeletal system, thereby reducing the number of workers who might develop work-related disorders (primary prevention); and
2. aid those already injured in returning to work with a reduced risk of recurrence (secondary prevention); this may be accomplished by identification of the stressors that aggravate a current medical condition.

The purpose of this chapter is to outline methods for assessing musculoskeletal risk factors present in dental workplaces. The chapter will address the methodological issues involved in ergonomic job analyses and examine their relevance to assessing stressors acting on the dental care provider.

What is a Job or Task Analysis?

A task or job analysis can be defined as a process by which information about work is collected and translated into a format that will represent the job, or some aspects of it, for the purpose of design and evaluation.[1] As the term refers to a process and a product, both need to be clarified.

Although the concept of analyzing human behavior at work is central to the field of ergonomics, the terms used have not been rigorously defined. In general, jobs are being viewed as composed of tasks and roles; however, the scope of what a task or role is varies. The lack of agreement on a common definition arises from the range of contexts in which a task can occur, since tasks are rarely defined in a way that would be applicable to all situations. For example, definitions that focus on physical and observable activity fail to account for tasks that are cognitive in nature. To allow a common approach to the issues of analysis, we will use the term "task" to mean an activity that

- has a defined goal and purpose,
- is achieved by a cognitive or physical action, and
- is defined in space and in time.[1,2]

The definition of the process also varies. Three broad categories are used to break down the information on work activity: job analysis, task analysis and task description. Job analysis addresses occupational issues by looking at overall duties and responsibilities within the total work context. *Task analysis* addresses more detailed work issues than job analysis. It looks at how individuals work and interact with each other, with equipment, and with the workplace environment. *Task description* is a statement of criteria; it documents the observable elements of behavior and concentrates on the physical level of the task, without making quantitative or qualitative judgments. Although it can be used in its own right, a task description often serves as a preliminary step in task analysis. In contrast, task analysis is both descriptive and prescriptive; it describes the task it analyzes, and then evaluates, specifies, synthesizes and interprets the information.[1]

Any analysis that aims to have some general application should consider the following dimensions:

- *Where*—physical location. Location can be defined by type (hospital clinic or private practice); environment (urban or rural); or functional space (reception, patient workstation, x-ray or lab, consulting office).
- *What*—description of tasks or job elements, such as the means of interaction or the ways in which tools and equipment are used. Tasks can be defined as specific dental procedures or types of care (conservative, prosthetic, or surgical).
- *When*—timing and sequence of actions. This dimension might address the duration and frequency of specific procedures (scaling, filling); activities (standing, sitting, talking); or functions (consulting, treating, administration, accounting).
- *How*—tools and equipment that are used. Examples are a patient chair, a caregiver stool, hand pieces, and mirrors.
- *Why*—the goal of the activity expressed as the end-result. For example, the hygienists task of dental cleaning is defined by the goal.
- *Who*—the performer of the task. This dimension might classify by function (dentist, dental hygienist, dental assistant) or by attributes (gender, age, experience).

This section has discussed the format and process of job and task analysis in general. The characteristics that are applicable to dental ergonomics will be addressed next.

What is the Ergonomic Analysis?

An ergonomic job analysis entails classifying work activity into its components and assessing their impact on the performer. In other words, it is an analysis of job or task demands. In this context, demands can be viewed as a set of factors that influence the body and mind of the worker. For example, physical work requires muscle activity for force exertions. This work can be assessed by measuring muscle tension or cardiopulmonary responses. In dental care, we focus on posture and force exertions. Visual and tactile stimuli are critical in all dental procedures, and we can measure the presentation of these stimuli and their impact on eye-hand coordination. Mental work activities require, among other things, the ability to sense patients' responses and adapt actions accordingly. Analytical abilities are required to translate patients' complaints into medical terms, and creativity is required to explain the findings and treatment to the patient. To provide a comprehensive view of the activities at work, we need to state the purpose of the activities, relate them to concrete objects or structures, and assess what affects the performance.

Work exposes us to a variety of demands. Conceptually we may differentiate between operational demands—mental (information processing) and physiological (peripheral and central processes)—that are innate or specific to the tasks performed and situational demands that arise from the circumstances under which the tasks are performed. Figure 1 presents a schematic framework for viewing the demands placed on the performer.

The application of the concept to dentistry is presented in Table 1. The operational demands are task specific. Every job requires processing of information, starting with sensory data (seeing, hearing, touching) and ending with some action such as eye-hand coordination or communication. Similarly, every job activity has some physiological requirements. Static work refers to activities that keep the body in a constrained position without movement. Dynamic work entails repeated muscular contractions. Every activity requires some limbs to work in a static way while others move dynamically. The physiological responses to these demands can either be limited to a

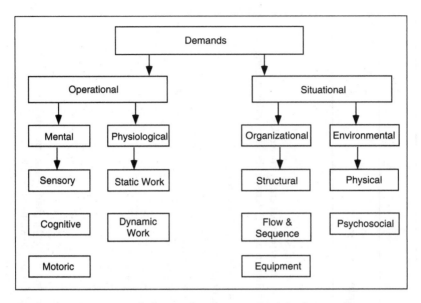

FIGURE 1.—Framework for analyzing ergonomic demands.

certain body part (localized demands), or involve whole body systems (systemic demands). Specific muscles will get fatigued in the first case, while the worker may get out of breath in the second case. As dentistry consists of fine motor activities, we can expect high visual, tactile, and manipulative demands. In activities that involve eye-hand coordination, we typically would expect most of the body to act as a static support for the upper extremities.

The situational demands are performance specific, as shown in Table 1. Work is structured in terms of duties, responsibilities, and skill requirements that will affect interactions with coworkers or patients. The flow and sequence of these interactions determine the duration and frequency of activities. In dental practices, for example, scheduling of patient caseload will determine the magnitude of the exposure to the task-specific processes. Equipment, such as the patient chair and the dentist's chair, and positioning with respect to the patient and the trays both determine performance in specific situations. As dentistry has high visual demands, we expect lighting to be a critical environmental factor. Many tasks

Table 1.—Application of the Job Analysis Framework to Dentistry

Type of Demand	Performance	Example
Task-specific (Operational)		
1. Information processing	*sensory perception:*	
	visual	presence of caries
	auditory	verbal reaction from patient or co-worker
	proprioceptive/tactile	tooth motion, reaching dense substance while drilling
	cognitive:	
	anticipation	medical history, lab diagnostics, x-ray
	decision making	treatment protocol
	perceptual-motor:	
	manipulation (eye-hand)	crown preparation
	communication	educating patient
2. Physiological		
2.1 Static work	upper extremity	preparation
	seated posture	all precision duties
	standing posture	
	(trunk, head, shoulders, elbow, wrist, fingers)	
	pelvis & lower extremities	
	(lower back, hip, knee, ankle)	
2.2 Dynamic work	local muscle work	extraction, root canal, change instruments
	finger, hand motion	all dental manipulations, use of tools
	whole body motion	move to improve visibility, rotate between workstation

Table 1.—*Continued*

Type of Demand	Performance	Example
	leg/foot motion	foot switches, changing of work stations
	trunk motion	reaching instrument trays
	force exertion	surgery, scraping, crown removal
Performance specific (Situational)		
3. Work organization		
3.1 Structure	duties	co-worker, dental lab
	responsibility for materials	
	comfort and health	patients, co-worker
	safety	occupational hygiene
3.2 Flow	time schedule	patient visits and breaks
	contacts with co-workers	
	coordination	use of supplies or lab work
	planning	order supplies, preparation, treatment protocol
3.3 Sequence	support	work materials and aids
3.4 Equipment	tools & instruments	handpieces
	machines	
	clinical practice	file cabinets, desks, chairs

Table 1.—*Continued*

Type of Demand	Performance	Example
4. Environment		
4.1 Physical	lighting	fixtures, task light
	noise	powered handpieces, suction
	vibration	powered handpieces
	facility layout	air flow
	climate	temperature, air quality, humidity
	communication relationship with co-workers	motivation, training, conflict resolution
4.2 Psycho-social	relationship with patients	calming patients

also make use of powered hand tools. The frequency, magnitude, and power spectrum of the vibrations transmitted to the operator are known to affect sensation and performance. The duration of the exposure may determine health outcomes such as the development of Raynaud's phenomenon, which can be caused by vibrating tools. Therefore, the exposure to vibration in various tasks is another environmental factor that we need to measure.

As in all situations in which the work object is another human being, interpersonal interaction is important. In most dental practices, work is conducted in teams; therefore, the number, frequency, and importance of communications with coworkers also influence the design of the facility.

The methods and techniques needed to describe or assess what is going on at work will be determined by the tasks and the circumstances of the performance. How can we measure and assess the work activities that put someone at risk for developing or aggravating musculoskeletal disorders?

Methods of Ergonomic Job or Task Analysis

Any analysis breaks down the job or the task into manageable units. In the context of prevention of musculoskeletal disorders, the ergonomic job or task analysis aims at assessing demands or occupational exposure to risk factors. The methods for measuring physiological, postural, and physical workload demands can be classified along a spectrum ranging from direct measurement; through observations, interviews, and diaries; to questionnaires and surveys.[3] Table 2 lists the various ergonomic methods that are employed to assess job demands. Direct and indirect techniques are noted together with some of the outcome measures.

Few of the methods of task analysis have been validated by formal studies, although many have gained a high degree of face validity through repeated use and application over a number of years and contexts. The accuracy of some instrumental measurements can be established, such as motion analysis or goniometers for measuring angles. Some observational techniques of posture analysis can be validated against

Table 2.—Methods, Techniques, and Outcome Measures Used in Ergonomics to Analyze Task and Work Activity Demands Relevant to the Development of Musculoskeletal Disorders, with Techniques Ranging from Direct to Indirect within Each Classification

Method	Technique	Outcome Measures
Physical workload	Biomechanical models	Moments & force calculations to compare with criteria
	Performance records, secondary or alternative tasks of psycho-motor performance, physical changes	Performance decrement
	Indirect observation (psychophysical techniques)	
Posture analysis	Biomechanical models	Subjective ratings (ability requirements, ratings of perceived exertion)
	Optical or electromagnetic methods (motion analysis, eye movement cameras)	Motion patterns in space Line of sight for visibility
	Observation (live, video)	Angular configuration data to compare with normative range of motion
	Self-rated questionnaires	
Physiological analysis —fatigue, stress, function	Cardiovascular demands (heart rate, blood pressure)	Direct or 'objective' that data need to be interpreted against norms or criteria
	Energy expenditure or consumption (O_2 uptake)	
	Muscle tension (electromyography EMG)	

Table 2.—*Continued*

Method	Technique	Outcome Measures
Mental workload	Direct observation of response to task	Performance decrement (reaction time, etc.)
	Indirect observation of response to task	Subjective rating of fatigue or concentration
	Indirect physiological responses (heart rate variability, tremor, galvanic skin response, eyelid blink rate)	'Objective' data that need to be interpreted against norms or criteria
Job and work attitude measurements	Indirect observation, special rating scales, informal group or individual interviews	Satisfaction, needs, important job characteristics
Archives, data base	Schedules or operation records of productivity or motion time studies	Standard times for procedures, case load
	Medical records, accident/injury reports	Incidence and severity of injuries and illnesses

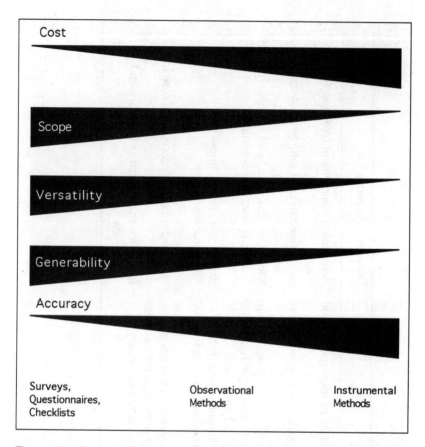

FIGURE 2.—Trade-off considerations in the selection of methods for job or task analysis.

instrumental measurements. In the absence of "gold standards," attempts to validate ergonomic methods are often limited to reliability testing. These studies examine, for example, the degree to which experts analyzing the same task independently of each other with the same method produce the same results. The methods that measure subjective issues such as job attitude require other types of validation, which go beyond the scope of this chapter.

It is unlikely that a single method will adequately capture all the dimensions of the actions and interactions at work. Several issues need to be considered in selecting the methods. The first issue is the level of detail we would like to have about the job. Secondly, we need to consider the techniques and procedures of the methods we employ (e.g., direct measurements of job behaviors or "indirect" measures such as checklists and surveys). Finally, we need to consider who is going to do the data collection and analysis (e.g., assessments by experts or by employees). The following discussion will show that these issues are interrelated.

The choice of a specific method is a trade-off among several considerations. The first consideration is feasibility. Figure 2 presents the relative merit of various techniques; indirect measures represent one end of a spectrum, instrumental or direct techniques the other end, and observational techniques fall somewhere in between. The relative merit can be expressed in several dimensions. These include cost, scope of the activities or job demands captured; the generality of the data versus its specificity; the versatility or the ability to apply it in different circumstances, and, last but not least, the accuracy of the assessment.[3] Direct technical measurements rely on instrumentation to provide information about the workload. Although measured data such as force still need to be interpreted against norms or criteria, investigators expect direct or instrumented measurements to provide the most accurate means of quantitatively assessing exposure to occupational risk factors. However, in view of the high cost and technical difficulty of direct measures, other less expensive alternatives with sufficient accuracy have to be considered.[4]

The expertise needed to collect the data and conduct the analysis is a related issue. Instrumented techniques invariably require considerable expertise. Checklists and other observational techniques require varying degrees of training. Questionnaires or surveys use the worker or a supervisor as a subject-matter expert on job demands and do not require training. Interviews use the worker as a subject-matter expert; however, they require training in data collection. Besides the ability to capture information from many subjects, questionnaires, surveys and interviews have the ability to capture data that are not immediately or readily observable. Instrumental and observational techniques, on the other hand, provide "snapshots"; that is, they are limited to current activity only.

One approach to increasing the robustness and comprehensiveness of the measurement is to use more than one method in any one study. Despite the comprehensiveness of this approach, three issues still pose major challenges to assessing the occupational impact of musculo-skeletal disorders:

1. how to assess nonstereotypical tasks,
2. how to account for past exposure to risk factors, and
3. how to account for the effects of nonoccupational activities such as sports or domestic chores.

So far, these challenges remain unanswered.

Ergonomic Job or Task Analysis in Dental Care

Several job and task analyses have been performed in dental care to establish cost, efficiency, and resource allocations. However, ergonomic task analyses for prevention of musculoskeletal disorders are few. In this section, we show examples of methods from general industrial settings that can be adapted to dental care tasks, as well as methods that have been developed specifically for dental care.

Task descriptions

The most cursory task analysis involves a description of process flow, using functional terms such as patient care, administration, counseling, or storage. The terms are appropriate for interviews, surveys, and review of archived material. This analysis may be sufficient for addressing layout of a facility.

To document the actions performed, a more detailed analysis is needed. The activities are described as writing, talking, lifting, turning, carrying, walking, standing, or sitting. Using such a classification in a survey, Shugars et al[5] found that dentists who spend about 80% of the time working in a seated position are more likely to report low back pain. The US Department of Labor has used similar terms, such as "standing," "sitting," "reaching," or "fingering," to describe job factors in the *Dictionary of Occupational Titles* .[6] This classification does not distinguish between gross body posture (e.g., sitting) and functional activity (e.g., writing). These terms can be used in combination with time measurements during observation of work activities, as well as in surveys, questionnaires, and interviews. This level of detail is sufficient when the whole body is engaged or when the metabolic demands of the job are of concern.

The Department of Labor is currently replacing the *Dictionary of Occupational Titles* with a new database called O*NET— The Occupational Information Network.[7] The new system contains over 1,000 descriptors organized in six domains (Experience Requirements, Worker Requirements, Worker Characteristics, Occupational Requirements, Occupation-Specific Requirements and Occupation Characteristics). Unlike the *Dictionary of Occupational Titles*, O*NET entails a more detailed and structured job analysis that conforms tot he framework described in Figure 1. However, we will not elaborate on this system, as it is not yet available to the public.

The job factors can be adapted to dental care. The activities of the dental caregiver may be sampled throughout the work day using a standard classification. For example, the keys may include working on the patient, working on something other than the patient, talking (to the patient or hygienist), or working out of the room. The classification can serve as a screening tool during observations of work activities, questionnaires, or surveys prior to a more detailed analysis. Table 3 shows that this classification can be used together with the observational methods described below.[8] Depending on the scope and purpose of the study, the investigator focuses on the activity of interest, e.g., working on the patient. Having narrowed the scope of the study, one can allocate more resources to study in depth some specific risk factors such as the posture used while sitting and working on the patient.

Observational methods to analyze task-specific demands

As awkward postures are considered a risk factor for developing musculoskeletal disorders, posture analysis has been used often to assess the risk in dental care. Most studies apply methods used in industrial settings. Such methods involve tracking the angular configurations of various body parts during the task of interest. At the simplest level, posture analysis entails classifying the postures by the degree of deviation from some standard configuration; this configuration is often the anatomical neutral position of a joint. An example for a classification key is provided in Table 3. All procedures view the activity as a series of frozen positions that are assumed during the job. This approach was used in observation of filmed,

---

Table 3. Example of a Classification for Coding Posture and Work
Activity in a Dental Care Environment

Work Sampling Key

Operator Status
P   working on the patient
W   working on something other than the patient
T   talking to the patient or hygienist
O   out of the room
Trunk Posture
1. Seated/Position

0	0 degree trunk flexion (forward bending)	B	sitting back on stool
30	30 degree trunk flexion (forward bending)	M	sitting in the middle of the stool
60	60 degree trunk	F	sitting forward in the stool

2. Standing
0   0 degree trunk flexion (forward bending)
30   30 degree trunk flexion (forward bending)
60   60 degree trunk flexion (forward bending)
Neck Posture
0   0 degree neck flexion (forward bending)
30   30 degree neck flexion (forward bending)
60   60 degree neck flexion (forward bending)
Shoulder Posture
0   0 degree shoulder abduction
30   30 degree shoulder abduction
60   60 degree shoulder abduction
90   90 degree shoulder abduction
Hand Position
S   hand is used for support
H   hand is holding something
G   hand is grasping or reaching for something
R   hand is resting

Source: Marklin & Cherney.[8]

---

photographed, or videotaped activities of dentistry as early as
1957.[9] Once the job has been broken down into its specific tasks,
the film or videotape is reviewed and the posture of the body
part of interest is documented on a form like the one shown in

Figure 3. These postures can be summarized over the workday so that various operations may be compared as to how often deviated postures occur. Using such a procedure, Marklin and Cherney[8] measured the gross posture of 10 dentists and 10 dental hygienists from videotapes. They found that dentists bent their neck at least 30° about 85% of the time while they were working on patients. The dentists also elevated their shoulders at least 30° about 50% of the time and maintained at least 30° of trunk flexion for about 60% of the time. Dental hygienists assumed postures similar to those of dentists.

Video observation is not a feasible means of gaining a dynamic and a three-dimensional assessment of the workplace—instrumentation is needed to facilitate the data collection. Automatic motion analysis systems keep track of the movement of markers placed on the body, either from videotape (passive systems) or from electromagnetic markers (active systems). These systems are useful for recording the movements of several body parts simultaneously. Another instrument is the electromechanical goniometer, a device that measures the angle between two body parts. This device is used when velocity and acceleration of particular body parts are of interest. In dental care, the postural configuration of several body segments is important. However, as the activities of most body segments are fairly static, motion analysis may be too expensive. Goniometers may be useful for wrist and hand motions, but the devices will interfere with patient treatment, so they might be practical only in simulated activities. Although practiced in industrial settings and sports, none of these methods have been applied in dentistry.

Suites of methods for analyzing task-specific demands of dental care workers

Using a battery or a suite of several methods gives us the ability to use both generic and job-specific methods to describe and assess the risks involved in dentistry. Rather than applying a standard general method to analyze postural demands, Kastenbauer[10] developed an observational procedure specific for dentistry. Using videotapes of dentists simulating 27 procedures, he identified 11 typical postural configurations adopted by dentists in standing and in seated practices. The investigator com-

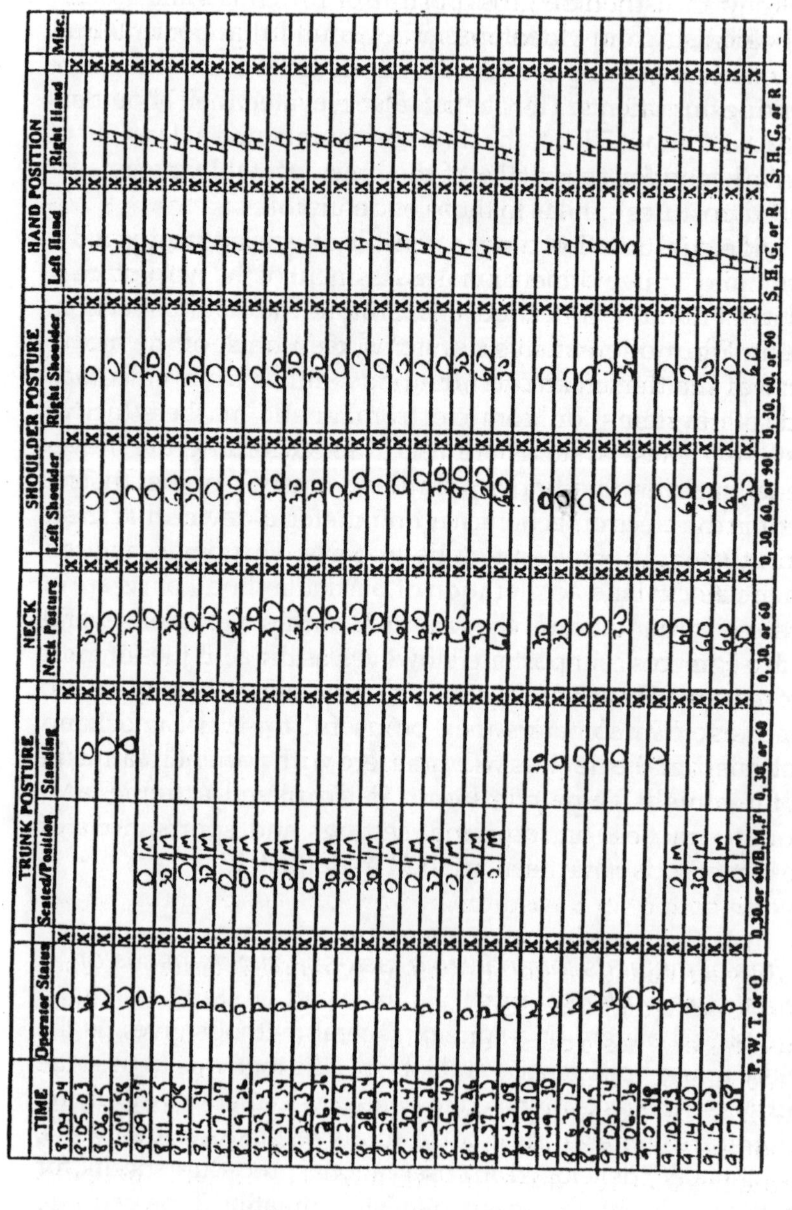

FIGURE 3.—An example of a data collection sheet for recording observed posture and general activity of a dentist and a dental assistant. (The key for the classification codes appears in Table 3.)

bined these observations with direct measurements of physiological responses in order to assess their physical demands. The physiological responses measured included the electromyography
(EMG) of neck, shoulder, arm and back muscles, heart rate, heart
rate variability, and blood pressure. One of the important findings of the study is that the physiological reactions are influenced
by the posture adopted for the task and the perceived "difficulty"
of the task.

An example of results from muscle activity measurements
is shown in Figure 4. This approach enables us to rank observed activities (postural alignment) according to effort
(physiological variables) measured directly by instrumental
devices. The analysis shows that the most demanding posture in Figure 4 entails bending the trunk forward, bending
sideways to the left and twisting, raising the arms up to 90°,
and rotating the shoulders forward (internally). In addition,
the elbow is flexed close to its maximal range of motion while
the forearm is rotated toward the thumb (pronated). The
EMG measurements revealed that this posture affected
mainly the right deltoid muscle, the right trapezius, and the
left erector spinae.

To rate the "difficulty" of the task, the dentists used a scale
of 1 to 5 for concentration, professional skill, and physical effort required in each of the clinical procedures they performed.
The most difficult task was a group of surgical procedures,
which included the extraction of a deeply impacted tooth and
root treatment. These procedures also required high back and
shoulder muscle activity. However, the study demonstrates
the difficulty we may encounter in interpreting the results of a
diverse battery of measurements or suites of methods. Thus,
the investigators characterized comfortable postures by low
cardiovascular stress (*low* heart rate or blood pressure), higher
muscle activity (*higher* EMG activity at the shoulder and back
muscles), and more dynamic trunk posture (*higher* accelerations
of the trunk). Conversely, uncomfortable postures were characterized by *low* muscle tension and *low* trunk acceleration,
denoting a static constrained posture, combined with *higher*
cardiovascular responses. In addition, comfortable postures
were characterized by shorter task duration, *lower* professional
demands, and *higher* concentration than the uncomfortable

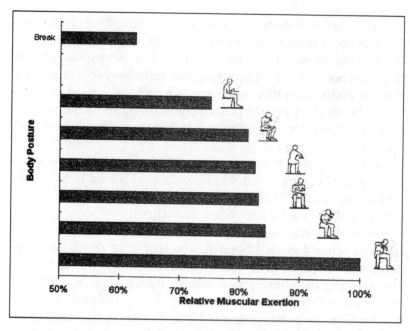

FIGURE 4.—Relative muscular exertion at different body postures. Exertion scores were derived from the sum of electromyographic (EMG) activity of the neck, shoulder, arm, and back muscles, and expressed as a percentage of the most demanding posture. Portions of this material are reprinted from Kastenbauer[10] with the permission of Quintessenz Verlag.

ones. To interpret these complex interactions, the investigators suggested that the lower the concentration and professional demand are, the more the dentist becomes aware of the physical demands.

While the perceived difficulty of the clinical procedure and the awkwardness of the posture account for some of the muscular and cardiovascular responses, the activity of the forearm muscles appears to depend mainly on the precision required in dental tasks.[11] Force may not have an impact on the EMG activity in any of the neck and shoulder muscles or the forearm. Although these results may be limited to the conditions tested in the laboratory, they suggest that the assessment of the risk of dental tasks should focus on the postural and mental demands of the fine motor skills required in some procedures.

Methods of describing fine motor activities

The description of the activities of the upper extremities is quite challenging. In many cases, it is sufficient to describe the task operationally as "grasp part" or "hold part." Micromotion studies may further describe the direction and range of the motion of the upper extremities, its duration, or its frequency. However, in formal engineering studies, fundamental operations are recorded for each hand (see Table 4). For example, among conservative treatment procedures, a subtask such as the application of fluoride will be described by the terms "hold tool," "position patient head," and so forth. This level of detail may be needed for identifying specific operations that we seek to improve. It is particularly useful for repetitive manual operations with short cycle times. The method is attractive because it is generic; it does not require us to develop a new methodology. The disadvantage of this approach is that the process and product of the analysis cannot be readily used by people not trained in ergonomics.

An example of a standard system that addresses the latter concern is presented in Table 5. Relying on an observational method, the Task Analysis/Performance Specification (TAPS) form is intended for people trained in dentistry, and it includes information on the concrete circumstances of the work.[12] However, it lacks information about risk factors for musculoskeletal disorders. Thus, data about posture, force exertion, repetitiveness, and task duration should be obtained during the observations.

Methods of analyzing situational demands

The information on the conditions under which the tasks are performed is important because it can help us to identify the possible causes of the risk factors present on the job. Table 6 lists some of the ergonomic parameters that could be relevant to dentistry. The reader should be aware that the list is not an exhaustive literature review. It is intended as a hypothetical framework for designing comprehensive studies of job demands; however, some of the specific examples have been mentioned in various studies. Several examples illustrate the methods that could be used to analyze these aspects of the job.

Table 4.—Gilbreth Table of Work Elements	
Element	Description
Search	Looking for something with the eyes or hand.
Select	Locating an object mixed with others.
Grasp	Touching or gripping an object with the hand.
Reach	Moving the hand to some object or location.
Move	Moving an object from one location to another.
Hold	Exerting force to hold an object at a fixed location.
Position	Moving an object in a desired orientation.
Inspect	Examining an object by sight, touch, sound.
Assemble	Joining together two or more objects.
Disassemble	Separating two or more objects.
Use	Manipulating a tool or device with the hand.
Unavoidable delay	Interrupting work activity because of factors beyond the worker's control.
Avoidable delay	Interrupting work activity because of some factor under the worker's control.
Plan	Performing a mental process that precedes movement.
Rest	Interrupting work activity to overcome fatigue.

Few studies investigated the interaction between awkward posture, force exertion, and visibility together with the design of the workstation, the tools, the position of the patient, the lighting, and so forth. Tables 4 and 5 provide a good start in recording some of these data. The International Standards Organization (ISO) also provides a card for recording information on the setup of the dentist workstation, using the clock

Table 5.—Example of a Standard Dental Task Analysis—The Task Analysis/Performance Specification (TAPS) form[12]

Task	Steps of Performance	Instruments/Materials
Procedure:		
Site:		

Process

			Doctor-Patient Relationship				
Step	Instrument	Performer's Position (o'clock)	Patient's Head Tilt (A/P)	Patient's Head Rotation (L/R)	Inter-maxillary Space (min/max)	Instrument Grip (1/2/3)	Intraoral Stabilization (Digit/Size) (3/4@ O/I/B/L)	View (D/I)

Table 6.—Ergonomic Parameters That May Be Associated with Risk Factors of Musculoskeletal Disorders Among Dental Care Providers

Ergonomic Parameter	Dentistry
Workstation design • affects posture, visibility and reach.	Layout and setup with respect to the patient
Tool design • affects posture and force	Dentist chair Mirror Hand piece size and shape Vibration of power tools Gloves (ambidextrous vs fitted)
Work object • affects visibility, posture and mental workload	Treatment site (jaw, quadrant) Patient fear and reaction during treatment
Work technique • affects force, posture, reach, mental workload	Use of mirror Breaks and pauses
Work organization • affects force duration and repetitiveness, and mental workload	Reassuring and calming the patient Scheduling and case load Piece rate payment Distracting phone calls and walkthrough traffic
Environment • affects force, sensation, visibility	Lighting Vibration

system with the patient's mouth as the reference point (ISO 4073, 119ß).[13] Four concentric circles around the center at a distance of 0.5 m (20 in) each enables to locate the position of the items of dental equipment. The reference plan also indicates the working place of the dentist and the assistant. Four standard positions for describing the layout of the workstations of a dentist and a dental assistant are shown in Figure 5.

The ISO system provides a way to investigate postural demands under different workstation layouts. Kastenbauer[10] observed the postures adopted most frequently in each layout. One of the results is shown in Figure 6. One posture (the third most awkward posture shown in Figure 4) was observed in 60% of the cases in ISO setup 4, which required the 11 to 12 o'clock position. This is an example of a constrained posture in a specific situation.

The patient can be viewed as the work object of the dental care provider. The treatment site (i.e., the jaw or the quadrant of the oral cavity) needs to be documented since it affects access and visibility and, consequently, the posture that needs to be adopted. In addition to positioning the patient's head, the dentist also has to react to the patient's behavior during the treatment. The patient's fear may add to the mental workload of the dentist. Currently, no standard questionnaires are available to measure this aspect of the work.

The discussion of the methods for measuring the demands of the other parameters is beyond the scope of this chapter. They are covered by the respective disciplines of engineering and psychology.

Conclusion

In one of the leading publications in the field, Putz-Anderson[14] specified two ways to conduct a job analysis. One is a task description that consists of a list of work methods. The second is a task analysis, which may consist of an ergonomic checklist that assesses the exposure to risk factors. This approach has been widely adopted by ergonomics practitioners and researchers. It has also been proposed in guidelines or standards initiated by the Occupational Safety and Health

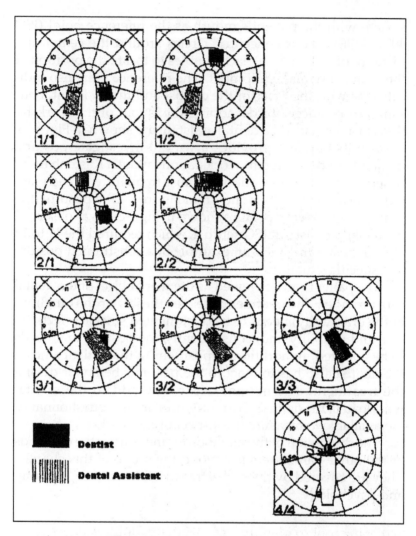

Figure 5.—ISO standard positions of the dentist's and dental assistant's instrumentation. Portions of this material are reprinted from ISO 4073:1980 with the permission of the American National Standards Institute. All rights reserved.

Administration (OSHA) or the American National Standards Institute (ANSI). In a working draft proposed to control cumulative trauma disorders, the ANSI accredited Z-365 committee outlined guidelines for job or task analysis.[15] The process starts with hazard surveillance that is intended as a

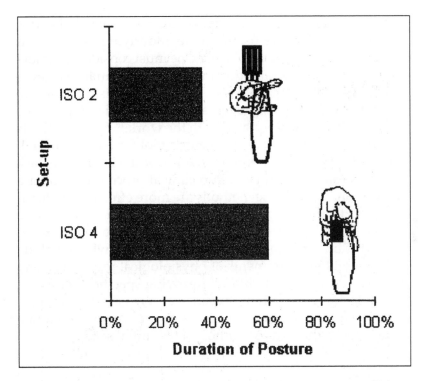

FIGURE 6.—An example of an ergonomic posture analysis: the duration of an akward posture, expressed as a percent of the observed work time in two standard workstation setups. Portions of this material are reprinted from ISO 4073:1980 with the permission of the American National Standards Institute. All rights reserved. Portions of this material are also reprinted from Kastenbauer[10] with the permission of Quintessenz Verlag.

screening tool to identify the jobs that require and justify attention. The tools used in this stage are checklists. Task analyses are then used to determine the part of the job that should be further evaluated. If risk factors are present and a quick fix is not readily found, a more detailed analysis may be needed to measure the exposure in ways that will help find solutions. This chapter has mainly addressed the methods used in the second stage by professionals trained in ergonomics, not the hazard surveillance stage.

Ergonomic evaluation techniques vary by the level of detail involved in the analysis, and the amount of information that can be gained about the risk of musculoskeletal disorder. The analysis is only as useful as the underlying assumptions or model of risk that is employed. One must consider the trade-off between the time and cost involved in the analysis. Gross analyses and workplace layout analyses are fast and easy to use but have not been proven effective in explaining a large amount of the risk associated with the work.[16] These methods may be sufficient only as a screening tool for hazard surveillance. Observational methods that break the job into its task elements—and in dentistry, into clinical procedures—offer a detailed analysis. These methods are more effective in identifying the factors associated with the risk, and in helping to control them; however, they are generally more complex and time consuming. The most detailed methods, which include instrumental measurements of physiological responses, may provide additional insight for improving specific operations, but these are also the most expensive. A reasonable compromise would be a suite of methods that covers in moderate detail specific hazards identified in the initial screening.

ACKNOWLEDGMENT

I am grateful to Dr Richard Marklin from Marquette University for his insightful comments and support.

REFERENCES

1. Rajan JA, Wilson JR. Introduction to task analysis. In: Nordin M, Andersson GBJ, Pope MH, eds. *Musculoskeletal Disorders in the Workplace.* St. Louis: Mosby; 1997:167–190.
2. Drury CG, Paramore B, Van Cott HP, Grey SM, Corlett EN. Task analysis. In: Salvendy G, ed. *Handbook of Human Factors.* New York: John Wiley & Sons; 1987:370–401.
3. Winkel J, Mathiassen SE. Assessment of physical work load in epidemiological studies: concepts, issues and operational considerations. *Ergonomics.* 1994; 37: 979–988.
4. Kilbom A. Assessment of physical exposure in relation to work-related musculoskeletal disorders—what information can be obtained from systematic observations? *Scand J Work Environ Health.* 1994; 20: 30–45.

5. Shugars DA, Williams D, Cline SJ, Fishburne C. Musculoskeletal back pain among dentists. *General Dentistry.* 1984; 32:481–485.
6. Department of Labor, Employment and Training Administration. *Selected Characteristics of Occupations Defined in the Dictionary of Occupational Titles.* Washington DC: US Government Printing Office; 1981: 9.
7. Peterson NG, Mumford MD, Borman WC, Jeanneret PR, Fleishman EA, Levin KY. *O*NET final technical report.* Salt Lake City, UT: Utah Department of Employment Security, 1996.
8. Marklin RW, Cherney KJ. *Design of a Stool to Improve the Working Postures of Dentists and Dental Hygienists.* Final report for project sponsored by The Brewer Co, Menomonee Falls, WI. Milwaukee, Wisc: Marquette University; 1995.
9. Eccles JD. Dental practice—a field for ergonomics research. *Appl Ergon.* 1976;7(3):151–155.
10. Kastenbauer J. *Zahnartz—ein Risikoberuf?* [Dentistry as a high risk job]. Berlin: Quintessenz Verlag; 1987.
11. Milerad E, Ericson MO. Effects of precision and force demands, grip diameter and arm support during manual work: an electromyographic study. *Ergonomics.* 1994;37(2):255–264.
12. Belenky M. Performance Logic in Clinical Dentistry. Baltimore, MD: Center for Human Performance in Dentistry, Dental School, University of Maryland, 1987.
13. *Dental equipment —Items of dental equipment at the working place: Identification system.* Geneva: International Standards Organization, ISO 4073E; 1980.
14. Putz-Anderson, V. *Cumulative Trauma Disorders.* London: Taylor & Francis; 1988.
15. American National Standards Institute. Accredited Standards Committee Z-365: *Control of Cumulative Trauma Disorder.* Draft. NSC\ANSI: Itasca, Ill; 1996.
16. Marras W. Task analysis. In: Nordin M, Andersson GBJ, Pope MH, eds. *Musculoskeletal Disorders in the Workplace.* St. Louis: Mosby; 1997:191–204.

Chapter 4

Stress in the Practice of the Art and Science of Dentistry

Edward Grace

Abstract

Dentistry, like other health care professions, can be very stressful physically and psychologically. The chief causes of professional stress in dentistry are the personality and temperament of dentists, practice and patient management problems, and problems in the actual delivery of dental services. This professional stress can be managed and reduced by a variety of means which are included under the following five general methodologies: 1) physical, 2) behavioral, 3) cognitive, 4) interpersonal and social, and 5) educational and skill acquisition. Developing insights into one's own stressors and gaining the knowledge and ability to eliminate or reduce those stressors should be an attainable goal for every dentist.

Dentistry and Stress

It is generally accepted that dentistry is a stressful profession. Recent dental and medical literature is replete with theories about the origins of this stress and methods of coping with it. Many of these theories and recommended coping mechanisms are general in nature and could be applied to many other professions, particularly other health professions such as medicine. When research focuses on the unique aspects of dentistry and dental practice, three general areas of stress that affect dental practitioners are usually identified. These are

1. the personality type and temperament of dentists,
2. practice management and patient management problems, and
3. the physical and psychological difficulties inherent in actually delivering dental care and performing dental procedures.

The first two areas have been researched extensively and are discussed quite often in the literature while the third area has received much less attention in the scientific literature. Only very recently has any significant amount of research been performed. This book is designed to remedy this situation and to stimulate new and much needed investigations into the delivery of dental care. I will review all three areas of stress in this chapter.

Personality Types

The personality and character traits of dentists and their effect on stress levels is a subject much written about (Joffe,1996; DiMattco et al, 1993; Grace, 1993; Katz, 1986).[1-4] Dentists have been described, in general, as hard working, perfectionistic, obsessed with detail, lacking in high self-esteem, and often not taken to sharing feelings or seeking help from others about personal problems.[1] Almost all the publications mentioned above, as well as and others (Swagger, 1986; Cooper and Di Baggio, 1995)[5,6] have found that dentistry attracts individuals with compulsive traits who tend to have unrealistic expectations of themselves and others who strive for unattainable standards of excellence. It should also be noted that many of these same characteristics are ones that we as patients would probably seek out in those individuals who provide our health care. Hard work, attention to detail, and striving for perfection are certainly admirable traits for those entrusted with the care of our health. The problem for dentists and other health professionals occurs when these same characteristics are detrimental to the health professional's own emotional and physical well-being. They also ultimately become hazardous to the best interests of their patients since these characteristics cause stress and can interfere with critical professional thinking and clinical judgment on the health professional's part.

Many of these same personality characteristics are also found in the now familiar designation of Type A personality which was first described by Friedman and Rosenman (1974).[7] Type A persons are characterized as always being time conscious, always being in a hurry, trying to do many things at once, being highly responsible people, thriving on challenge, and constantly feeling as if they have to do more and do it better than others. Many of us will recognize ourselves in that profile, but then, doing well in dentistry often makes us aware of time constraints, the challenges of patient diagnosis and treatment, and the many "things" that we are required to do every day to enable us to practice our profession successfully. We therefore are "damned if we do and damned if we don't."

Fortunately, there are many physical, cognitive and behavioral stress management techniques (Roskies, 1986; Christen and McDonald, 1986; Atkinson et al, 1991; Grace, 1996),[8–11] which can help in greatly reducing the negative effects of these tendencies and traits while enabling the dentist to retain positive characteristics that help in the management of a successful life and a successful practice and in the reduction or elimination of tendencies or traits that cause physical and emotional stress. One change that is often needed is the willingness and ability on the dentist's part to learn good patient and practice management techniques. This is also our second area of stress etiology, as mentioned previously.

Practice Management

Dentists who have not learned the skills, art, and science of patient and practice management and who have the adverse personality characteristics mentioned above are almost certainly experiencing high levels of stress and dysfunction both professionally and personally. The need to manage the business and professional demands of a practice as well as personal interactions with patients and staff is one of the chief sources of anxiety and stress mentioned by dentists.[4]

Practice management problems usually revolve around financial considerations and time related pressures. The time-related problems can be remedied by pre-planning or organizing the style and type of practice. All practitioners must decide for themselves what their philosophy of practice is and what type of service they can deliver with efficiency and quality and without undue stress. As Freeman et. al. (1995a) state, "The key words are organization, efficiency and a realistic approach."[12] Dentists who plan their patient time carefully so that they control the flow of the day, the week, and the month are infinitely more successful and less stressed than those practitioners who are controlled by time and scheduling constraints and poor planning. Strawn has written an excellent article on time management for dentists. In it, he stresses four aspects of time management practices for dentists. The first aspect is planning or setting up realistic and attainable goals, objectives, and outcome measures. Thought must be given to what you are going to do and how you are going to do it. The second aspect is to prioritize tasks in the order in which they need to be done, while the third is to organize office personnel and material to accomplish the desired goals and objectives. Finally, and sometimes this is most difficult for dentists to do, there must be delegation of authority and responsibility to office auxiliaries.[13]

Financial stresses can be avoided or at least diminished by obtaining expert help with financing of office setup and expenses as well as with accounting and bookkeeping practices. Too many dentists try to save on initial expenses by doing it themselves when they are not properly trained and are not really capable of doing it well. It is imperative, though, that the dentists themselves set up the goals and objectives of the practice at the outset and that they be comfortable with these goals and objectives. Experts can only be helpful to you when they are informed of your reasonable and well-thought-out plan for the future and of your present needs. Getting expert advice and determining long- and short-term financial needs and goals can reduce the potential conflict between the need to earn money, the satisfaction of doing a good job, and patient treatment planning. Many patients are wary of the veracity of some treatment plans, especially when they do not have pain or do not perceive a personal dental need. Articles in the popular press, such as the one in *Reader's Digest* (February, 1997) in which the same person was given treatment plans for his oral condition ranging from $0 to over $42,000, reinforce in the public mind the image of dentists who put their own financial situation first rather than the patient's interests. While most dentists disagree with and question many "facts" contained in the article and some of the conclusions that were reached, the general public has already formed its own opinion. Good time management and good financial planning can maximize a dentist's interests as well as the patient's interests and needs and helps to foster patient confidence and trust.

Personal interactions with patients, staff, and even with family members can be a cause of stress. To be effective and have a successful practice as well as an enjoyable and satisfying home life, the dentist must be able to communicate effectively with others. Developing good communications skills requires practice, patience, and the desire to hear and understand the other person's point of view. Essentially it is by communication that change is brought about in human beings, and it is the process by which we learn to understand each other.

The first skill to be learned is how to be a good listener (Grace, 1996).[11] Many health care professionals have learned the art and skill of talking and imparting information but are not as skilled at listening to others and hearing what they have to say. Research has shown that most malpractice claims and most dissatisfied patients are a result of a lack of proper communications and a lack of understanding and trust between doctor and patient.[14,15] The more the patient's needs and expectations are understood by the dentist and the more the patient understands the dentist's practice philosophy and aims, the better that dentist/patient relationship will be.[16] This understanding leads to better compliance with professional recommendations, greater acceptance of treatment plans, and increased satisfaction with dental care. All of which leads to reduced doctor and patient stress.

Similarly, stresses that arise from dentist/staff relations are often based on poor communications and a lack of rapport. Staff members who feel that they are an integral and valued part of the office team perform better and help to reduce stress on the dentist. All staff members should have realistic and well-defined job descriptions that delineate their duties and responsibilities. Staff should also be part of regular office meetings that are aimed at sharing information as well as improving the office interpersonal atmosphere and the working conditions for doctor, staff, and patient. While many offices are quick to blame someone for poor performance, praise for a job well done is often less forthcoming. Yet research has shown that positive reinforcement of good performance is most often associated with better productivity and lessened office distress.[17]

Delivery of Dental Care

The third area of stress in dentistry is the emotional and physical strain of delivering the dental care itself—that is, the actual work of dentistry. This area has received much less attention than the others, and the answers to these problems are not as numerous nor are they as clear-cut. Presently, many other health professions, such as medicine[18] and nursing,[19] are investigating and researching the interactions between their health professional workers and their work system. In dentistry, it has been demonstrated that those dentists who learn how to "practice smart" or in a way that is compatible with their physical and emotional makeup can reduce the effects of stress on themselves. Dentists who have ergonomically correct offices designed or adapted for them (e.g., based on size, vision adaptation, working style, and complexity of practice) and who learn to practice dentistry in a way compatible with their physical and emotional makeup have fewer backaches, headaches, and other physical complaints and are more relaxed at the end of the day.[20,21] Every dentist should learn to practice in the manner that is best for him or her as an individual, not for the average dentist. Recent studies have demonstrated that dentists and dental hygienists who learn to practice in a manner that helps them to achieve optimum access, visibility, comfort, and control have fewer musculoskeletal disorders[22] and deliver better dental services and work products.[23]

Some of the more common sources of stress in the dental working environment that emanate from the delivery of dental care are poor working posture from the utilization of dental equipment that is not designed for proper posture or from the improper utilization of properly designed dental equipment; noise from drills; poor and strained visibility (see Photo 1); and problems with gaining easy access to the working area. The difficulty in quickly and efficiently delivering esthetically and biologically acceptable dental care in a compassionate, patient-centered manner while observing strict asepsis in a confined space in a small working area (the mouth) that is filled with saliva on a patient who probably wishes to be elsewhere can be challenging, to say the very least. Colangelo and Belenky state, "Fatigue caused by this physically stressful approach to the delivery of dental care undoubtedly adds to the overall stress of practicing dentists."[24]

Stress Management in Dentistry

While dealing with the various causes of stress in dentistry may, at first glance, seem insurmountable, many studies have demonstrated that these stresses can be overcome and that dentistry can be practiced in a manner that is healthy, enjoyable, and profitable for both dentist and patient.

The basic differences between a healthy, low-stress dental practice and an unhealthy, high-stress one are usually made apparent by the presence of methods used for stress reduction or stress elimination. The following categories are the most common general areas in which stress can be identified, reduced, and/or eliminated:

1. physical,
2. behavioral,
3. cognitive or mental,
4. interpersonal and social, and
5. educational and skill acquisition.

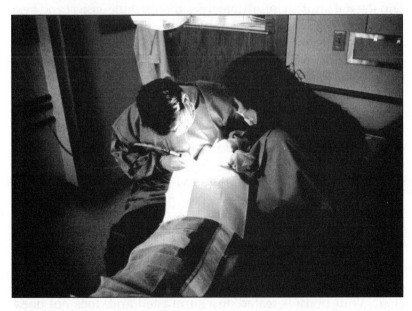

PHOTO 1.—Strained visibility.

Physical Methods

Stress reduction methods that come under the heading of physical methods include general health maintenance approaches such as incorporating improved diet and exercise into daily life. New scientific data are available about the reduction of fats, sugars, salt, and cholesterol in diets, increasing fiber content, and limiting total calorie intake. Research clearly links diet to emotional stress and physical dysfunction.[25] There are enough commercially available publications, audiovisual materials, lectures, advice-givers, and so forth to help anyone who is serious about improving his or her health through dietary changes.[25,26] Similarly, exercise has been studied and researched extensively enough that we know its contribution to overall health. First, it is important to incorporate light exercise, such as walking and stretching exercises, into a daily routine. More intense exercise, such as running, treadmills, aerobics, and so forth, should be done at least three times a week for 45 minutes at an intensity level that increases one's heart rate to somewhere between 70% and 80% above the resting heart rate. These two simple forms of exercise, when included as part of a routine life style, together with adequate sleep and rest on a daily basis and a proper diet, are the most basic and essential aspects of increasing physical and mental health. Unfortunately, sometimes the easiest and best known strategies are the least utilized.

Other physical approaches to stress reduction are the ability to relax physiologically and mentally. There are many different theories about relaxation and a myriad of approaches to learning this skill. One of the most recommended books about relaxation and one that I highly recommend, *The Relaxation Response,*[27] describes a simple five-step muscular relaxation process that most people can learn in a very short time.

These very simple steps involve

1. a convenient place—select a quiet restful place to practice relaxation;
2. a quiet environment—ensure that no disturbances will occur for the time period (15 minutes to 1 hour) during which you will practice;
3. a comfortable position—sit or lie down in a place where your body is rested and supported and does not need to be "held in place";

4. a mental device—clear your mind of extraneous thoughts by concentrating on a "blank screen" in your mind or by reciting or chanting to yourself the word "one" or a nonsense word that has no meaning but that will help clear your mind of the usual distractions of life that can be stressful; and
5. a passive attitude and calm breathing—breathe slowly and calmly from the abdomen rather than from the chest and adopt a "let it happen" rather than "make it happen" attitude.

When practiced on a regular basis, this exercise can bring on physical and emotional rest as well as relief from stress. What often happens, though, is that the skill is learned but is not practiced and is eventually lost. If one learns and practices relaxation regularly and well, it becomes a natural part of one's reaction and coping systems and occurs automatically.

A variety of other relaxation methods have been recommended. These include mental imagery,[28] Jacobsen progressive muscle relaxation,[29] autogenics,[30] meditation or yoga, and even simple diaphragmatic breathing exercises.[31] Each individual should choose the technique or method that seems to be the most useful and effective for him or her. Every public library and book store has a large selection of books, videotapes and audiotapes from which to choose.

Behavioral, cognitive, and interpersonal approaches to stress management frequently overlap, and different authors place certain methods under different categorical headings. For simplicity, we will use the following classification:
- behavioral approaches—time management and practice management;
- cognitive approaches—cognitive restructuring, realistic problem solving, and goal setting; and
- interpersonal and social approaches—improving communication skills, utilizing social support systems and increasing good social and professional interpersonal relationships.

Behavioral Methods

Time management and practice management are inevitably linked together. The first step in good practice management is the efficient management of your time. In dentistry, as in other professions, time is money. Inefficiency and waste lead to poor time usage, which creates financial problems, interpersonal stresses, and a decrease in quality of care. The goal of effective time management is to find the harmony or balance in the use of time that serves productive, professional needs but still meets personal needs of caring, sharing, and growing. Hans Selye, one of the earliest researchers on stress, believed that the right amount and type of work was essential for a stress-free life. Too little or too much work can cause stress, as can inadequate working conditions or poorly managed workplaces, according to Selye.[32]

To manage time efficiently, it is important to set priorities for the day, week, month, and year. These are established by setting goals for what one wants to accomplish and identifying the steps needed to reach those goals and the order in which they should be done to reach the desired results. Other time management principles include all of the methods described in the following paragraphs.

Time should always be set aside in the daily schedule for emergencies, and if the emergencies don't occur, then there is more time to accomplish identified long-term tasks. Thus, something is constantly being accomplished. Schedules should be organized both at work and at home to avoid unnecessary interruptions or distractions. Use answering machines to screen telephone calls or post "do not disturb" or "not available" signs on your private office door. Delegate tasks to others whenever another person can just as competently complete that task and thus free up your own time. Dentists frequently dislike giving up control and delegating tasks to others, even though it is a proven time saver.

Besides learning to effectively manage time in our personal and professional lives, we also need to be good business managers of our dental practices. Most rules for good managers can be simplified to a few basic guidelines. The first rule is to determine your priorities and your values for your practice and your life. Try to arrange your personal and professional time to reflect these values. All dentists should have both short- and long-term plans that will, it is hoped, allow them to fulfill their life's aspirations.

Next, inform and train your staff to help you implement these plans. They should know what your philosophy is, what you want done, and what their duties are in that "game plan." The more your staff understand what is needed and what their role is, the more they will take pride in and feel "ownership" of the practice. Frequent short meetings are needed to elucidate your vision and to receive staff input into that vision. Treat your staff as you would like to be treated and reward those who are part of the solution, not the problem. Good office personnel always refer to the dental practice as "our office," not "the doctor's office" because they feel respected, valued, and needed, and they want the practice to succeed. This feeling is infectious and is transmitted to your patients, who also come to value your practice and who become your best assets and referral sources.

Cognitive Methods

The principal cognitive methods, setting goals and objectives as well as realistic problem solving, have been discussed already. These can be accomplished by the use of many different techniques, one of which is called cognitive restructuring, whereby we change our approach to problem solving and rational thinking by the use of logic, positive reinforcement, and cognitive conflict resolution. The first step of the cognitive conflict resolution method is to identify the results that are desired from your actions or behavior. Next, list those behavior patterns that are not helping to produce those results and identify the reasoning behind those beliefs and actions. Lastly, recognize the poor results or negative behavior that has and will continue to result from those beliefs. This should lead to the recognition and implementation of actions or behaviors based on beliefs that will produce the positive results that are desired and the elimination of the negative actions. This "mental rehearsal" or mental "what if" exercise should enable a person to know what it is he or she really wants and how to get it.

Interpersonal and Social Methods

Two very important stress reduction strategies fall under this heading. These are acquisition of good communication skills and increasing the quality and quantity of our social support systems. Effective communication requires foremost that we develop the ability and willingness to listen to others and try to understand their viewpoints. Frequently, people are rehearsing their answers or thinking of ways to deliver their own message rather than listening to the other person. Listening skills are developed by paraphrasing in your own words or feeding back to the other person the message they are attempting to send to you. If you haven't heard the other person correctly, that person will often repeat the message for you in order to help you understand. The more people have to repeat a message, the greater the frustration level will be, and the less effective the communication will be. Good listeners rarely have to have the message repeated, and good listeners find that their own stress and that of the other person are greatly reduced because there has been a proper conveying of accurate information. While agreement may not have been reached, understanding has begun.

Effective communications are essential for relationships between members of families and office staffs, and among doctor, staff, and patients. Start developing good communication skills by asking a staff member to give you his or her ideas on a particular office task or problem while you sit and actively listen. You may be surprised by their reaction to your wanting to hear their ideas and by your being able, through feedback, to demonstrate that you did hear their ideas. Poor listening skills on the dentist's part and an inability and unwillingness to listen are some of the major stressors identified in surveys of dental office staff personnel.[33]

The other interpersonal stress reduction technique is to develop a social support network system to enhance one's mental and physical health. Research by Lynch[34] and Greenblatt[35] demonstrated that strong interpersonal relationships and social support are essential for mental and physical health. In *The Broken Heart: Medical Consequences of Loneliness* Lynch reviews the findings from his own and other's studies, which show that loneliness and the absence of support, love, and affection from others is one of the best predictors of ill health, poor physical responses to medical and surgical therapy, and to increased stress and emotional difficulties.[34] Dentists must take the time to search for and nurture meaningful and mutually satisfying relationships that affirm the uniqueness of each individual and the importance of each of us to the other. This is important in our homes, offices, and all of our relationships.

Education and Skill Acquisition

A dentist's confidence in his or her knowledge of the dental profession and in the fact of being well trained and educated can reduce stress. When one feels unsure of one's existing professional skills and training and of one's ability to diagnose and treat oral disease and to perform dental procedures, burnout sets in. Brod coined the term "technostress" which he defined as " a condition resulting from the inability of an individual or organization to adapt to the introduction and operation of new technology."[36] Health professionals are particularly vulnerable to technostress because of the amount and diversity of knowledge needed to be competent and because the knowledge base in health sciences is always growing and changing. A dentist must learn to be a lifelong learner and must acquire this skill early in his or her career.

Education of dentists and dental students as well as of hygienists in the principles of good work-related ergonomics is still at a very early stage. Most practitioners have not been trained, nor have they developed the skills and knowledge necessary to practice in a manner that is correct for them. This lack of training is partly due to the need for more research and partly due to the need for better teaching tools and better informed and trained teachers. Part of the blame for the lack of training also is attributable to the magnitude of the task. Peate puts the issue into perspective by stating,

The successful management of occupational disorders must account for workplace conditions (ergonomic and work practices), psychosocial factors, diagnostic uncertainties and the need for active modalities (exercise and activity) rather than passive (bed rest, traction and medication). Prevention is more important than treatment.[37]

Prevention is indeed more important than treatment, especially when it involves mental, emotional, or physical stress. Preventing or eliminating the various stressors mentioned in this and other chapters in this text is easier than having to deal with the treatment process and damage caused by the sequelae of those stressors. But the key is to learn the right way to practice and deliver dental services at the beginning of a career or to intervene as early as possible. The longer bad habits persist, the more resistant they are to change. Becoming educated about practice management, developing skills to overcome stress, and learning how to deliver dental services in a manner that is ergonomically correct are essential for effective and stress-free dentistry.[24]

Education is particularly important when learning the "way" to practice dentistry. The dentist must learn to practice in a physically centered manner in an ideal environment to increase efficiency and reduce physical and mental stress. Practicing "smart" and ergonomically correct, which is the core message of this book, is one of the first steps that a dentist must take to reduce stress in his or her life. Reducing our physical and psychological stress in performing dentistry and increasing the quality of our work in a more efficient manner are results of correct ergonomic practices. This book is the beginning of the fulfillment of the need for information and research into the art and science of the actual practice of dentistry. It is hoped that there will much more to come in the future.

Summary

Dentistry can be a stressful profession but it can also be a very rewarding profession that benefits both practitioners and patients. By identifying those aspects of dentistry that are uniquely stressful to each of us and by following simple steps that can reduce stress and increase emotional and physical health, dentists will enjoy their professional and personal lives more and will become better dentists and better individuals in their personal relationships.

REFERENCES

1. Joffe H. Dentistry on the couch. *Australian Dental Journal.* 1996;41(3):206–210.
2. DiMattco M, Shugars D, Hays R. Occupational stress, life stress and mental health amongst dentists. *Journal of Occupational and Organizational Psychology.* 1993;66:153–162.

3. Grace M. A friend in need. *British Dental Journal.* 1993;174:151–154.
4. Katz C. Stress factors operating in the dental office environment. *Dental Clinics of North America.* 1986;30:S29–S36.
5. Swagger G. The Type A personality: overwork and career burnout. *Dental Clinics of North America.* 1986;30(4, October Special Issue): S37–S53.
6. Cooper T, DiBaggio J. Understanding the effects of stress in dental practice. *PreVue.* 1995;Fall:4–10.
7. Friedman M, Rosenman R. *Type A Behavior and Your Heart.* New York: Knopf Publishers; 1974.
8. Roskies E. *Stress Management for the Healthy Type A: Theory and Practice,* New York: Guilford Press; 1986.
9. Christen A, McDonald J. Management of stress in the dental practitioner. *Dental Clinics of North America.* 1986; 30(4, October Special Issue):S67–S78.
10. Atkinson J, Millar K, Kay E, Blinkhorn A. Stress in dental practice. *Dental Update.* 1991;18:60–64.
11. Grace E. Dentistry, stress, and substance abuse. *Maryland State Dental Association Journal.* 1996;39(2):77–79.
12. Freeman R, Main J, Burke F. Occupational stress and dentistry: theory and practice. Part I—recognition. *British Dental Journal.* 1995;178:214–217.
13. Strawn C. Time management practices for the dentist. *Dental Clinics of North America.* 1986;30(4, October Special Issue):S107–S116.
14. Ingersoll B. *Behavioral Aspects in Dentistry.* New York: Appleton-Century-Crofts; 1985.
15. Chambers D, Abrams R. *Dental Communication.* Norwalk, Ct: Appleton-Century-Crofts; 1986.
16. Freeman R, Main J, Burke F. Occupational stress and dentistry: theory and practice. Part II—assessment and control. *British Dental Journal.* 1995;178:218–222.
17. Dana A. Practice management. *Maryland State Dental Association Journal* 1995;38(4):54–56.
18. Bergeur R. Ergonomics in the O.R. *American Journal of Surgery.* 1996;171(4):385–387.
19. Hignett S. Work-related back pain in nurses. *Journal of Advanced Nursing.* 1996;23(6):1238–1246.
20. Shugars D, Miller D, Williams D. Musculoskeletal pain among general dentists. *General Dentistry.* 1987;34(4, July/August):272–276.
21. Colangelo G, Belenky M. Performance logic: a key in improving dental practice. *Journal of Dental Practice Administration.* 1990;7(40, October):173–177.

22. Rudcrantz B, Johnsson B., Moritz U. Occupational cervico-brachial disorders among dentists: analysis of ergonomics and locomotor functions. *Swedish Dental Journal*. 1991;15(3):105–115.
23. Catovic E, Kraljevic K. Effect of work on the body posture in dental team members. *Acta Stomatologica Croatica*. 1990;24(1):39–43.
24. Colangelo G, Belenky M. Performance logic: a new horizon in the delivery of dental care. *Dentistry*. 1989;9(2, April):12–15.
25. Ornish D. *Stress, Diet and Your Heart*. 3rd ed. New York: Signet Books; 1994.
26. Benson H. *The Relaxation Response*. New York: William Morrow Co; 1975.
27. Rice P. *Stress and Health: Principles and Practice for Coping and Wellness*. Monterey, Calif: Brooks/Cole Publishing Co; 1987.
28. Miller L, Smith A. *The Stress Solution*. New York: Simon and Schuster Inc; 1993.
29. Jacobsen E. *Progressive Relaxation*. 2nd ed. Chicago: University of Chicago Press; 1938.
30. Linden W. *Autogenic Training: A Clinical Guide*. New York: Guilford Press; 1990.
31. Pelletier K. *Healthy People In Unhealthy Places*. New York: Delacorte Press; 1984.
32. Selye H. *The Stress of Life*. 2nd ed. New York: McGraw-Hill; 1980.
33. Locker D, Burman D, Otchere D. Work related stress and its predictors among Canadian dental assistants. *Community Dentistry and Oral Epidemiology*. 1989;17:263–266.
34. Lynch J. *The Broken Heart: The Medical Consequences of Loneliness*. New York: Basic Books Inc; 1977.
35. Greenblatt M, Beccera R, Serafetinides E. Social networks and mental health: an overview. *American Journal of Psychiatry*. 1982;139(1);977–984.
36. Brod C. Managing technostress: optimizing the use of computer technology. *Personnel Journal*. 1982;61:753–757.
37. Peate W. Occupational musculo-skeletal disorders. *Primary Care*. 1994;21(2, June):313–327.

Chapter 5

Vibration and Dental Equipment

Martin Cherniak

Abstract

Vibration has been associated with several characteristic hand disorders in workers using industrial tools. These include injury to the nerve endings in fingertips, heightened vascular reactivity to the cold, and an increased level of carpal tunnel syndrome. A similar profile of symptoms and clinical signs has been detected in dental workers and other biomedical personnel using dental and surgical instruments. Because dental instruments operate at frequencies that are much higher than those recognized from industrial tools, the etiology that produces clinical disease is unclear. There is a compelling need for further research before an adequate preventive strategy can be developed.

Introduction

Almost any vibrating source can cause adverse health effects to the hand and arm if the source is sufficiently intense and if the exposure is sufficiently long. The frequency ranges can induce damage or altered function in susceptible tissues. In the workplace literature, sufficient exposure times have ranged from as little as 1 month to more than 30 years, depending on intensity, tissue injury, and an identified frequency range—usually between 4 and 5000 Hz.[1]

Many commonly used air-powered and electrical instruments produce significant forces in these frequency ranges. Of interest to dental professionals, electric tooth brushes and plaque removers usually deliver peak forces at the lower range, below 100 Hz, whereas dental drills are effective at the higher-end frequencies and may exceed 10 000 Hz (see Photo 1).

Workers who use vibratory tools, that are either air powered, such as grinders and impact wrenches, or reciprocating,

129

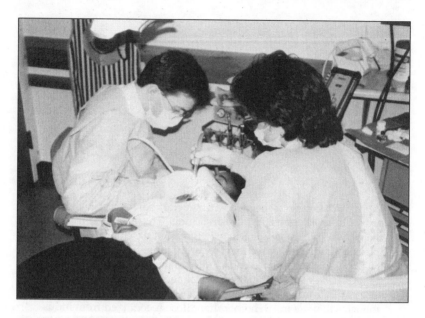

PHOTO 1.—Vibration frequencies of dental drills may exceed 10 000 Hz.

such as chainsaws, commonly experience upper-extremity symptoms. With some notable exceptions in the very-high-frequency range,[2] generally above 5000–10 000 Hz, the findings are remarkably consistent, independent of the type of tool used and the manner in which it is employed. Many of the signs and symptoms associated with exposure to vibration are distinct and the etiologic association with particular hand held tools quite reproducible. Accordingly the medical diagnostic and regulatory controversies that surround other work-acquired upper extremity disorders, such as carpal tunnel syndrome and repetitive strain injury (RSI), are less common around vibratory exposures. For one thing, because vibration has distinct and measurable physical characteristics, hazards associated with tools and instruments can be quantitated in the laboratory, and there is less need to define discrete correlates of "trauma."

Characteristic findings are blanching of the digits upon exposure to cold, referred to as vibration white fingers (VWF); deep, radiating forearm pain; dysesthesias and paresthesias of the hands; perceived weakness in the absence of grossly demonstrable nerve or muscle pathology; and a focal pattern of neuritic dysfunction and discomfort. The latter presentation does in fact initiate some overlap with more general categories of cumulative trauma disorders. Several authors have noted that there are sometimes complicated differential diagnoses, since some of the symptoms associated with vibratory exposure require differentiation from (and sometimes an inclusion within) more common diagnoses affecting peripheral nerves.[3,4] These include entrapment of the median nerve at the wrist (carpal tunnel syndrome), entrapment of the ulnar nerve at the elbow or in the forearm (cubital tunnel syndrome), and irritation in the neck of spinal nerves that innervate the arm and hand (cervical myelopathy).

The control of adverse health effects from vibration has been approached by international organizations for more than 20 years through standards such as International Standard (ISO) 5349[5] and British Standard (BS) 6842.[6] Their primary purpose is to curtail vasospastic disease (vibration white fingers) in workers through the standardized measurement of frequency-weighted acceleration as an approximation of hand-transmitted vibration exposure. The standards, which have evolved out of a consensus approach, are intended to limit the prevalence of vascular symptoms to 10% of an exposed working population through time-dependency adjustments, so that "energy equivalents" and allowable exposure time are inversely related. For example, ISO 5349 predicts that 10% of a working population exposed to vibration will develop vibration white fingers in 3 years if the tool accelerations (the most common measure of exposure) are $10 m/s^2$, but the same 10% of the workforce will develop the disease much more gradually in 15 years (five times longer) if exposures are reduced by 80% to $2 m/s^2$.

The key elements of standard setting are a quantitation of allowable limits on exposure time as a function of vibratory force, usually measured as tool acceleration. Because hand tools, unlike tuning forks, produce oscillations over a wide spectrum of frequencies, standard setting has also involved an attempt to segregate more damaging frequencies from those presumed to be less injurious to hand and arm tissues. In practice, this has meant greater caution towards tools and instruments that generate frequencies on the lower end of the spectrum—usually less than 100 Hz. This has considerable importance for the types of instruments used by dental personnel, with which transmitted frequencies, as noted, are usually much higher—in excess of 5000 Hz. However, an adverse consequence is that the sizable volume of investigation that has occurred around lower-frequency tools, such as chain saws, is not necessarily transferable to dental instruments. Accordingly, the effective preventive strategies that have lowered vasospastic disease in tree loggers are not particularly applicable to clinical medical and dental work.

Hand Tools and Neurological Injury

In recent years, there has been a growing recognition that nerve dysfunction caused by vibration could coexist, often independently, with the better known vasospastic effects. These *sensorineural* afferent defects, which often involve altered sensation or perception, have been most notable in the fingertips, at the source of tool contact and maximum vibration absorption. They appear to be caused by pathologic damage to mechanoreceptors, thermoreceptors, and nocioreceptors of the skin. While finger blanching remains the most characteristic clinical sign, Raynaud's syndrome, or so-called cold induced vasospasm, is principally a problem of colder climates and is associated with outdoors work. Neurological symptoms are potentially more ubiquitous and broadly disabling, because of the wider range of jobs at risk. Accordingly, the bulk of current work, particularly for instruments producing higher frequencies, has been on nerve fiber abnormalities, which are more prevalent, more quantifiable, and more subtle in their distribution than Raynaud's syndrome. This is a change in emphasis from earlier investigative work which primarily involved vascular-related observations on outdoor workers in heavy industry. However, much of the occupational medicine literature and the approach to standard setting reflects this earlier orientation toward vascular abnormality and toward work with larger industrial tools.

These differences in focus have implications for determining case definition and for clinical staging. The concentration on vascular presentation reflected the predominant recognition of the dramatic and qualitative clinical sign of skin blanching, which could be characterized with instruments no more complex than an ice bath, a thermometer, and a questionnaire. Sensorineural injury to small organelles in the hands and fingertips requires a reliance on quantitative sensory testing. While this offers enhanced tools for the clinical investigator, there is less consensus on the overall definitions of abnormality and disease.

The more sophisticated capacity for diagnosing vibration-related disease has had a parallel in the enhanced measurement tools available to the engineer for measuring physical characteristics of tools and instruments. In the past 20 years, accessible computer power and small accelerometers weighing a few grams that can be attached directly to tools have revolutionized measurement. The availability of Fourier spectrum analysis and recording in the 1970s, and low mass spectrometers, have made it possible to simultaneously measure a range of frequencies generated by a tool or instrument from 1 to 20 000 Hz. Only a quarter of a century ago, exposure measurement relied on machine-specific measures such as rpms or the production of unpleasant symptoms. Currently, standardized approaches to vibration measurement, as outlined in the ISO standard,[5] are internationally accessible. Vibration is markedly distinguished from other risk factors associated with work-related musculoskeletal disease in the sophistication and precision of applicable measurement.

The concentration on hand function and perception in the finger tips reflects a more subtle emphasis than the crude vascular symptoms that are characteristic of industrial tool use. Nevertheless, there is no overall approach to dental tools, which are lighter, smaller, and operate at much higher frequencies than are seen in the industrial milieu. Before the clinical implications of small electrical and air-powered tools are considered, it is first necessary to consider characteristics of vibration from hand-held tools as a matter of exposure.

Exposure Considerations

The basic dose-response approach to exposure evolved out of the work of Miwa, which linked subjective appreciation of discomfort with exposures measured as m/s² and plotted as a continuous variable for *octave center band* frequencies from 3 to 300 Hz.[7,8] A linear *weighting curve* was developed, its shape reflecting greatest adverse effect at 8 to 16 Hz (this expressed as unity) and declining rapidly, so that a weight of 0.10 would apply at 100 Hz. It was this basic weighting approach that was adapted by the British Standards Institute (BSI) in 1975,[6] and included in standards of the International Standards Organization (ISO 5349) in 1986.[5] Although the range of measured frequencies in these more modern scales has been extended beyond 1000 Hz and there were adaptations to the dose-response curves for both specific frequencies and duration of work, the basic tenets established in the 1960s for measurement and weighting have still applied. Common assumptions included the following:

1. a weighted, linear response curve;
2. measurement in three axes (x, y, z) with exposure taken from the dominant single axis; and
3. exposure measured in daily hours as root mean square (rms) acceleration for center octave bands.

The assumptions behind this standard approach would appear to have little application to dental tools. One reason is that standardized weighting almost entirely discounts force contributions over 150 Hz, whereas dental tools have acceleration peaks that are in the range of several thousand Hertz. In particular there has been almost a decade of controversy over the implications of down-weighting higher frequencies. The American National Institute for Occupational Safety and Health (NIOSH) recommends no weighting.[9] It is generally acknowledged that Miwa's approach was based on physical symptoms, consistent with the jarring of a large tool, rather than occult and organ-specific effects.

Many hand-held tools produce peak accelerations in a range from 100 to 300 Hz, generating a ten- to twenty-fold downward rating for the most impulsive portion of the acceleration curve. Moreover, there is some medical evidence suggesting that fingertip neurological injury occurs most prominently at 150 to 350 Hz and vascular injury above 100 Hz.[9,10] Recent work has substantiated these observations. Whereas frequencies over 50 Hz are unattenuated up to the elbow, the digit acts as a rigid body up to 250 Hz, so that tissue injuries related to higher-frequency tools would be necessarily limited to structures in the fingers. In the case of many hand-held appliances, finger rather than palmar gripping is a principal mechanism of contact and control, amplifying the interaction of biological exposure surface and higher proximally translated frequencies. It is also increasingly recognized that grip force, as well as frequency, can be an important factor in hand transmission. While this has not been a major factor with larger inertial industrial tools, it is very relevant to exposures from small instruments.

Vibration from Hand-Held Dental Tools: A Risk to Practitioners?

An answer based on known physiology and dental tools characteristics would seem to suggest that the frequencies associated with dental tools should be above the threshold of nerve or small-vessel injury. Nevertheless, there is an incumbent body of studies and case reports suggesting that dental workers who use vibrating tools have a variety of deficits that cannot be explained entirely by biomechanical factors such as awkward postures and untoward forces.

Pneumatic and electrical tools operating at considerably higher frequencies have been adapted to uses in surgery and dentistry as drills and saws. Use is intermittent, and frequency crests have exceeded a range usually thought to be physiologically problematic. Abnormalities in temperature and vibration recognition thresholds among dentists and dental technicians using high-speed hand-held instruments have indicated injury to at least two different types of fibers.[2,11] Elevated vibrotactile thresholds have also been documented among physical therapists using ultrasound devices.[12] In a prospective 3-year study of dental hygiene students, an expected occurrence of carpal tunnel syndrome was not observed, but an unexpected and very marked shift in vibrotactile threshold was observed.[13] This is characteristic for injury to fingertip nerve receptors. In only one study has significant vasospasm been demonstrated with this type of high-frequency tool, and that was among bone harvesters.[14] This was an unusual setting with potentially high feed forces and frequency damping, so it is not strictly comparable with work in the human mouth. In each of these cases, peak accelerations were from 10 to 40 kHz, considerably higher than from industrial tools. However, exposures were more transient and finger gripping more prominent.

It is sufficient to say that small-fiber finger tip injury from very high frequencies seems quite plausible, but that the results are inconclusive, particularly as to whether the problem lies with peak accelerations in the highest range or cumulative effects from lower frequencies. The studies are too numerous and consistent to be ignored, but the mechanism remains unclear.

Dental Tools and Carpal Tunnel Syndrome

Carpal tunnel syndrome has been recognized as a consequential occupational hazard for dentists and dental hygienists.[15,16] This has usually been attributed to biomechanical factors, including awkward posture, repetition, and force. Conrad's prospective study raises the possibility that peripheral sensory dysfunction in the fingertips may be misclassified as carpal tunnel syndrome, a significant problem of differential diagnosis which is pertinent to many classes of employment in which vibratory tools are used.[13] However, in addition to the recognized small fiber injuries caused by vibration, there is also good evidence from exposure to larger pneumatic tools that vibration produces an excess of carpal tunnel syndrome (CTS), with generally poor recovery characteristics.[5,17] In fact, vibratory exposures have been associated both with median nerve abnormalities in the absence of characteristic CTS symptoms and with a broader array of axonopathic abnormalities.[18,19] Functional abnormalities also have been noted in digital nerves well distal to the wrist, potentially affecting digital nerve function directly.[20] Pathoanatomic corroboration of nerve fiber injury has come through biopsy examination of peripheral digital nerves in vibration-exposed industrial workers[21] and in the peripheral limb nerves of experimental animals exposed to vibration.[22] Other work has suggested that even short exposures of vibration cause nerve swelling and potential susceptibility to mechanical injury.[23,24] These laboratory observations have their clinical correlations in the industrial work setting, where the concomitant exposures to biomechanical stresses and to vibration seem to intensify the occurrence of CTS.[25]

In some quarters, the presence of numbness and tingling in the fingers linked to a probable work exposure almost automatically leads to a requisite inclusion of carpal tunnel syndrome on the list of most probable etiologies. Yet there is evidence that clinico-epidemiologic case definition, when applied to workplace exposures, is only modestly confirmed by independent and more detailed medical evaluation.[26] To consider a more applied example, vibratory exposure has been linked to carpal tunnel syndrome through a common mechanism of increased grip, synovial injury, and external compression.[27] In this setting, vibration is an indirect or confounding factor eliciting or associated with conventional biomechanical causes of nerve entrapment. Yet Burstrom's careful and elegant models for measurement of hand-arm impedance suggest that with the resultant alteration of vector forces, increased grip may play a minor role in augmenting the actual transmission of resonant exposure to the contacting surface on the hand (28,29). Stated slightly differently, does the occurrence of vibration as a risk factor in studies of carpal tunnel syndrome indicate an independent influence of vibration on the median nerve, or is the vibratory signal lost in the noise of repetitive and stressful work?

While it is tempting to postulate that CTS in dental workers is a combination of misclassified digital neuropathy and an interaction between biomechanical stresses and myelinated nerve fibers made susceptible to injury by vibration, it is also true that there are major problems with the hypothesis. Since vibration frequencies above 150 Hz are not transmitted beyond the level of the wrist, there is no straightforward mechanism which can explain a purely vibration-related injury to the median nerve as it passes through the carpal canal.

Injury Plausibility and High Frequency Tools

The issues that surround vibratory exposure of dental workers are curiously understudied. Conceptually, it is difficult to explain such evident levels of disease from vibratory peaks occurring at frequencies that are in a range that would seem to overlap with driving a car or mowing a lawn. Other explanations may not require so extensive a divergence from conventional understanding of the frequencies likely to cause tissue injury in the fingers and hands. It is indeed possible that the damping of small tools through forceful contact against bony surfaces transmits much lower frequency to the hands.

There would seem to be a feasible avenue of clinical research that would link the transmission of vibration from dental tools into the hands and fingers. The interplay with tight-fitting synthetic gloves presents still another permutation of exposure. Even thin plastics may attenuate very-high-frequency vibration. It is perhaps surprising that this work has not been sponsored. In some respects, the greater attention that has been addressed to carpal tunnel syndrome, with associations with poor arm posture and repetitiveness, has masked the interesting and complex questions that involve strictly vibratory components of exposure, as well as potential interplay with biomechanical factors.

Preventive Measures

For industrial tools, a variety of preventive strategies have developed. Most important is limiting the time of exposure. From an engineering perspective, antivibration mounts and bushings or absorbent handles have effectively lowered exposure for some tools. Absorbent gloves also offer margins of protection. In fact, absorbent or elastomeric rubbers are highly effective in filtering out vibration levels over 800 Hz, presumably the range most pertinent for dental tools. However, personal protection is probably not an option in dental work. Before solutions are advanced, there needs to be a far better understanding of cause. Because neither the exposure nor etiology has been characterized, it is difficult to devise either preventive measures or effective tool adaptation.

A different situation arises around instruments such as plaque removers. These do vibrate at much lower frequencies, well below 1000 Hz. Although short duration of use probably shields most patients, dental hygienists and technicians may encounter potentially more serious problems. Antivibration wraps are available for customizing around industrial tools and can be adapted to barrel-type handles.

Conclusion

The weight of the evidence supports the conclusion that vibratory tools do produce nerve receptor injuries in the fingertips of regular users of dental tools and similarly contoured surgical instruments. The question of whether vascular problems will arise under usual circumstances of work requires more conjecture. While prevention and tool redesign would seem to be logical and even relatively straightforward remedies, the entire issue has earned such minimal attention that it is virtually impossible to devise an effective strategy. This is an area that urgently needs further investigative work.

REFERENCES

1. Pelmear PL, Taylor WT. Hand-arm vibration syndrome. *J Fam Prac.* 1994;38:180–185.
2. Hjortsberg U, Rosen I, Orbaek P, Lundborg G, Valogh I. Finger receptor dysfunction in dental technicians exposed to high-frequency vibration. *Scand J Work Environ Health.* 1989;15:339–344.
3. Juntunen J, Matikainen E, Seppalainen A, Laine A. Peripheral neuropathy and vibration syndrome. *Int Arch Environ Health.* 1983;52:17–24.
4. Koskimies K, Farkkila M, Pyykko I, Jantti V, Aatola S, Starck J, Inaba R. Carpal tunnel syndrome in vibration disease. *Br J Ind Med.* 1990;47:411–416.
5. ISO Mechanical vibration—guidelines for the measurement and the assessment of human exposure to hand-transmitted vibration. ISO 5349-1986: International Organization for Standardization (ISO); 1986.
6. *British Standards Institution Guide to the Evaluation of Exposure of the Human Hand-Arm System to Vibration.* BS DD43, 1975.
7. Miwa T. Evaluation methods for vibration effects: Part 6. Measurements of unpleasant and tolerance limit levels for sinusoidal vibrations. *Ind Health.* 1968;6:18–27.

8. Miwa T. Evaluation methods for vibration effects: Part 4. Measurements of vibration greatness for whole body and hand in vertical and horizontal vibrations. *Ind Health.* 1968;6:1–10.
9. NIOSH. Criteria for a recommended standard. Occupational exposure to hand-arm vibration. DHHS #89-106. 1989.
10. Rawlinson R. Are we assessing hand-arm vibration correctly? *J Low Freq Noise Vib.* 1991;14:53–60.
11. Lundstrom R, Lindmark A. Effects of local vibration on tactile perception in the hands of dentists. *J Low Freq Noise Vib.* 1982;1:1–11.
12. Lundstrom R. Effects of local vibration transmitted from ultrasonic devices on vibrotactile perception on the hands of therapists. *Ergonomics.* 1985;28:793–803.
13. Conrad JC, Conrad KJ, Osborn JB. Short-term, three-year epidemiological study of median nerve sensitivity in practicing dental hygienists. *J Dent Hyg.* 1993;67:268–272.
14. Cherniack M, Mohr S. Raynaud's phenomenon associated with the use of pneumatically powered surgical instruments. *J Hand Surg.* 1994;19A:1008–1015.
15. Gerwatowski LJ, McFall DB, Stach DJ. Carpal tunnel syndrome: risk factors and preventive strategies for the dental hygienist. *J Dent Hyg.* 1992;66:89–94.
16. McFall DB, Stach DJ, Gerwatowski LJ. Carpal tunnel syndrome: treatment and rehabilitation therapy for the dental hygienist. *J Dent Hyg.* 1993;67:126–133.
17. Hagberg M, Nystrom A. Recovery from symptoms after carpal tunnel syndrome surgery in males in relation to vibration exposure. *J Hand Surg.* 1991;16A:66–71.
18. Chatterjee DS, Barwick DD, Petrie A. Exploratory electromyography in the study of vibration-induced white finger in rock drillers. *Brit J Indus Med.* 1982;39:89–97.
19. Farkkila M, Pyykko I, Janntti V, Aatola S, Starck J, Korhonen O. Forestry workers exposed to vibration: a neurological study. *Brit J Indus Med.* 1988;45:188–192.
20. Sakakibara H, Kondo T-a, Miyao M, Yamada S. Digital nerve conduction velocity as a sensitive indication of peripheral neuropathy in vibration syndrome. *Am J Indus Med.* 1994;26:359–366.
21. Takeuchi T, Takeyama M, Imanishi H. Ultrastructural changes in peripheral nerves of the fingers of three vibration-exposed persons with Raynaud's phenomenon. *Scand J Work Environ Health.* 1988;14:31–35.
22. Ho ST, Yu HS. Ultrastructural changes of peripheral nerve induced by vibration: an experimental study. *Brit J Indus Med.* 1989;46:157–164.

23. Lundborg G, Dahlin LB, Danielsen N, Hansson HA, Necking LE, Pyykko I. Intraneural edema following exposure to vibration. *Scand J Work Environ Health.* 1987;13:326–329.
24. Lundborg G, Dahlin LB, Hansson HA, Kanje M, Necking LE. Vibration exposure and peripheral nerve fiber damage. *J Hand Surg.* 1990;15A21:346–351.
25. Wieslander G, Norback, Gothe C-J, Juhlin L. Carpal tunnel syndrome (CTS) and exposure to vibration, repetitive wrist movements, and heavy manual work: a case-referent study. *Brit J Indus Med.* 1989;46:43–47.
26. Moore J. Clinical determination of work-relatedness in carpal tunnel syndrome. *J Occup Rehab.* 1991;1:145–157.
27. Radwin R, Armstrong T, Chaffin D. Power hand tool vibration effects on grip exertions. *Ergonomics.* 1987;30:833–855.
28. Lundstrom R, Burstrom L. Mechanical impedance of the human hand-arm system. *Int J Ind Erg.* 1989;3:235–242.
29. Burstrom L. Measurement of the mechanical energy absorption in the hand and arm while using vibrating tools. *J Low Freq Noise and Vib.* 1990;9:1–14.

Chapter 6

Musculoskeletal Problems among Dental Hygienists:

A Canadian Study

Gary M. Liss, MD, MS, FRCPC, and Evie Jesin, RDH, BSc

Abstract

This chapter summarizes an investigation of musculoskeletal problems conducted among dental hygienists in Canada. We conducted a questionnaire survey of all 2142 dental hygienists belonging to the Ontario Dental Hygienists' Association, and a referent group of 305 dental assistants, who do not scale teeth. The response rates in the two groups were identical. Seven (7) percent of the dental hygienists had been told by a physician since starting work that they had CTS. Compared with the dental assistants, after adjusting for age, the dental hygienists were 5.2 times more likely to have been told they had CTS and 3.7 times more likely to meet a CTS case definition. The dental hygienists were also more likely to report hand/wrist, shoulder, and neck problems in the past 12 months but were less likely to report low back trouble. Internal analyses among dental hygienists using logistic regression models showed that the number of heavy-calculus patients per day, "clock" position around the dental chair, and years in practice were significant predictors of CTS. Days worked per week, time with the trunk rotated, and years of practice were significant predictors of reported shoulder trouble in the past 12 months. With more than 11 000 dental hygienists in Canada and about 100 000 in the United States, these findings suggest an important public health problem. They highlight the need to inform dental hygienists during training and continuing education about musculoskeletal problems in general and CTS in particular. Attention should be directed to areas such as work station design, posture, treating patients with heavy calculus, and scheduling (rest periods).

Introduction

Occupational hazards in dentistry in the past have focused in large part on exposure to mercury or safe handling of anesthetic gases. With 15 600 dentists and 11 500 dental hygienists in Canada, the current focus includes the recognition of risk factors and treatment and prevention of occupational injuries. Ergonomic problems have been noted among the hazards in the dental workplace.[1] Two surveys from the United States have suggested that dental hygienists may suffer inordinately from carpal tunnel syndrome (CTS)[2,3] as well as other musculoskeletal problems.[4] The prevalence of CTS reported by dental hygienists was 7.0% in one study,[3] and 8.4% in the other, but the associated questions that followed were answered by only 6.4%, suggesting to the authors that some responses were "self-diagnosis."[2] These studies also found associations of reported symptoms with various work factors.

However, there was no indication in these studies of whether the analyses were limited to CTS diagnoses occurring after starting work. Moreover, these studies did not use validated questionnaires or control for potential confounders such as age. In order to further examine whether dental hygienists are at risk for CTS and other upper extremity problems, the Ontario Ministry of Labour (MOL), in cooperation with the Ontario Dental Hygienists' Association (ODHA), conducted a questionnaire survey of ODHA members. In this chapter, we present a summary of that investigation including
1. a comparison of the prevalence of reported symptoms, diagnosed CTS, and modified activity among dental hygienists with among a referent group; and
2. internal analyses among dental hygienists examining work-related factors associated with upper-extremity problems.

Materials and Methods

Development of Questionnaire
For questions about work factors, we obtained and adapted the survey instruments from both U.S. studies. The Standard-

ized Nordic questionnaire[5] was used as the basis for asking about musculoskeletal symptoms during the past 12 months and the past 7 days (hand/wrist, shoulder, neck, and low back difficulties).

Information was obtained regarding work-related characteristics including which hand was used for scaling; years of practice; days practiced per week; number of patients and number of heavy-calculus patients seen per day; primary type of practice; type of instruments used (most frequently, second most frequently, and third most frequently); shape of instrument handles; "clock" position used most often relative to the patient when operating; and percent of time that the trunk was in a rotated position relative to the body when operating. Heavy calculus was defined on the questionnaire as subgingival or supragingival calculus covering at least 50% of tooth surfaces of maxillary molars and lower anteriors. We asked whether the respondents had been told that they had certain musculoskeletal conditions including CTS. Enquiry was also made regarding demographic and personal factors, including age and medical history.

Other Possible Confounding Exposures

We asked about possible CTS risk factors such as whether the respondents had been told by a physician that they had diabetes mellitus, fracture of the wrist, or hypothyroidism. For women, we also asked about oral-contraceptive use, estrogen replacement after menopause, and pregnancy in the past 12 months. Leisure activities that could be associated with upper-extremity problems that were listed in the questionnaire included playing piano or other musical instruments, tennis, other racquet sports, bowling, and gardening.

Pilot Testing and Distribution of Questionnaire

The questionnaire was pilot tested, revised, and then distributed to all 2142 ODHA members in the August 1992 ODHA newsletter. Local society presidents reminded their members to respond. Final returns considered in the analysis arrived in February 1993. There was a 50% response rate. The analyses here involves 951 dental hygienists currently practicing who indicated their primary type of practice as a clinical setting (Table 1).

Referent Group

In March 1993, an identical questionnaire (with respect to symptoms, medical history, hobbies, and leisure activities) was distributed to a sample of dental assistants in Ontario. This questionnaire was pilot-tested prior to distribution to improve clarity and change confusing wording. The questionnaire was distributed to all 305 members of three affiliate associations of the Ontario Dental Nurses and Assistants Association. Dental assistants were considered an appropriate referent group since they are demographically similar to dental hygienists, they work in dental practices, they may handle instruments, but they generally do not scale teeth. As Table 1 indicates, the response rate was 50.5%, equivalent to that of dental hygienists. After exclusions identical to those used for dental hygienists, there were 109 dental assistants currently working in clinical settings for analysis in comparison with dental hygienists.

Analyses

1. Determination of CTS

First, we asked whether the respondent had ever been "told by a physician that you had CTS." Second, because most practice variables reflect recent conditions (past 12 months), we also derived a questionnaire-based definition of CTS, referred to as CTS(Q), similar to that used by Silverstein et al.[6] CTS(Q) was considered to be present if all the following conditions were met:

1. Wrist or hand trouble had occurred during the last 12 months.
2. The total length of time of wrist/hand trouble was more than 7 days.
3. Specific symptoms during the past 12 months included numbness and tingling or pain or burning in the distribution of the median area (a diagram of hand with median nerve distribution was provided on the questionnaire).

Table 1.—Questionnaire Eligible for Analysis		
Subgroup Characteristics	Dental Hygienists	Dental Assistants
Total Distributed	2142	305
Total Received	1066 (50%)	154 (50.5%)
Returned too late	5	—
Not usable	7	1
Not working due to health problem	15	2
Not working but not due to health problem	45	21
Not primarily engaged in providing active patient care (e.g. public health, administration)	43	21
Primarily in clinical practice (eligible for analysis)	951	109
% Female	99.6%	100%
Average Age	33.2	29.0
Age Distribution, %*		
20–24	8.4	34.9
25–29	27.9	27.5
30–34	25.0	17.4
35–39	20.7	12.8
> 40	18.0	7.3

* Age Distributions are significantly different $P < .001$

4. Night pain or numbness in hands was present.
5. Negative response was given to the question "Have you ever hurt your wrist/hand in an accident?"

2. COMPARISONS OF DENTAL HYGIENISTS AND DENTAL ASSISTANTS

We present crude comparisons of reported symptoms and reduced activity among dental hygienists and dental assistants and age-adjusted odds ratios, comparing dental hygienists with dental assistants. We hypothesized in advance that dental hygienists would have more reported CTS and shoulder trouble, likely associated with scaling activities but that dental assistants, who may stand for much of the day (while dental hygienists sit on stools), might tend to report more back problems (see Photo 1).

3. COMPARISONS AMONG DENTAL HYGIENISTS

We present two types of internal analyses. First, factors associated with or possibly predictive of CTS(Q) and problems of shoulder *used for scaling* were examined. Work-related, medical, and demographic factors were examined initially in univariate analyses. Unconditional logistic regression models were used to obtain estimates and 95% confidence intervals (CIs) for measures of association among dental hygienists relating outcomes [symptom or CTS(Q) status] and various work-related factors while treating age as a covariate. In the

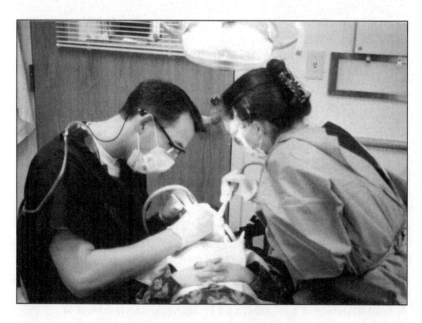

PHOTO 1.—A dental assistant (on right) stands with forward flexion of the back, while the dentist or dental hygienist scales the patient's teeth.

model building, variables that were associated with a significant change (at the traditional $P < .05$ level) in univariate analyses were included in the full multivariate models, with age retained in all models, and were dropped one at a time, retaining in the final models those associated with a change in the likelihood ratio test at $P < .1$. Two-way interaction terms among significant main effects variables were also examined. If the model did not converge with interactions between two categorical variables (e.g., duration of practice categories), the models were rerun with one as a continuous variable. The influence of other potentially confounding terms on the change in the regression coefficients was then examined and retained if inclusion was associated with a change of greater than 10% in the odds ratios of the other main effects. Only multivariate analyses are presented here.

Second, we made *internal comparisons* of the prevalence of symptoms in the scaling versus nonscaling hand—that is, each dental hygienist was compared with herself. Statistical comparisons for this used a matched analysis (McNemar test).

STATISTICAL ANALYSIS

Most analyses were conducted in PC-SAS; True Epistat was used to compute trends, some Mantel-Haenszel stratified analyses, and McNemar tests.

Results

Participation and Demographic Characteristics of Hygienists and Assistants

The response rates in the two groups were identical (Table 1); the dental assistants were all female as were all but four dental hygienists. The dental hygienists were on average 4 years older than the dental assistants, and the age distributions were significantly different. Over one third of dental hygienists were under 30, and less than 20% were older than 40. Over one third had worked less than 5 years, and almost 20% had worked more than 15 years (mean ± SD, 8.6 ± 7.0 years). Almost 90% indicated general practice as the primary type of practice.

External Comparisons of Dental Hygienists to Dental Assistants

Table 2 shows the crude proportions of dental hygienists and dental assistants 1) reporting that they had been told by a physician that they had CTS; 2) meeting the case definition of CTS(Q); and 3) reporting wrist/hand, shoulder, neck, and low back "trouble" in the past 12 months and in the past 7 days. Age-adjusted odds ratios (ORs) comparing dental hygienists to dental assistants are also shown. Dental hygienists were 5.2 times more likely to have been told they had CTS and 3.7 times more likely to meet the CTS(Q) case definition. Dental hygienists also reported significantly more wrist/hand, shoulder, and neck trouble, while the dental assistants were slightly more likely to report low back trouble. The ORs for the past 12 months were unchanged if a positive response was restricted to those reporting symptoms for more than 7 days in the past 12 months.

Table 3 shows the crude proportions (and age-adjusted ORs) of dental hygienists and dental assistants *among those with symptoms in the past 12 months*, who reported that they had to modify or reduce their work, household or social activity, or that they had seen a physician or health care worker because of this trouble. There was little difference in the proportions of symptomatic dental hygienists and dental assistants who modified their activities or saw a physician due to wrist/hand, shoulder, or low back trouble. Dental hygienists who reported neck difficulty were significantly more likely to report modifying or being unable to work at some point ($P<0.05$), or to have seen a physician or health care worker during the last 12 months ($0.05 < P < 0.1$). No dental assistants reported that they were *unable to work* (as opposed to simply *reducing their activity*), while some dental hygienists did (data not shown).

Table 2.—Prevalence of Reported Carpal Tunnel Syndrome and Symptoms

Condition	Hygienists (n = 950)[a] % Reporting	Assistants (n = 108)[a] % Reporting	OR[b] (95% CI)	Hygienists % Reporting Symptoms for more than 7 Days in Past 12 Months	Assistants % Reporting Symptoms for more than 7 Days in Past 12 Months	OR (95%CI)
Told that had CTS[c]	7.0	0.9	5.2 (0.9, 32)[d]			
Questionnaire-Based CTS	11.1	3.0	3.7 (1.1, 11.9)[f]			
Hand/Wrist						
Past 12 mths	47.5	26.9	2.5 (1.6, 3.9)[g]	28.3	12.0	2.7 (1.5, 4.9)[g]
Past 7 days	21.2	8.4	2.6 (1.3, 5.3)[f]			
Shoulder						
Past 12 mths	49.8	26.9	2.8 (1.8, 4.4)[g]	34.1	16.7	2.4 (1.4, 4.2)[g]
Past 7 days	24.7	11.1	2.5 (1.3, 4.7)[f]			
Neck						
Past 12 mths	69.1	56.5	1.8 (1.2, 2.7)[f]	42.8	29.6	1.7 (1.1, 2.6)[e]
Past 7 days	31.5	18.7	2.1 (1.2, 3.4)[f]			
Low Back						
Past 12 mths	65.0	67.0	0.9 (0.6, 1.4)[h]	38.3	45.0	0.8 (0.5, 1.2)[h]
Past 7 days	26.9	29.4	0.9 (0.6, 1.4)[h]			

[a] Total reporting varied slightly from condition to condition
[b] From logistic regression, adjusted for age; OR = Odds Ratio; CI = Confidence Interval
[c] CTS = Carpal Tunnel Syndrome
[d] $P < .1$; [e] $P < .025$; [f] $P < .01$; [g] $P < .001$; [h] $P > .2$

Table 3.—Prevalence of Reported Reduced or Modified Activity During Last 12 Months

	Hygienists % of Symptomatic	Assistants % of Symptomatic	OR (95% CI)[a]
Wrist/Hand			
• Modify or unable to work at some point	21.3	27.6	0.6 (0.3, 1.5)
• Modify household responsibilities	24.0	24.1	0.9 (0.4, 2.1)
• Modify social/recreational activities	28.0	34.5	0.7 (0.3, 1.5)
• Saw doctor or other HCW[b] because of trouble during last 12 months	34.4	31.0	1.1 (0.5, 2.5)
Shoulder			
• Modify or unable to work at some point	22.4	20.7	1.1 (0.4, 2.7)
• Modify household responsibilities	26.9	31.0	0.8 (0.3, 1.7)
• Modify social/recreational activities	27.5	27.8	0.9 (0.4, 2.7)
• Saw doctor or other HCW because of trouble during last 12 months	53.3	44.8	1.3 (0.6, 2.8)
Neck			
• Modify or unable to work at some point	24.5	11.5	2.4 (1.1, 5.4)[c]
• Modify household responsibilities	22.2	19.7	1.1 (0.5, 2.1)
• Modify social/recreational activities	26.6	21.3	1.3 (0.7, 2.4)
• Saw doctor or other HCW because of trouble during last 12 months	51.2	36.1	1.7 (0.97, 2.93)

Table 3.—*Continued*

	Hygienists % of Symptomatic	Assistants % of Symptomatic	OR (95% CI)[a]
Low Back			
• Modify or unable to work at some point	25.3	32.9	0.7 (0.4, 1.2)
• Modify household responsibilities	35.9	41.1	0.6 (0.4, 1.1)
• Modify social/recreational activities	35.1	30.1	1.1 (0.6, 1.8)
• Saw doctor or other HCW because of trouble during last 12 months	45.3	34.3	1.5 (0.9, 2.4)

[a] From logistic regression, adjusted for age; OR = Odds Ratio; CI = Confidence Interval
[b] HCW = Health Care Worker
[c] *P* < .05

Physician-Diagnosed Conditions:

In all, 71 (7.6%) of 940 completing this section indicated that they had been told by a physician that they had had CTS; after excluding those diagnosed with CTS before starting hygiene practice, the prevalence was 65 (7.0%). Of these, nine (14%) had had surgery for CTS, and only one had received worker's compensation for this condition. The crude proportions of dental hygienists and dental assistants reporting that they had been told by a physician that they had tendonitis of the hands/wrists were 12.2% and 7.5%, respectively, for deQuervain's syndrome (tenosynovitis of the thumb) the proportions were 1.5% and 0.9%, respectively.

Comparisons Among Dental Hygienists

Questionnaire-Based Definition of Carpal Tunnel Syndrome

For the hand used for scaling, the CTS(Q) case definition was met by 100 (10.9%) of 916 hygienists with data available for all components of the definition.

MULTIVARIATE ANALYSES

The simultaneous influence of variables showing associations with CTS(Q) at the 5% probability level was examined in logistic regression models. The risk of CTS(Q) increased by 2% per year of age. Table 4 shows the final model among the 897 respondents with data available for these variables. Together the three "exposure" factors contributed significantly ($P < .0005$) to Model II compared to Model I containing only age (Table 4). None of the six possible two-way interactions were significant. The addition of possible confounders, diabetes and, among females, hormone replacement therapy and pregnancy in the past 12 months, provided little change in -2 log likelihood (all $P > .1$), and inclusion in the model was associated with little change in the above "exposure" variables (ORs changed less than 10%). The strongest predictors of CTS(Q) thus appeared to be seeing three (OR 2.4) or four or more (OR 2.3) heavy-calculus patients per day, operating most

Table 4.—Predictors of CTS(Q) in Scaling Hand: Multiple Logistic Regression Analysis (n = 897)

Model predictor	I Odds Ratio (95% CI)	II Odds Ratio (95% CI)
Age (year)	1.02 (0.99, 1.05)	1.02 (0.97, 1.06)
Patients with heavy calculus/day:		
None		1.0
1		1.7 (0.6, 4.8)
2		1.2 (0.4, 3.4)
3		2.4 (0.9, 6.8)
4 or more		2.3 (0.8, 6.5)
Clock position		
8:00, 9:00 or 11:00		1.0
10:00 or 12:00		2.0 (1.3, 3.1)
Years Practice		
< 5		1.0
5–14		1.8 (1.0, 3.2)
> 15		1.0 (0.4, 2.6)
–2 Log Likelihood	606.147	578.121[a]

[a] Predictors added to model: $P < .0005$

often in the 10 or 12 o'clock position (versus other positions) (OR 2.0), and 5 to 14 years of practice (OR 1.8).

Shoulder Trouble in Past 12 Months (Scaling Arm)

This section summarizes responses to the question "Have you had shoulder trouble during the last 12 months?" (S_{12}). Overall, 408 (42.9%) of 950 dental hygienists responded affirmatively for the scaling arm.

MULTIVARIATE ANALYSIS

In logistic regression analysis, the number of heavy-calculus patients ($P > .2$) and number of patients per day ($P > .1$)

which were significant in univariate analyses, were not significant. The variables retained in the final model are shown in Table 5. Together the latter four "exposure" variables contributed significantly ($P < .0001$) to Model IV, compared with Model III, which contained only age and history of shoulder

Table 5.—Predictors of S_{12} in Scaling Arm: Multiple Logistic Regression Analysis (n = 939)

Model predictor	III Odds Ratio (95% CI)	IV Odds Ratio (95% CI)
Age (per year)	0.98 (0.96–1.00)	0.99 (0.97–1.02)
History of shoulder injury:		
No	1.0	1.0
Yes	2.4 (1.4–4.2)	2.1 (1.2–3.8)
Type of Practice		
General		1.0
Other		1.8 (1.2–2.8)
Days per week		
2 or less		1.0
3		0.9 (0.5–1.64)
4		1.8 (1.0–3.0)
5 or 6		1.8 (1.1–3.2)
Percent of Time trunk rotated relative to lower body		
1–20%		1.0
21–40%		1.5 (1.0–2.2)
41–60%		1.5 (1.0–2.4)
61–80%		2.8 (1.9–4.3)
81–100%		3.1 (1.9–4.9)
Years Practice		
< 1		1.0
1–14		3.9 (1.9–7.9)
15		2.1 (0.9–5.1)
–2 Log Likelihood	1266.043	1176.964[a]

* Predictors added to model: $P < .0001$

injury. Other than a history of shoulder injury, the strongest predictors of S_{12} appeared to be type of practice other than general (OR 1.8), working 4 or more days per week (OR 1.8), spending 61% to 80% or 81% to 100% of the time with the trunk rotated (ORs 2.8 and 3.1, respectively), and practicing for 1 to 19 years (OR 3.9) or 20 or more years (OR 2.1), compared with less than 1 year.

Scaling Hand versus Nonscaling Hand

Table 6 shows the prevalence of various conditions according to scaling side (or both sides), nonscaling side (or both sides), scaling side only, and nonscaling side only, after excluding 23 dental hygienists who reported scaling with both hands. The matched analysis indicates that no subjects met the CTS(Q) definition in the nonscaling hand; symptoms were reported 10 to 17 times more frequently in the scaling hand only than in the nonscaling hand only, and 2.7 times more frequently in the scaling shoulder only compared with the nonscaling shoulder only.

Discussion

We have obtained estimates for the reported prevalence of wrist/hand and other musculoskeletal problems from this population-based sample of dental hygienists in Ontario. We first discuss the findings and then discuss the limitations of this investigation.

Suitability of Dental Assistants as a Comparison Group

Was the choice of dental assistants as the referent group appropriate? Both groups work in the same offices, both are almost entirely female, and the socioeconomic backgrounds are relatively similar. The validity of the comparisons is also supported by identical response rates in the two groups (Table 1). The dental hygienists are somewhat older, but age has been included as a covariate in comparisons between the groups.

Table 6.—Prevalence of CTS(Q), Wrist/Hand, and Shoulder Trouble, Scaling versus Nonscaling Side[a]

Prevalence (%)	Scaling (or both)	Nonscaling (or both)	Scaling only	Nonscaling only	OR (95% CI)[b]	P value
CTS(Q)	10.9	3.0	7.8	0	–	–
Wrist/Hand Trouble Past 12 months	45.7	10.3	37.7	2.3	16.6 (10.7–25.8)	$P < 10^{-8}$
Wrist/Hand Trouble Past 7 days	19.7	4.3	17.1	1.7	9.9 (5.9–16.5)	$P < 10^{-8}$
Shoulder Trouble Past 12 months	42.6	31.0	18.7	7.0	2.7 (2.0–3.5)	$P < 10^{-8}$

[a]After excluding those reporting scaling with both hands
[b]Matched analysis, McNemar's Test

Comparisons with Dental Assistants

There was very high symptom reporting by dental hygienists (greater than 40% to 60% in the past 12 months and greater than 20% to 30% in the past 7 days), somewhat greater than that found among other working groups surveyed using the Nordic questionnaire (previous prevalence estimates provided by Dr Claire Dickinson, Health and Safety Executive, United Kingdom).

COMPARISON OF SYMPTOMS

After adjusting for age, dental hygienists reported significantly higher rates than dental assistants for CTS(Q), wrist/hand, shoulder, and neck trouble. The magnitude of the increased risk was large, about 2 to 3 times higher (Table 2). The dental hygienists reported low back trouble slightly less frequently than the dental assistants, which was consistent with our prior hypothesis; perhaps this was related to longer periods of standing among dental assistants.

PREVIOUS DIAGNOSIS OF CTS

We observed that 7.0% of dental hygienists had been diagnosed as having CTS after starting work as dental hygienists, a finding that is very similar to that reported in the two US questionnaire surveys of dental hygienists. If one assumes that all cases of CTS had occurred among the dental hygienists who responded, then the prevalence of previously diagnosed CTS was, at a minimum, 3.5%. There are no established values for the population prevalence of CTS, but our findings can be compared with several estimates. Fewer than one percent of the population is expected to suffer from CTS during their lifetime; the 1989 National Ambulatory Medical Care Survey in the United States (unpublished data from the 1989 National Ambulatory Medical Care Survey data tape) found that the prevalence of CTS was 3.8 per 1000 office encounters; and among family/general practitioners it was 1.95 per 1000 office encounters. Second, among the dental assistants in our survey, the prevalence of having been told that they had CTS was 0.9%. The dental hygienists had an age-adjusted CTS prevalence 5.2 times greater. Finally, Tanaka et al[7] found in the 1988 US National Health Interview Survey that the rate of "medically-called" CTS among "recent workers" (adults who worked any time during the past 12 months) was 0.53%. Among our dental hygienists, 27 (2.9%) had been diagnosed as having CTS in the past 2 years.

COMPENSATION FOR CTS AND MUSCULOSKELETAL PROBLEMS

It should be noted that the proportion of respondents diagnosed with CTS who applied for compensation is rather low. Apparently, most dental hygienists are not eligible for workers' compensation because the dentists for whom they work are not required to provide this benefit; this may be an area for future discussion. Because most dental hygienists do not qualify for workers' compensation coverage, many in the profession take out disability policies from insurance companies. To explore this aspect, we contacted the five insurance carriers covering the majority of dental hygienists in Canada. In recent years (about 1993), several of the companies downgraded dental hygienists to a higher-risk class, resulting in higher premiums, while one company has not yet done so. This has resulted in the expected movement of dental hygienists between companies. The data provided by these companies indicated that in 1996, a total of 2613 dental hygienists held disability policies (range, 40 to 2034). Historical data over 5 years were available at two companies. At one (which had downgraded the profession), the number of policies decreased from 138 in 1991 to 65 in 1996. The company that had not downgraded dental hygienists now covers the vast majority in Canada (447 in 1991 versus 2034 in 1996). Data on claims made by dental hygienists were only provided by one company, the largest carrier. The number of claims (for all causes) increased from five in 1991 to 32 in 1996. Of the five claims in 1991, one was for musculoskeletal injury, two were for musculoskeletal noninjury (which includes repetitive strain injuries and CTS), and one was for back sprain/strain. The 32 claims in 1996 included one musculoskeletal injury, eight musculoskeletal noninjuries, and six back disorders/diseases.

VALIDITY OF EXTERNAL COMPARISONS

The validity of these external comparisons, which suggest an excess of upper-extremity trouble among dental hygienists, is supported by several observations. First, the dental assistants appeared to be a reasonable referent group, as discussed. Second, those dental hygienists with symptoms appeared to be disabled to an extent similar to dental assistants as far as can be ascertained by the extent to which they reported decreased activity or having to see a health care worker within the past 12 months (Table 3). Third, with respect to wrist/hand problems, as more stringent criteria were applied—from 12 months reported wrist/hand problems to CTS(Q), to the more objective criterion of having been diagnosed by a physician as having CTS, the prevalence of the outcome *decreased* (as expected) but the *age-adjusted ORs* comparing dental hygienists with dental assistants *increased* (Table 2). Fourth, the dental hygienists did not report all symptoms more frequently; rather, the dental assistants reported more low back symptoms. Finally, the findings are consistent with the few other surveys conducted among dental hygienists, as reviewed below.

Comparisons Among Dental Hygienists—Predictors of Carpal Tunnel Syndrom

QUESTIONNAIRE-BASED DEFINITION OF CTS

We found a cross-sectional prevalence, based on our CTS(Q) definition, of 10.9% in the past 12 months. Silverstein et al[6] observed a similar CTS prevalence of 9.6% in the high-force, high-repetition group of industrial workers *on interview alone* (5.6% on interview and exam). However, unlike those authors, we did not exclude respondents who had worked for less than 1 year, among whom the prevalence was lower.

PREDICTORS OF CTS(Q)

In the analysis of CTS(Q) in the scaling hand, age was not a significant predictor, but there was a weak positive association with CTS(Q) (increase of 2% per year). In fact, our regression coefficient (0.012) and OR (1.02) are very similar to those reported by Silverstein et al[6] of 0.0258 and 1.03, respectively. Osborn et al[3] also did not find hand (CTS-like) symptoms to be significantly related to age. Macdonald et al[2] observed, as did we, that both symptoms and a CTS diagnosis were correlated with the number of heavy calculus patients but not strongly with the number of patients per day. It is plausible that a dental hygienist would "work harder" (i.e., use more force) to scale the teeth of such patients; the trend with increasing number of heavy calculus patients may also reflect *the frequency* of these stressful maneuvers.

We found that the 5- to 14-year duration-of-practice category was a predictor of CTS(Q). Macdonald et al[2] also reported significant correlations of some CTS-like symptoms (nocturnal pain or numbness, hand weakness, and CTS) with years worked, although it is not clear if these were adjusted for age. However, Silverstein et al[6] reported that years *on the current job*, as a continuous variable, was not associated with CTS. Because the risk may change over time, the association may be masked as a continuous variable. These investigators pointed out that their finding that CTS was negatively associated with years on the job supported the possibility of underestimating CTS prevalence. The decline in CTS(Q) prevalence beyond 15 years that we observed may represent a survivor effect or a learning effect, in that dental hygienists in practice for longer periods may have adapted to their jobs. In a retrospective cohort morbidity study of food processors,[8] we found that the standardized morbidity ratio for having had a CTS *operation* was highest in the period 5 to 9 years after hire, consistent with our current findings among dental hygienists.

Certain clock positions reported by the dental hygienist as used most often relative to the patient appeared to be significant predictors of CTS(Q). Dental hygiene textbooks suggest that the operator position should change depending on the areas of the mouth being treated,[9,10] with the 8 o'clock position close to the front of the patient taken as the baseline or "ideal" one. Positions moving further from 8 o'clock may require increased flexion or deviation of the wrist. The two positions that we observed to be high-risk positions (10 and 12 o'clock) represent two of the three positions furthest from 8 o'clock; these are most awkward for the scaling hand. It should be emphasized, however, that the two positions showing increased risk were combined *a posteriori*. Although this finding should be confirmed elsewhere, it suggests the need for education regarding the implications of wrist postures as the dental hygienist moves about the patient.

PHYSICIAN DIAGNOSED CTS VERSUS CTS(Q)

The comparison of these two markers of CTS indicated that our case definition of CTS (referring to the past 12 months) had moderate sensitivity and high specificity for having been diagnosed previously by a physician as having CTS.

Comparisons Among Dental Hygienists—Predictors of Shoulder Trouble in Past 12 Months

The prevalence for S_{12} of 43% that we observed is very close to that reported by Osborn et al[4] among Minnesota dental hygienists (39%) over the same time period. Shoulder and neck disorders have been associated with overhead work and static muscle load.[11]

In our study, a history of previous shoulder injury was associated with a doubling of the risk of reporting shoulder problems, analogous to prior back injury, which is recognized as a predictor of future low back problems.[12] We found, as with wrist/hand problems, that the reported prevalence of S_{12} increased sharply after the first year but then remained relatively constant. Unlike our observations for CTS(Q) and wrist/hand problems, the *number of heavy-calculus patients* per day was *not* a significant predictor of shoulder problems although *the number of days worked per week* was. Osborn et al[4] found that those reporting shoulder pain practiced more hours per week than those without pain, which is consistent with our finding.

The fact that heavy calculus was not significant suggests that factors other than the scaling activities themselves, such as trunk posture, that are a function of the number of days worked or that may affect *both shoulders*, may be important predictors of shoulder problems. The matched analysis comparing the S_{12} prevalence in the scaling shoulder only to that in the nonscaling shoulder only (Table 6), yielded a much lower OR than that observed for hand/wrist problems. This is also compatible with a role for factors other than scaling.

POSITIONS AND POSTURES OF DENTISTS AND DENTAL HYGIENISTS

Dental hygienists (and dentists) perform work with the shoulders above the neutral (elbow) position. We have observed that some dental hygienists, particularly while avoiding indirect vision with the mirror, work with "poor" posture and forward trunk flexion. The right shoulder becomes elevated compared with the left shoulder (for a right-handed dental hygienist); this may predispose the worker to neck and shoulder discomfort.

Being in a practice other than general (mainly orthodontics and periodontics) was associated with an increased reported prevalence of shoulder trouble. Patients seen in periodontal practices may require more instrumentation procedures and/or longer treatment periods. Dental hygienists working in orthodontic practices perform repetitive motions requiring considerable force during the placing and removal of orthodontic brackets.

Limitations and Advantages

We should consider the limitations and possibility of bias in this study. There was only a moderate response rate of 50%, although self-administered mail questionnaire studies routinely can be expected to yield a response rate of about 30%.[13] Although we attempted to increase the response by follow-up reminders, the nonresponders could not be contacted directly; this likely limited the response. It is possible that dental hygienists with symptoms were more likely to respond, yielding an overestimate of risk. It should be noted that the response rate among dental hygienists was identical to that among dental assistants in our study.

The fact that we observed, for example, a pattern for CTS(Q) indicating no or a weak association with days worked per week or number of patients seen per day but a strong (and significant) association with *the number of heavy-calculus patients* per day where more force is required to scale teeth, suggests that the symptomatic subjects were not responding to all possible practice factors.

This survey is limited by the cross-sectional design: those now working may demonstrate a "survivor bias," which may lead to an underestimation of risk.[14] Although we determined whether CTS started after commencing work, we did not determine this for symptoms; they may have preceded dental hygiene work in some instances. Our investigation is also limited by failure to capture all explanatory variables—including psychosocial stressors; further studies should incorporate these variables. A recent review[15] noted that studies of the role of job satisfaction and stress in upper-limb musculoskeletal disorders have, as yet, been inconclusive. However, Bongers et al[16] suggested that several aspects, including low control on the job, lack of social support by colleagues, monotonous work, high perceived work load, and time pressure are related to musculoskeletal symptoms.

Another limitation is that only symptoms are considered; because physical examinations or electrodiagnostic tests were not performed, the reporting is subjective and thus may overestimate the prevalence of syndromes such as CTS. For example, nocturnal CTS symptoms have been shown to have only moderate sensitivity and poor specificity compared with neurophysiologic diagnoses.[17] Silverstein et al[6] reported that the proportions of subjects meeting the criteria for CTS on both physical exam and interview was 2.1%, or just above half of that on interview alone (3.8%).

The previous surveys of dental hygienists did not use a standardized questionnaire, nor did they consistently adjust for confounding factors such as age. Advantages of our study include the external comparison group, the use of a standardized questionnaire, reasonable study size, multivariate analyses including control for age, and the incorporation into the questionnaire of an explicit definition of heavy calculus.

Conclusions

Public Health Significance

There are more than 11 000 dental hygienists in Canada and approximately 100 000 in the United States. Given the large population at risk, and a moderate (doubling) of CTS and other musculoskeletal problems associated with work, our findings suggest an important burden of illness attributable, at least in part, to the workplace. Possible recommendations include that preventive sessions be initiated to inform dental hygienists about musculoskeletal problems in general and CTS in particular. A number of specific preventive strategies aimed at the CTS risk factors of repetitiveness, posture, force, and mechanical stresses were summarized by Gerwatowski et al.[18] In our experience, the dental hygiene profession is now keenly interested in protective strategies. Without these strategies, an increase in disability claims by dental hygienists will likely occur. Protective strategies of the 1990s include techniques to modify the operator/patient position; modified grasp and fulcrum; and the emergence of ergonomically designed instruments, handpieces, and gloves. However, the effectiveness of these techniques must be demonstrated.

Dental hygiene and continuing education courses should include awareness of the implications of work-related factors including

- awkward postures such as flexion or deviation of the wrist from the neutral posture, which may be related to clock position;
- height of the dental hygienist relative to the patient; and
- posture or rotation of the trunk relative to the lower body when operating.

Attention should be directed to the design of the work station; design of chair and lumbar and arm support; equipment such as dental instruments and mirrors; and training in posture and technique. Finally, there should be increased awareness about the implications of treating patients with heavy calculus, as well as duration of treatment and rest periods (scheduling), for work-related conditions.

Extrapolation to Dentists

While it is assumed that many of the awkward postures and maneuvers performed by dental hygienists apply to dentists as well, we have had difficulty in getting the attention of the dental society in Ontario to communicate our findings.

ACKNOWLEDGMENTS

The assistance of the ODHA, Elizabeth Craig, Kathleen Feres Patry, Barb Gibb, and the local society presidents, is appreciated. We thank Irene Rule and Rose Pagliaro for data entry; Marlene Vaz, who produced the tables; and the contacts at the insurance companies who provided data on numbers of disability policies. Mary Lou Fischer and Jeff Miller from the Ontario Dental Nurses and Assistants Association helped in the development and distribution of the questionnaire. I thank my wife, Gwen Liss, for initially suggestng that we do this study.

Portions of this chapter appeared in the *American Journal of Industrial Medicine* as Liss GM, Jesin E, Kusiak RA, White P, "Musculoskeletal Problems among Ontario Dental Hygienists," 1995.

REFERENCES

1. Macdonald G. Hazards in the dental workplace. *J Dental Hygiene.* 1987;61:212–218.
2. Macdonald G, Robertson MM, Erickson JA. Carpal tunnel syndrome among California dental hygienists. *J Dental Hygiene.* 1988;62:322–328.
3. Osborn JB, Newell KJ, Rudney JD, Stoltenberg JL. Carpal tunnel syndrome among Minnesota dental hygienists. *J Dental Hygiene.* 1990;63:79–85.

4. Osborn JB, Newell KJ, Rudney JD, Stoltenberg JL. Musculoskeletal pain among Minnesota dental hygienists. *J Dental Hygiene.* 1990;63:132–138.
5. Kuorinka I, Jonsson B, Kilbom A, et al. Standardised Nordic questionnaires for the analysis of musculoskeletal symptoms. *Applied Ergonomics.* 1987;18:233–237.
6. Silverstein BA, Fine LJ, Armstrong TJ. Occupational factors and carpal tunnel syndrome. *Am J Ind Med.* 1987;11:343–358.
7. Tanaka S, Wild DK, Seligman PJ, Cameron L, Behrens VJ, Putz-Anderson V. The US prevalence of self-reported carpal tunnel syndrome: 1988 National Health Interview Survey data. *Am J Public Health.* 1994;84:1846–1848.
8. Liss GM, Armstrong C, Kusiak RA, Gailitis MM. Use of provincial health insurance plan billing data to estimate carpal tunnel syndrome morbidity and surgery rates. *Am J Ind Med.* 1992;22:395–409.
9. Nield JS, Houseman GA. *Fundamentals of Dental Hygiene Instrumentation.* 2nd ed. Philadelphia: Lea & Febiger; 1988.
10. Woodall IR, Dafoe BR, Young NS, Weed-Fonner L, Yankell SL. *Comprehensive Dental Hygiene Care.* 4th ed. Toronto: CV Mosby Company; 1993.
11. Gerr F, Letz R, Landrigan PJ. Upper-extremity musculoskeletal disorders of occupational origin. *Annu Rev Public Health.* 1991;12:543–566.
12. Snook SH. Approaches to the control of back pain in industry: job design, job placement, and education/ training. *Occup Med: State of the Art Reviews.* 1988;3(1):45–59.
13. Williamson YM. *Research Methodology and its Application to Nursing.* New York: John Wiley & Sons; 1981.
14. Checkoway H, Pearce NE, Crawford-Brown DJ. *Research Methods in Occupational Epidemiology.* New York/Oxford: Oxford University Press; 1989.
15. Armstrong TJ, Buckle P, Fine LJ, et al. A conceptual model for work-related neck and upper-limb musculoskeletal disorders. *Scand J Work Environ Health.* 1993;19:73–84.
16. Bonger PM, de Winter CR, Kompier MAJ, Hildebrandt VH. Psychosocial factors at work and musculoskeletal disease. *Scand J Work Environ Health.* 1993;19:297–312.
17. Katz JN, Larson MG, Sabra A, et al. The carpal tunnel syndrome: diagnostic utility of the history and physical examination findings. *Ann Int Med.* 1990;112:321–327.
18. Gerwatowski LJ, Bailey McFall D, Stach DJ. Carpal tunnel syndrome: risk factors and preventive strategies for the dental hygienist. *JDH,* 1992;65:89–94.

Chapter 7

Instruments Used in Dentistry

Richard Fredekind, DMD, MA
and Eve Cuny, CDA, RDA

Abstract

Human beings excel at being adaptable, but tools and machines are adept at repetition. When the human body is required to repeat a given motion, the effects on the musculoskeletal system can be deleterious. The design of dental instruments and the body mechanics of the operator influence the prevention or generation of these effects, often known as repetitive strain injuries. There are a number of risk factors for repetitive strain injuries, including the number of repetitions, the force applied, mechanical stress, operator posture, vibration, and temperature. These risk factors combine with characteristics inherent in every piece of dental equipment to produce their effect on the body. Instrument size, handle diameter, shape, and weight are examples of such tool characteristics. This chapter will examine these attributes in detail, explaining the nature of an ideal dental instrument and how, with proper use and maintenance, such an instrument can reduce the chance of injury to the two primary anatomic sites, the back and wrist.

Introduction

Repetitive strain injuries have a significant impact on workers in all fields. Nearly two-thirds of all workplace illnesses in the United States in 1994 (332 000) were attributed to repeated trauma. The number of these injuries experienced a 10% increase over the corresponding figures for 1993. Because these types of injuries can last years, and even a lifetime, they create a tremendous burden in terms of workers' compensation claims, not to mention the personal impact to the injured worker. The dental field is not immune to repetitive strain injuries, such as carpal tunnel syndrome.[1] The design of hand instruments and

169

other devices, placement and type of operating equipment, and body mechanics play an important role in controlling these injuries.

As a rule, human beings excel at being adaptable. They are less adept at repetition. Machines, by contrast, are seldom very adaptable, but they can repeat a given movement consistently over many months or years. Repetitive strain injuries, or cumulative trauma disorders, are insults to the body caused by repeated or chronic movements that result in inflammation to the musculoskeletal system, including muscles, tendons, ligaments, and bony structures.[2] Holding a part of the body in a certain position for an extended period of time also may cause repetitive strain injury. This is called static loading. The upper trapezius muscles are especially susceptible to injury as a result of the elbows being held out from the body.[3] It is not uncommon for practitioners to deviate from the ideal of no more than a 20° abduction of the shoulder.[4] Often, more than one factor is responsible for the injury. Experiences outside the dental office combine with those in the office to produce the deleterious effect.[5,6] For instance, spending hours playing computer games while at home, then going to work and cleaning teeth all day may have a cumulative effect on the hand and wrist.

All members of the dental team are susceptible to repetitive strain injury. Published studies have indicated that hygienists have a high rate of these injuries.[7] This is most likely due to the lack of variety in their job as well as their tendency to stay in one operatory all day. Hygienists are most susceptible to repetitive strain injury in the hand and wrist, otherwise known as carpal tunnel syndrome. Dentists are also affected, but less so, probably because of the variety of movements they make during the course of a day. Because of inattention to proper posture and the need to see into areas with limited visual access, dentists are most prone to neck and shoulder strain resulting from static loading.[8] Assistants seem less prone to repetitive strain injury than either hygienists or dentists. However, it remains important for assistants to monitor posture, move frequently, and provide enough variety of movements in the day to avoid repetitive strain injury.

This chapter will examine the instruments used in dentistry and how they can contribute to or help eliminate repetitive strain injury. An instrument is broadly defined as any tool, appliance, or apparatus used to do work.[9] In the context of the dental office, the term "instrument" includes manual hand instruments, automatic handpieces of all types, dispensing implements, drill bits, chairs, carts, lights, hand-held equipment such as intraoral cameras, and accessory items such as computer keyboards. These instruments are designed according to three primary criteria: ergonomic efficiency, cost, and user demand. Manufacturers need good reasons to redesign a given instrument, and the reason most likely to initiate redesign is user demand. Whether the redesigned instrument will actually be constructed has much to do with the cost involved and the potential for profit.

Guidelines for Ergonomic Tool Design and Use

All instruments should be designed and used with some basic concepts in mind. First, a number of risk factors are involved in the development of repetitive strain injury, including the number of repetitions, the force applied, mechanical stress, posture, vibration, and temperature.[10,11] The risk factors can be affected by many characteristics of the instruments we use daily in dentistry.[12,13] These include

- size of the entire instrument,
- diameter of the instrument barrel or handle,
- surface configuration where the instrument contacts the fingers,
- overall shape,
- weight of the tool including attachments,
- the balance and alignment of the tool,
- maneuverability of the instrument in space,
- how well moving parts of the tool can be manipulated, and
- maintenance of the working edge of any tool used to cut or remove tissue.

Instruments should be able to provide ease of use in an ergonomically efficient posture for the entire body, including the hands, and they should be simple to maintain that way. Most instruments are manufactured with angled handles that place the operator's hand in a relatively consistent neutral posture. It is important that these tools be used in the manner that maintains this position.

Instruments should be maintained in proper working order. Keeping tools with moving parts well lubricated will reduce the amount of force exerted by the operator.[14] Tools that are used to remove tissue typically have a cutting edge, which must be maintained. It is essential to keep scalers, periodontal curettes, hoes, and other cutting hand tools well sharpened. This means beginning a procedure with sharpened edges and resharpening during the procedure. The amount of force and number of repetitions required to produce a result will be greatly reduced through proper maintenance of the cutting edge. The importance of this maintenance in hygiene cannot be overstated because the variety of movements in this discipline is so limited.[14]

The force needed to operate any equipment or instrument should be minimized. It has been found for hygienists that the amount of force exerted is more likely to cause carpal tunnel syndrome than the number of repetitions.[14] Therefore, any tool with a cutting edge should be kept as sharp as possible during the entirety of the operation. When possible, automatic instruments should replace hand instruments. However, because injuries are associated with vibration, neither hand instruments nor automatic instruments should be used exclusively. Repetitive strain injuries associated with vibration are discussed in Chapter 5, "Vibration and Dental Equipment."

The combination of tool design and the body mechanics of the dental worker contribute to injuries involving the wrist/hand area and the shoulders, neck, and back. Generally, a bent wrist (either flexed or extended) should be avoided and a neutral wrist posture encouraged.[15] A neutral wrist position occurs when a line can be extended along the long axis of the radius bone extending down through the long axis of the second metacarpal.[4] Figure 1 illustrates the neutral wrist position in contrast to a flexed position. Excessive flexion or extension will reduce grasp power, manipulation effectiveness,

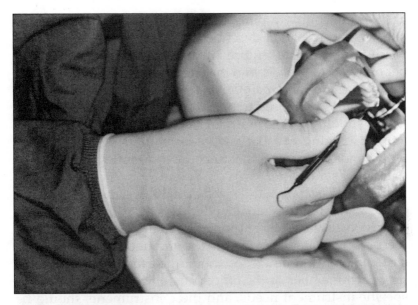

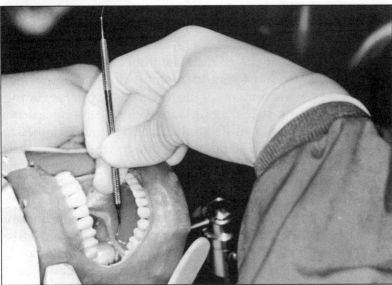

FIGURE 1.—The figure on the top illustrates the neutral position of the lower arm, wrist, and hand. The figure on the bottom illustrates the wrist in deep flexion, a position that can cause inflammation in the carpal tunnel if maintained or repeated.

and/or the ability to pinch and hold.[15] Injuries to the hands and wrist, most often described as carpal tunnel syndrome, result from the force required in a given movement, the number of repetitions used, and the hand posture. Therefore, tools should be made and maintained to reduce the amount of force and repetition required to produce the work. In addition, the hands should be held without flexion or extension. For example, working at a flat keyboard requires ulnar flexion of both hands, a position that encourages development of carpal tunnel syndrome.[16]

Another issue is hand size.[4] Generally, males have larger hands and longer fingers than females. At issue here is overextension and underextension of hand muscles. Either one of these extremes may lead to muscle strain. Because of this, instruments of different sizes should be available in every office. Each member of the office must have specific jobs with specific instrument needs, and these instruments should be sized to fit the hand of the operator. This arrangement will require changes in how instruments are manufactured and purchased by dental offices.

Elbow, hand, or finger rests are important too. Pivoting the entire arm from the shoulder joint is tiring and provides less accuracy of movements at the fingertips. Upper arms and elbows should be at rest against the sides of the operator's body, with forearms parallel to the floor. The more closely to the work site one can stabilize the fingers, the less work is done, especially by the shoulder muscles. Just as importantly, more precise movements can be accomplished with the fingers when a rest is provided.

Variety of movement throughout the day is an important aspect of repetitive strain injury prevention. Dentists and assistants are likely to move from room to room during the work day. Hygienists tend to remain in a single treatment room. There are a number of ways to provide variety at the worksite. Make sure to change positions often during a procedure. Classic four-handed dentistry, which encourages the dentist to move the elbow, wrist, and fingers (avoiding shoulder, neck, and back movements), should continue to be used for efficiency. Periodic posture changes, including micropauses, are encouraged, as is alternating sitting and standing for some procedures.[14]

The back, neck, and head should be aligned along a straight axis.[17] The vertebral column is healthiest when held in a vertical stack. Any tool that requires flexion or extension, especially at the neck, will encourage inflammation in the area.[18] If the inflammation affects the brachial plexus, nerve conduction and muscle function can be diminished in the hand and wrist. Just as important, static loading of any musculoskeletal group will cause strains and sprains in the area. The most common occurrence of this phenomenon in dentistry is in the upper trapezius.[8] Certain postures, as when the elbows are held out from the body (a position often used in dentistry) will require constant tension in the trapezius muscles. The weight of any tool held in the hand will add to this tension. Therefore, tools should be made, maintained, and used to reduce the amount of static loading in the neck area.

Hand Instruments

Hand instruments are manual tools, often double ended, that are used throughout dentistry. They include scalers, curettes, hoes, chisels, scalpels and other knives, explorers, probes, and grasping instruments like cotton pliers and needle holders. Most have working edges used to incise, scrape, or plane. All of these motions require a sharp working edge. The edge should be resharpened when dull or disposed of if sharpening is not possible. Increasing the amount of work the tool does may minimize the strain on the musculoskeletal system.

Instruments that are lightweight and well balanced require the muscles to do less work.[14] Any tool that is heavier at one end than the other requires more work in the shoulder, arm, and hand to overcome this imbalance. Hollow tools are more ergonomically sound than solid ones.[14] The material of which these tools are made is important too. Some instrument handles are now made of resin materials that are lighter yet larger in diameter than metal handles. Carbon steel is preferable to stainless steel for instruments with a cutting edge, because carbon steel stays sharper when exposed to heat sterilization. In grasping and other hinged instruments, cheaper materials break down sooner at the hinge, causing more friction and therefore more work for the hands. Spending more money on properly made tools will save time, money, and possibly injury.

Among dental instrument manufacturers, no industry standard exists for the size and shape of the handles. The traditional dental instrument handle approximates the size and shape of a number two pencil. In response to concerns about the pinching effect associated with these small diameter handles, manufacturers are developing a greater variety of handle sizes, shapes, materials, and textures. Larger handles reduce the pinching effect and distribute forces over a larger area. Some of the newer handles, such as the Hu-Friedy Advantouch™, are a full 50% greater in diameter than traditional handles. These handles are constructed of resin, resulting in a weight decrease of 0.7 grams.[19]

Endodontic instruments tend to be quite small in diameter and manipulating them therefore requires a more extreme pinching posture. File, reamer, and broach handles should be wider to reduce the pinching effect of these small-diameter instruments, or avoid their use when possible. For example, long-handled finger pluggers might be substituted for finger pluggers. Just as importantly, these cutting instruments must be replaced when dull. Recent advances in file taper appear to reduce the amount of time spent filing.[20] Time can also be saved if automatic instruments are used, like Gates-Glidden drills and endodontic handpieces.

The surface of instrument handles is significant as well. Holding and manipulating smooth handles require more pinching force.[21] Handles with shallow, circumferential grooves allow somewhat better friction with the fingers and grasping them requires less pinching force. The best surface is knurled[14] or cross-cut[4,22] and is becoming increasingly available from manufacturers. The handles of tools which are old tend to become smooth with use and should be replaced.

Grasping instruments include cotton pliers, crimpers, needle holders and hemostats, extraction forceps, rongeurs, and orthodontic pliers, among others. Scissors are included in this category. As with other instruments, these should be selected to fit the size of the hand using them. An interhandle distance of 5 to 8 cm provides the most grip strength, and 11 cm should never be exceeded.[22] Grasping handles set too close or too far apart will understretch or overstretch the muscles of the fingers, making work more difficult, causing fatigue, and increasing the potential for strain. The handles should be knurled or cross-cut for grip. They should be used for appropriate jobs so that excessive force is not required by the fingers using the instrument. Let the tool do the work. The tools should also have properly loaded spring openers that move the handles apart without the fingers having to do so.[4]

Automatic Handpieces

Whenever possible, an automatic handpiece should be used instead of a manual hand instrument. When the quality of the product is the same, let air-driven, belt-driven, or electric tools do the work otherwise provided by the human body. The term "handpiece" refers here to high-speed and slow-speed dental drills, belt-driven drills used in the lab, lasers, ultrasonic scalers, endodontic handpieces, autocondensers for amalgam placement, and electrosurgical units.

Handpieces should have many of the ergonomically sound characteristics we look for in hand instruments. Figure 2 shows two different handpiece styles. Hand pieces should be as light as possible and well balanced. Too much weight at either end of a tool will require the hand and wrist to counteract this force and therefore to do more work. Handpiece weight also should be minimized because of the extra work involved in supporting additional ounces. At this point in their evolution, handpieces require hoses that feed water and air to them. These hoses have weight and therefore require more exertion from the muscles of the shoulder and arm. Placement of the hose or cord for operator convenience and patient comfort can also be a struggle. Whenever possible, instruments with hoses or cords should be avoided.[4]

Handpieces should be well lubricated and kept in good working order. Leaks in hoses that provide air to a turbine-driven handpiece should be repaired so that the proper amount of power is available to the unit. Whenever appropriate, a handpiece should be used at maximum power to reduce the amount of time the hand and wrist have to

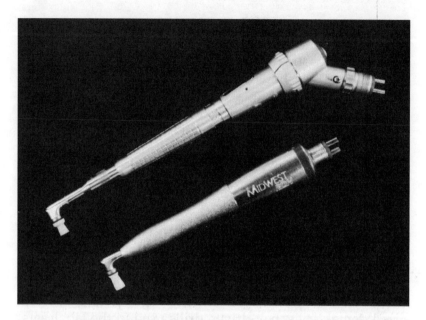

FIGURE 2.—The bottom handpiece illustrates a wider, shorter profile: weight balancing; and contour that help to relieve hand and wrist strain. The handpiece on the top has contrasting characteristics that tend to require the hand and wrist to work more.

support it. Keeping appointments short or incorporating micropauses during a long appointment will keep dental care workers from maintaining a static position for extended periods of time.

Hose length and pliability are also important in handpiece use. Hoses should be of adequate length to allow the practitioner to place the handpiece into an appropriate position that maintains an ergonomically sound posture. Pulling on a short hose or repositioning the body into an injury-provoking position must be avoided.[4] Hose material is important too. It should be strong and thick enough to last, but not so much so that the body has to work harder to put the tool into the proper working position. Coiled hoses may cause the hand and wrist to do more work if the coils have too much resistance to deformation. Some hose management systems use retractable mechanisms to get the hoses out of the way when not in use. These systems are very useful, but care must be taken to keep the locking mechanism in good working order. Otherwise, the hand and wrist will have to exert more force to counteract the retraction force of the unit.

Handpieces have hold and release mechanisms for attachment of drill bits. These mechanisms must be strong enough to hold the bur securely in place while allowing the practitioner to remove and replace the bur easily. The mechanisms may be buttons, levers, or knobs which can be rotated. Autochuck units are now available for high- and slow-speed handpieces. These allow the operator to release the bur with one push, rather than trying to place and rotate a very narrow wrench into the head of the handpiece. Occasionally, excessive force is required to activate these mechanisms, especially considering that the force exerted by the thumb opposes the other four fingers. This isolates force to the thumb, setting it up for strain in the flexor tendons.[23] Ideally, the mechanism should be easy to activate; little force should be required to engage it. Also, the mechanism should not require multiple applications of force; one application should activate it. Finally, the mechanism should be large enough so that the operator can avoid a pinching motion, which encourages inflammation in the wrist.

As with hand instruments, the diameter of a handpiece should be relatively large to reduce the pinching effect. The contour must fit the hand—larger at the base, maintaining a large diameter in the middle, and narrowing quickly at the working end. Less force is required to hold a knurled or cross-hatched surface than a smooth surface or one with shallow, parallel grooves.

Finally, the operator must be able to rotate and turn the handpiece with minimal effort and be able to hold it in the new position easily. This requires a pliable hose and a swivel mechanism in the barrel of the handpiece that rotates with minimal effort.

Curing lights used in the placement of composites and glass ionomers deserve mention here. Again, they should be manufactured with the same ergonomically sound characteristics discussed above. Unfortunately, an ideal curing light does not yet exist. The ideal light would be readily accessible to both the dentist and assistant. It should be lightweight and maneuverable. Cordless lights are available now but tend to be somewhat heavy.

Syringes

A syringe is any instrument that extrudes material out of a narrow-gauge tip when a plunger is forced with the thumb. Typical extruded materials include local anesthetics and certain impression materials.

The movement of these materials through the needle is identical to the movement of any fluid through a tube, and is described by the following equation:

$$\frac{\text{Volume of Fluid}}{\text{Time}} = Av$$

where A is the lumen cross-section and v is the speed of fluid at the cross-section.[24]

If the cross-section (A) of the needle is reduced (as in a 30-gauge needle), the volume of fluid dispensed must decrease or the length of time increase. Attempting to keep the volume the same or greater will require the operator to reduce the time, which can only be done by increasing the force applied by the thumb to the plunger. This can lead to inflammation in the carpal tunnel. It is ergonomically sound, then, to dispense materials through the largest lumen size possible or to extend the length of time. For patient comfort during injections, the latter option is most sensible.

As with any tool, syringes must be kept free of material that will increase the force required to extrude. This is especially true of impression material syringes, which tend to collect material on the inside walls of the syringe barrel. Also, latex glove material can sometimes get caught where the plunger enters the barrel, thus clogging the plunger mechanism and requiring the thumb to exert more force. Finally, the smaller the lumen at the tip is, the larger the force needed to depress the plunger. Cutting back the plastic syringe tip used in prosthodontics will increase lumen diameter.

Placement techniques for local anesthesia deserve special consideration. Self-aspirating syringes for placement of local anesthesia are preferred because they reduce the work exerted by the thumb. Also, certain techniques require additional force at the plunger. The periodontal ligament injection, the interdental papilla injection, and the intrapulpal technique used in endodontics require placement of the needle tip into dense tissue. Much force exerted over an extended period of time is needed to get the anesthetic solution into the tissue. This results in greatly increased pressure to the thumb flexors for a relatively long time period, thus setting it up for inflammation, especially at its base.[24] Therefore, use of syringes like the Ligmaject® or the Wand® is encouraged, since these syringes do most of the work.

Location of force application must also be considered. Most dental schools teach placement of the syringe plunger loop in the ventral pad of the thumb. This technique provides optimum control. We must realize, however, that the technique also increases force generation to the base of the thumb. This dilemma is a further argument for the use of large lumens and clean barrel walls as a way of reducing the force required of the thumb.

The air-water syringe tip combines the characteristics of both a syringe and a dispenser. All four fingers touch the handle relatively close to the base of each digit, and the instrument therefore mimics a dispenser. It also, however, requires placement of the tip of the thumb on the air-water buttons and therefore mimics a syringe. This physiologic relationship is similar to another injection technique, the thumb grasp. For both of these issues, the thumb is isolated. To reduce exposure of the thumb to excessive forces, the operator should apply force slowly and as gently as possible. This is especially precarious in the thumb grasp injection technique, which is used precisely because it can generate more force. Also, the very narrow 30-gauge needle is often used in this technique. When using this technique, then, the operator should attempt to place the syringe ring as far away from the tip of the thumb as possible. Again, lumen size should be as large as possible. All parts of the instrument should be kept clean and in good working order, and parts should be replaced as they wear out.

One more syringe system is the acid etch dispenser, which is typically a plastic syringe attached to a very narrow-gauge replaceable needle. It is important to dispense slowly because of the force needed to push the etchant through the needle lumen. If the etchant begins to dry out and thicken, the force needed to expel it will increase significantly, potentially causing tendon inflammation in the carpal tunnel. Therefore, etchants that are too thick should be discarded.

Lighting

This is a critical part of any job. Mistakes are more likely to occur if the operator has difficulty seeing the work site. In dentistry, significant improvements have been made through the use of fiber optics. High-speed handpieces can now be purchased through most manufacturers with fiberoptic light sources at the base of the handpiece. A fiber-optic bundle carries the light to the working end of the handpiece. This construction allows the operator to place light right at the work site without having objects in the way. While the overhead operator's light is still indispensable, the operator's head often obstructs the light. As a result, the options are moving the light, placing the operator's head in a less ergonomically sound position, or working in the dark. None of these options is desirable. Repositioning can place excessive force on the trapezius and cervical spine, thereby leading to neck and shoulder problems. An additional lighting system is described in the section entitled "Personal Protective Equipment."

The light switch on the overhead light must be readily accessible to the dentist, the hygienist, and the assistant. The switch should have a mechanism that moves with a minimum of effort. Switches with long handles tend to require less force from the operator's hand.

While high-speed handpieces are now readily available with fiber optics incorporated, other handpieces are not. Great benefit will be realized when slow speed handpieces, lasers, and ultrasonic units can be purchased with fiber-optic light incorporated.

Hand mirrors also can be used to provide light to an intraoral worksite. As with all other hand instruments, the handle should be hollow, with a large barrel and a knurled surface. Double-sided mirrors are encouraged as they have two surfaces from which light or images can be reflected. Some mirrors are available with lights mounted on the head, which improve visibility, but managing the cords is awkward.

Personal Protective Equipment

Personal protective equipment consists of those items used to reduce the spread of infection in the dental operatory, including gloves used intraoperatively or for cleanup, masks, glasses, caps, and gowns. All of these items influence ergonomic efficiency.

Glasses should be lightweight, well-fitted to the head, and clean. Of primary importance is the use of magnification. Magnifying lenses set to the proper focal length help the operator not only see better, but require the operator to maintain a more ergonomically sound posture. This is most important in reducing flexion of the neck and injury to the cervical spine. Magnification systems are also available with small lightweight head lamps to improve lighting to the operating site. Their use is encouraged.

Gowns and caps should fit loosely. In fact, no clothing, whether used in the office or outside, should cause the musculoskeletal system to do more work. Clothing should be lightweight, pliable, and as thin as possible while still providing protection.

The use of protective gloves intraoperatively and during preparation and cleanup is now standard operating procedure.[25] These gloves should be sized properly. If an exact size match cannot be obtained, they should be slightly larger than the hand. Gloves that are too small will cause strain and inflammation in the wrist. Also, ambidextrous gloves should be avoided because they cause the muscles and tendons in the wrist to do more work. Well-fitted, right- and left-handed gloves are strongly recommended. They better fit the static and functional anatomy of the hand and reduce the force necessary to open (or extend) the fingers.[14] While this type of glove is more expensive, the long-term benefits are significant. Gloves should be lightweight and extremely pliable. They should fit the hands well and never be too small. Gloves that are stiff or too small are more likely to cause carpal tunnel syndrome. Glove material probably has some effect on user comfort as well. Some of the nonlatex materials used by people with latex sensitivity seem to be less pliable than their latex counterparts. All of these issues are more important for workers susceptible to hand and wrist injuries.

Material Dispensers

Instruments are now available that provide convenient holding and dispensing of numerous materials, including composites, bases, buildup materials, temporary prosthodontic material, and impression materials. Material dispensers are defined here as those tools that deliver a dental material through a grasping, or handgun, mechanism. Such tools often have two barrels, which hold the base and catalyst and which combine into one barrel where the base and catalyst are mixed before placement. Material dispensers differ from syringes in that they spread out force generation to multiple fingers.

All four fingers are used in grasping a dispenser while the handle engages the skin between the thumb and index finger. With a syringe, the tips of the index and middle fingers are used to counteract the force generated by the tip of the thumb. As with any lever, forces applied at the end of the lever (here represented by the tip of any digit) generate significantly more force at the base of the lever. Dispensers are preferred because they use more digits and forces are applied closer to the base of the digits.[26] At the same time, it is important that the distance between the two arms of the handle not be too great. Too much distance requires excessive force at the distal phalanx of the fingers. Forces generated here can be two or three times greater than force generated at the middle phalanx.

The same evaluation criteria can be used in examining dispensers. They should be kept clean and free from hardened material. If the material is old enough, it may also set up without being exposed to the catalyst. As a result, more force will be required to extrude it. As with syringes, lumen size should be as large as possible. Material thickness has a significant effect on force generation too. For example, some provisional material dispensers combine two detrimental effects: the use of relatively thick material dispensed out of a significantly narrow lumen tip. To counteract these cumulative effects, the operator should apply force slowly while keeping the dispenser handle as close as possible to the base of the digits.

The dispenser handles should fit the size of the hand.[27] The handle surface is best gripped when it is knurled or cross-cut.

Some instrument handles have finger profiles, which are usually shallow indentations where the fingers are supposed to fit. If the hand size is just right, these profiles can be helpful. Profiles that are set too close or far apart, however, cause the fingers to be placed in positions that potentiate fatigue. Generally, instrument handles with finger profiles should be avoided.[28]

Evacuators

Evacuators are the instruments and mechanism by which fluids and other materials are removed from the operative site. They include the suction generating mechanism, hoses, on/ off controls, and suction tips. There are two primary concerns in the use of evacuators. The first concerns hoses. They should be light-weight, pliable and of sufficient length that they can easily be manipulated into position. The concern here is the potential for static loading, usually in the dental assistant.

The other problem location is the on/off mechanism found on the attachment module between the end of the hose and the suction tip. The mechanism may be a switch that can be moved forward and back, or a button that is rotated. In either case, the switch or button should move with minimal effort. It must be maintained this way as well. Occasionally, materials become incorporated into the mechanism, causing it to become more resistant to movement and requiring more force application by the operator. As usual, too much force or repetition of movement may lead to carpal tunnel syndrome. As with light switches, an on/off switch with a relatively long handle requires less work by the operator.

One other hose system that should be discussed here is gas delivery. Nitrous oxide sedation, which is used in many offices, is an example. Typically, this system has rubberized hoses that drape down and behind the patient's head. Two issues are pertinent here. First, the hoses should be of adequate length for easy access, and the hose material could be lighter and less likely to catch on surfaces that touch it. Second, the operator often must position his/her legs around the hoses. A delivery system that placed the hoses away from any part of the operator's body would be preferable.

Ambidexterity

Mention must be made about hand dominance and ambidexterity. The vast majority of people prefer to use their dominant hand when performing manual operations. Dentistry is no different. Repeated use of one hand will help that hand become more proficient in its performance of a given task. At the same time, we have seen that repetition is one of the primary causes of carpal tunnel syndrome. All dental personnel should attempt to switch hands when possible.[14] Using the nondominant hand will feel awkward at first. Additionally, it could be dangerous if attempted without consideration to the task at hand. When the task cannot injure the operator, assistant, or patient, attempts can be made to use the nondominant hand. Through repeated use, this hand will become more proficient and can be used to share the workload with the dominant hand. Special accommodations to the standard four-handed technique will have to be considered. Switching hands while relying on an assistant to deliver instruments may increase the risk of puncture injury to the dental team members.

Patient Chair

The patient chair, also known as the dental chair, has a number of ergonomic requirements. The first is patient comfort. It should provide proper support for the patient's entire body in every position.

The other requirements concern the dental personnel. The chair must be easily movable in every direction, so that the operators do not strain in adjusting its position. It is important here to note that constant attention must be paid to moving the patient chair, and the patient, to positions that allow ergonomically sound postures for the operators. Controls for chair movement should be readily accessible to both the dentist and the assistant. The chair should move automatically whenever possible, so that dental personnel do not have to adjust or lift.

The chair back and headrest must combine strength with thinness. Classic four-handed dentistry usually places the patient's head in very close proximity to the dentist's abdomen. The operative site, usually the mouth, should be placed at the level of the elbow when the operator is seated in an upright posture. This means that there are about 6 to 8 inches between the elbow and the top of the legs. The chair back and patient must fit into this space, so chair thinness is essential.

While most procedures are performed using classic four-handed techniques, (operator and assistant are seated and the operator is at the 11 o'clock position), they should not be limited to this style. Variety is critical to an ergonomically sound treatment approach. Depending on the procedure being performed and the length of time needed to complete it, positions should vary during the course of a patient appointment as well as the course of a treatment day. Alternating standing and sitting is encouraged. Selecting certain procedures to routinely perform standing, such as taking impressions, will enable the operator and/or the assistant to include this variation in position. Important here is the ability of the patient chair to move up and down to accommodate operators of differing heights. Adjusting the chair back to different angles is also encouraged to spread the work load to different muscles, tendons, and bones. At the same time, patient positions that require the operator to torque his or her body must be avoided. The operator's center of mass should be maintained at its optimal point, approximately the level of the navel centered in the abdomen. This position minimizes torque and static loading. As discussed previously, properly-adjusted glasses, with magnification system attached, will place the operator's head, neck, and back at this optimal position. Again, it is critical that the dental team be sensitive to changing positions, and it must be easy to place the dental chair into these positions.

Conclusion

We have discussed a number of issues relating to sound ergonomic design of dental instruments, including the importance of variety in product design and use, risk factors for injuries, ideal characteristics of an instrument, maintenance of moving and cutting parts, and appropriate instrument use. Unfortunately, sound scientific studies examining these issues are scarce. Without the science, observation of current practices, and feedback from the practitioner, the prevention of repetitive strain injury is hampered. It is important, therefore, that studies be conducted and the results forwarded to the users of dental instruments, so that they can request appropriate design changes from the product manufacturers. A combination of better equipment design, training of the practitioner, and attention through professional journals and continuing education programs are the keys to preventing injuries.

REFERENCES

1. *Annual Occupational Injury and Wellness Report: Workplace Injury and Illness Summary.* US Department of Labor, Bureau of Labor Statistics; 1996.
2. Macdonald G. Hazards in the dental workplace. *Dent Hyg.* 1987;61(5):212–218.
3. Bjelle A, Hagberg M. Sjukdom, alder och belastning pa muskulaturen orsaker till skulder-back-besvar hos industriarbetare. *Lakartidningen.* 1984;81:1419–1422.
4. Johnson SL. Ergonomic design of handheld tools to prevent trauma to the hand and upper extremity. *J Hand Therap.* 1990;3(2):86–93.
5. Birbeck MQ, Beer TC. Occupation in relation to the carpal tunnel syndrome. *Rheum Rehab.* 1975;14(4):218–221.
6. McDermott FT. Repetition strain injury: a review of current understanding. *Med J Aust.* 1986;144:196–200.
7. Macdonald G, Robertson MM, Erickson JA. CTS among California dental hygienists. *Dent Hyg.* 1988;62(7):322–328.
8. Rundcrantz BL, Johnsson B, Moritz U. Cervical pain and discomfort among dentists. Epidemiological, clinical and therapeutic aspects. Part 1. A survey of pain and discomfort. *Swed Dent J.* 1990;14:71–80.
9. Morehead A, Morehead L. Ed. *The New American Webster Handy College Dictionary.* New York: New American Library; 1972:246.
10. Armstrong TJ. Ergonomics and cumulative trauma disorders. *Hand Clin.* 1986;2(3):553–565.
11. Armstrong TJ. *An Ergonomics Guide to Carpal Tunnel Syndrome.* Akron, Ohio: AIHAI Ergonomic Guide Series; 1983.
12. Meagher SW. Human factors engineering. *Contemp Orthop.* 1987;8:173–180.

13. Meagher SW. Tool design for prevention of hand and wrist injuries. *Hand Surg.* 1987;12A:855–857.
14. Strong DR, Lennartz FH. Carpal tunnel syndrome. *Cal Dent Assoc J.* 1992;20(4):27–42.
15. The Zenith Insurance Company. Preventing strains, sprains in the dental office. *Insurance Insights, The Dentists Insurance Services.* 1996;11(3):4.
16. Rossignol AM. Video display terminal use and reported health symptoms among Massachusetts clerical workers. *J Occup Med.* 1987;29:112–118.
17. Goldman HS, Hartman KS, Messite J. Eds. *Occupational Hazards in Dentistry.* Chicago: Year Book Medical Publishers; 1984:138.
18. Nordin M, Ortengren R, Andersson GBJ. Measurement of trunk movements during work. *Spine.* 1984;9:465–469.
19. Handle Comparison Chart. Chicago: Hu-Fridey Manufacturing Co; 1997.
20. Buchanan S. The files of greater taper. *Dent Today.* 1997;16(1):51.
21. Comaish S, Bottoms E. The skin and friction: deviations from Amton's laws and effects of hydration and lubrication. *Br J Dermatol.* 1971;84:37–43.
22. Gowiztke BA, Milnar M. *Understanding the Scientific Basis of Human Movement.* 2nd ed. Baltimore: Williams and Wilkins; 1980:95.
23. Cailliet R. *Hand Pain and Impairment.* 3rd ed. Philadelphia: Davis; 1982.
24. Breuer H. *Physics for Life Science Students.* Englewood Cliffs, NJ: Prentice-Hall; 1975:120–127.
25. Centers for Disease Control and Prevention. *MMWR.* May 28,1993; 41(RR-8): 12.
26. Lindquist B. *How to Design Tool Handles and Triggers for Low Physical Load: Ergonomic Tools of Our Time.* Stockholm: T.R. Tryck; 1986:24–31.
27. Meagher SW. Human factors engineering. *Contemp Orthop.* 1987;8:73–80.
28. Tichauer ER: *The Biomechanical Basis of Ergonomics.* New York: Wiley Interscience; 1978:41–43, 69–70.

Chapter 8

Surgical Magnification:

Posture Maker or Posture Breaker?

Lance M. Rucker, DDS

Abstract

Surgical magnification has been widely promoted as an underused dental technology. A wide range of loupes, telescopes, and surgical microscopes is available to dentists and dental hygienists. Unfortunately, it is often assumed that just having or wearing surgical magnification is bound to improve the quality of treatment. As with most equipment, even more important than *whether* it is used is *how* it is used. Properly selected and adjusted, surgical magnification can support balanced musculoskeletal ergonomics, but *improperly selected or adjusted surgical magnification will support, or even create, poor working postures*. This chapter discusses how to ensure that the surgical magnification system fits the specific balanced musculoskeletal ergonomics of the intended user.

Introduction

The past several years have seen an explosion of interest in surgical magnification in dental operatories. Formerly assumed to be part of the realm of older practitioners and eccentrics, dental telescopes and loupes have now acquired a rapidly growing following among practitioners and clinical lecturers with international reputations.[1] A recent survey of practicing dentists in the United States estimates that about half of them use magnification while operating.[2]

Many dental schools and faculties are recommending surgical telescopes or loupes to their dental students.[3,4] Most of these university programs are suggesting that students acquire a particular brand for clinical applications; a few of them recommend telescopes for preclinical and simulation exercises as well. More often than not the selection of magnification system is based on the recommendation of an influential faculty member who has been especially satisfied with a particular brand.

A small but growing number of hygiene programs are also recommending surgical magnifiers to dental hygienists.[5] Some zealous clinical lecturers are recommending magnification for dental assistants who are licensed to perform expanded duties involving primary operating functions. In particular, orthodontic assistants spend much of their time placing and removing bands, appliances, arch wires, and so forth. Such tasks are ideally suited for surgical magnification.

Most clinicians embark on their explorations of the world of surgical magnification in hopes of seeing more clearly and achieving greater accuracy and accountability in diagnoses and restorations.[6] A few users are lured primarily by hopes that the telescopes' working-distance limitations will force them into better and more comfortable postures, but such ergonomically oriented practitioners are the exceptions.[7]

Some professional course presenters and clinicians, in their zeal to promote surgical magnification as an underused modern dental technology, have declared that any dentists who are not using surgical magnification in their practices are falling short of fulfilling their professional responsibilities. The presentations emphasize the use of surgical magnification as if *use alone* were sufficient, as if merely having and wearing surgical magnification of some sort were bound to improve the quality of treatment. As with most equipment, even more important than *whether* it is utilized is *how* it is used. Properly selected and adjusted, surgical magnification can support balanced musculoskeletal ergonomics, but *improperly selected or adjusted surgical magnification will support, or even create, poor working postures.*[8,9] Hence, it is important to make certain that the surgical magnification system fits the specific balanced musculoskeletal ergonomics of the intended user.

Types of Surgical Magnification Available

Several distinct categories of surgical magnifiers are on the market, from very expensive, large units to the smallest, inexpensive units (see Figure 1):

1. Stationary (fixed) microscopes (Figure 1a) have the following characteristics:
   • wall mounted or ceiling mounted,

- very useful for high magnification (6x to 20x),
- confined field at high magnification, and
- very limited depth of field at high magnification.

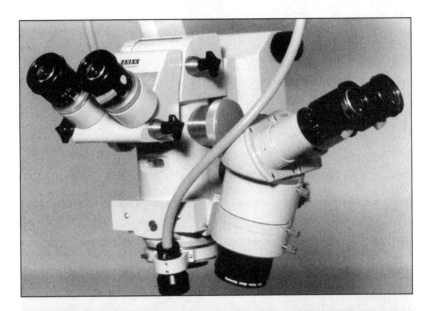

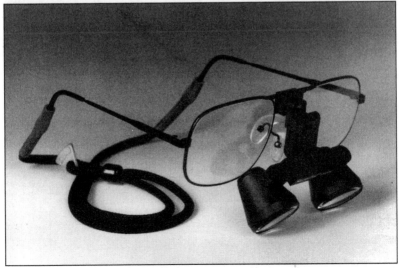

FIGURE 1.—Types of surgical magnification.

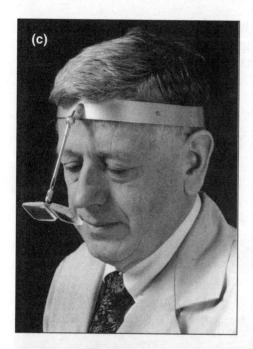

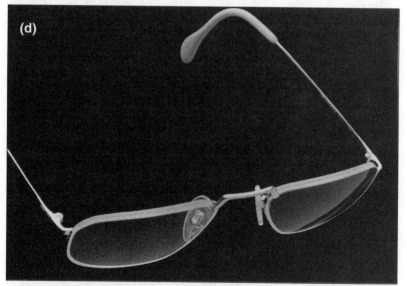

Figure 1.—*Continued*

2. Low magnification multi-lens systems (Figure 1b) have the following characteristics:
- spectacles-mounted or headband-mounted telescopes,
- very portable and convenient, and
- low to medium magnification range (2x to 5x).

3. Single-lens loupes and magnifiers (Figure 1c) have the following characteristics:
- headband mounted or spectacles clip-on,
- low magnification, and
- limited depth of field and working distance.

4. Prescription lenses and reading glasses[10,11] (Figure 1d) have the following characteristics:
- low magnification and
- limited depth of field and working distance.

Key Issues and Features of Surgical Magnification and How They Affect Operator Posture and Clinical Ergonomics

The various categories, brands, and models of surgical magnifiers can be properly compared and evaluated only when certain key issues and features are considered in relationship to the ergonomics of clinical dentistry. The following features will be discussed:
1. working distance;
2. depth of field;
3. declination angle;
4. convergence angle;
5. degree of magnification;
6. magnification scotoma ("blind zone");
7. coaxial alignment of telescopes and sightlines, including chromatic aberrations and diffractive viewing effects;
8. "flip-up" capability;
9. contact/cross-contamination potential;
10. need for adequate light;
11. subjective concerns such as flatness of field, weight, stability during use, and physical comfort; and
12. learning curve for using surgical magnification.

Working Distance

In the simplest terms, the working distance is the distance between the operator's eye and the working site (Figure 2a). Consideration of your musculoskeletal requirements as well as any unavoidable limitations of your working field will dictate the nearest and furthest working distances at which you must customarily perform clinically. If the existing operatory layout imposes limitations on your preferred working distance, consider modifying the layout (see Chapter 12, "Optimizing Dental Operatory Working Environments").

If there is a mismatch between the optimal working distance of the operator and the surgical magnification system, the operator may be forced to work with arms and neck over-extended (Figure 2b), or with back hunched and/or neck overflexed (Figure 2c).

You can have an assistant measure your nearest working distance (Figure 2d) and your furthest working distance (Figure 2e). From these can be calculated your mean working distance. All three of these measurements are useful for telescope selection and evaluation.

Restrictions of your surgical magnification system should *not* be the determining factor for your working range. Rather, the depth of field and working distance of your surgical telescopes should accommodate *your* working range.

Depth of Field

Depth of field is the range over which you are able to achieve visual resolution (discrimination). It is determined by the combination of your vision and the surgical magnification system. It is recorded in terms of the nearest and furthest extremes of distance from the surface of your eye to the object observed (e.g., a depth of field from 13 inches to 18.5 inches). Depth of field may also be recorded in terms of the difference between these extremes (e.g., a 4-inch depth of field). Most manufacturers rate their magnification systems for a specific range (e.g., 13 inches to 19.5 inches).

A well-centered depth of field of 3 inches (7.5 cm) is the minimum sufficient for visualization of structures from the nearest point (central incisors) to the farthest (a reflected view of a distal molar) in the average adult mouth. Less depth of

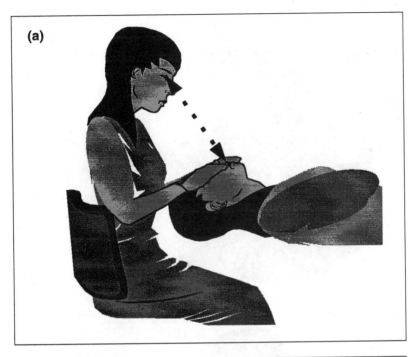

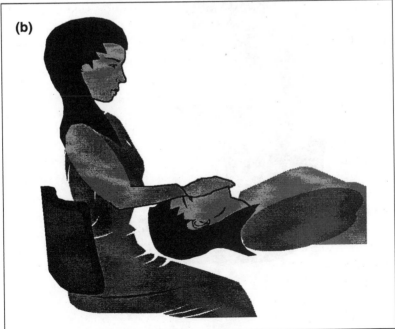

FIGURE 2.—Working distance issues.

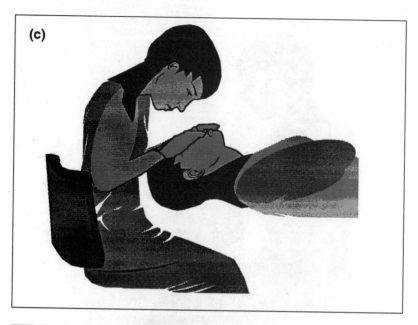

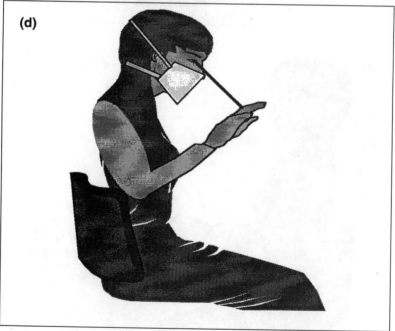

FIGURE 2.—*Continued*

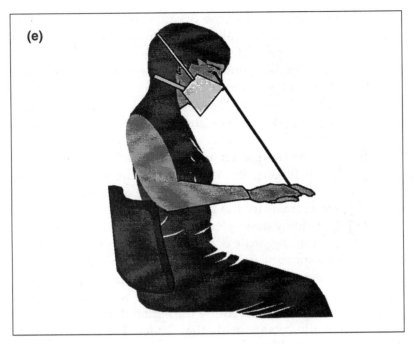

FIGURE 2.—*Continued*

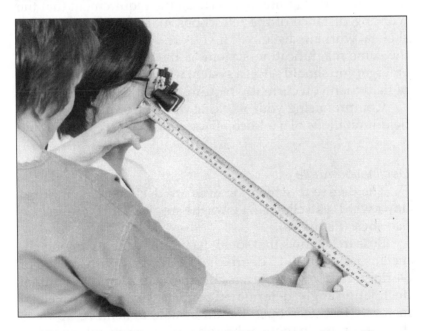

FIGURE 3.—Measuring the depth of field of a surgical magnifier.

field will certainly require the operator to tip the head forward or backward to visualize some areas of the oral cavity.

When the extremes of the operator's depth of field (a visual characteristic) are not well matched to the operator's musculoskeletal needs, much the same problem prevails as with mismatches between operator working distances and telescope working distances—and with identical deleterious ergonomic effects.

You should test surgical magnifiers by looking at a fine grid or at your own fingerprint to determine the system's actual depth of field for you. It is easiest to have an assistant with a measuring tape measure the near and far extremes at which you can comfortably make clear visual resolution (Figure 3).

Be aware that regardless of what the manufacturer indicates in the supporting documentation manuals or brochures, you may experience an entirely different depth of field based on your own visual status or age, so it is wise to check any prospective device to determine the actual depth of field you experience while you are using that device. The older you are, the greater the likelihood that you will experience a reduced depth of field, and the more crucial the requirement that the working distance of the telescopes matches your musculoskeletal working distance.[12] If you are young and wish to use the same magnification system as the effects of presbyopia emerge, you should select a system which has a broader depth of field than you currently require.

Compromising your working distance to meet depth-of-field limitations of a telescope system is not acceptable.

Declination Angle

The degree to which the eyes are declined (i.e., inclined downward) as a clinician views the surgical site is the *declination angle* (Figure 4a).

Research shows that ideal declination angles among clinicians range from 15 degrees to 44 degrees, with a mean of 34 degrees. However, each clinician has a unique optimal declination angle, determined primarily by musculoskeletal factors. Most telescopes should be able to achieve up to 45 degrees of declination, although until recently all manufacturers arbitrarily set the declination angles between 10

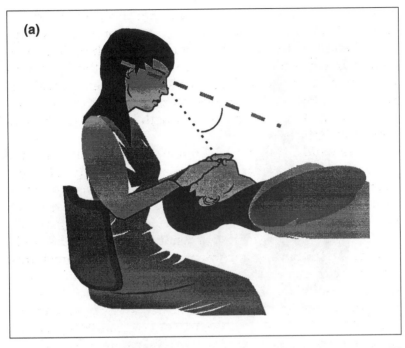

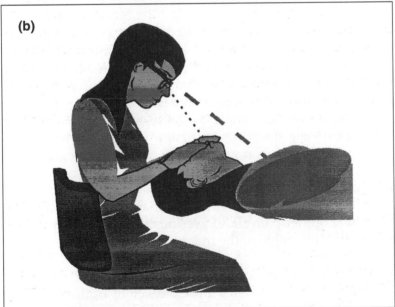

FIGURE 4.—The ideal declination angle for a telescope is one that exactly matches the musculoskeletally optimal declination angle of the operator.

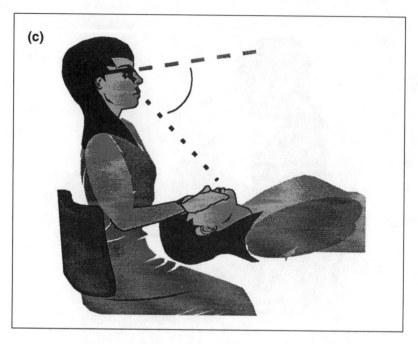

FIGURE 4.—*Continued*

degrees and 22 degrees. In the absence of a specification by the buyer, most manufacturers still use an arbitrary setting. Many adjustable telescopes (flip-ups) are unable to achieve greater than 34 degrees of declination. Each different system must be tested by the perspective user as described below.

If the declination angle of the telescope is less than or greater than the surgeon's optimal musculoskeletal declination angle, the surgeon will have to tip the head excessively downward (Figure 4b) or excessively upward (Figure 4c), depending on the mismatch. This introduces added risk of neck strain and/or back strain. Any surgeon who suffers back, neck, and/or shoulder pain should seriously consider inappropriate declination angle of the magnification system among the potential causes.

The ideal declination angle for a telescope is one that exactly matches the clinician's muscloskeletally optimal declination angle. Otherwise, the clinician will be forced to compromise to adapt to the equipment. Technically speaking, the optical declination angle is defined as the angle between the support axis of an operator's spectacles-mounted system and the actual line of sight chosen by the operator. The reference support axis for an operator's spectacles-mounted system is the SAC–Bridge of Nose Line. SAC is an abbreviation for superior auricular crevice, where the temple piece of spectacles rests on the ear. The bridge of the nose, for purposes of this discussion, is the weight-bearing part of the nose that supports the nose pads of the spectacles (Figure 5). This same reference is used for headband-mounted telescope systems or loupes, even though they do not bear upon the nose.

Determination of the declination angle is best accomplished in your treatment setting. For the needed patient simulation, use a mannequin head mounted in your dental chair, or enlist the help of someone in your office who will assume the role of a patient for the purposes of these measurements.

Assume your most balanced operating position. With your head in its least-strained posture and *without concern for focal distance or resolution*, open your eyes and look at the maxillary central incisors. Keeping the eyes on this point, tip the head forward and downward until musculoskeletal strain in the neck and/or back is felt. Raise the head until strain is felt in the ocular musculature (i.e., as you peer down at the control point over

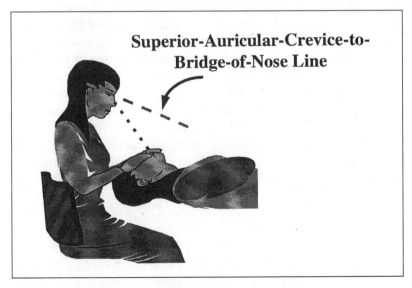

Figure 5.—Determining the optimal declination angle.

your lower eyelids). These two postures are the extremes of the range of head positioning that will allow you to achieve visual contact with the operating site. Keeping your eyes on the control point, tip the head forward and backward a few times through this range until you determine your *optimal* balanced head position. You may use a protractor to measure your declination angle, or you may simply establish the suitability of the surgical magnification system you are evaluating.

Once you've determined your preferred declination angle, you can use this information to assess the appropriateness of various optical devices. Carefully maintaining your balanced operating position (including the balanced head position derived above), place and secure the optical device you wish to assess. Notice whether the entire field of the oral cavity (or magnified portion of the oral cavity) is visible in the field of view offered by the optical device without requiring any turning or tipping of your head. The field of view should be centered on the intraoral control point. If you must tip or raise your head to see the working field, the optical device does not accommodate your needs in its current configuration and must either be modified or rejected.

In general, the further an operator is forced to tip the head forward and downward to see through telescopes, the greater the risk of strain to musculature of the head, neck and shoulder areas. Most operators, however, prefer a certain degree of forward and downward tipping of the head to minimize strain on the intrinsic and extrinsic eye musculature that is attendant to any extreme downward casting of the eyes. The declination angle, then, represents a balance between the extremes of eyestrain (when there is no downward tipping of the head—as in Figure 4c) and neck strain (when there is no declination of the eyes—as in Figure 4b). This balance is critical.

Convergence Angle

Convergence relates to the horizontal alignment of magnifying oculars so that their sight lines converge correctly on the object being viewed (see Figure 6). This is a more obvious feature of concern with multilens systems. Some tele-

FIGURE 6.—Magnifying oculars must be horizontally aligned so that sight lines converge correctly on the object being viewed.

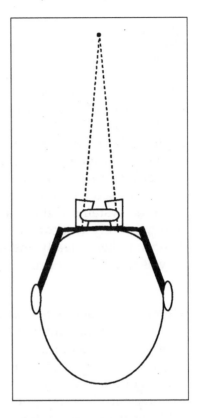

scopes allow for pivotal axis adjustment of convergence angles, and others try to address this issue in conjunction with lateral adjustment of the interpupillary distance (the distance between the oculars). If the convergence angle and interpupillary distance are not correctly aligned, eyestrain and poor visual resolution may result. This adjustment is similar to what most people have experienced as the primary adjustment for binoculars and opera glasses. Most operators easily recognize problems in this category. The alignment of telescopes in the vertical direction relative to each other is very important. The misalignment of telescope oculars in the vertical direction (called dipvergence) creates double images in the vertical direction and creates severe eyestrain. As the magnification power increases, the vertical alignment becomes more critical. Therefore through-the-lens telescopes having higher magnification should not be mounted on lightweight frames because a slight twist of the frames can produce significant dipvergence.

Degree of Magnification

A power of magnification of 2x to 3.5x is suggested for most dental applications. More than that will greatly reduce depth of field. For some endodontic and oral surgical applications, a stationary (fixed) microscope may be required for greater magnification. However, if more than 5x of magnification is used in either spectacles-mounted or headband-mounted systems, difficulties with stabilizing the field of vision are likely to occur. The objects being viewed may be difficult to keep steady and in the center of the field, particularly as the operator tires.

Magnification Scotoma (Blind Zone)

Magnification scotoma is the on-field-off-field blind zone created by your surgical magnification system. By virtue of the fact that surgical magnification systems often magnify only a portion of the total field of vision, a certain blind zone occurs whenever an object is carried from the peripheral unmagnified field toward the magnified center of the field. In general, the greater the power of magnification is, the greater the absolute size and proportion of the scotoma (blind zone).

The magnification scotoma is also enlarged by bulky design of the telescope oculars or the device(s) on which they are suspended in the field of vision. In general, flip-up telescopes, because of the hinging mechanism located in the visual field, have the potential to produce a larger scotoma than through-the-lens systems.

A large blind zone usually encourages the operator to turn the head sharply to one side to eliminate its effects during instrument movements and exchanges. The greatest distress related to the magnification scotoma is the risk of poor control when instruments are being moved into (or out of) the magnified field of view. The dangers both to clinicians and to patients are evident as instruments are passed through this blind zone. Most clinicians learn to compensate through some combination of 1) moving the telescopes aside until the instrument is placed and established with proprioceptive fulcrum at the operating site and/or 2) guiding the instrument to the operating site with any sharp points or edges guarded with gloved finger(s) until the instrument is under visual control in the magnified field of view.

Some degree of magnification scotoma is always present for magnifying systems, but the general rule of surgical magnification in dentistry is to use the least magnification required so as to minimize the scotoma.

Coaxial Alignment of Telescopes and Sight Lines

Chromatic aberrations are color deviations of lens systems. The observer senses anything from a subtle halo of color at the edges of observed objects to wild light shows that may interfere with resolution in the field of view. These aberrations are usually the result of defective optics or poor coatings on single-lens magnifiers or multiple-lens systems.

However, chromatic aberrations may also result from viewing targets through telescopes when the line of sight is not coaxial to the cylinder of the telescope oculars (see Figure 7). This is a common result of telescopes for which the declination angle has been increased without a commensurate overall lowering of the oculars relative to the pupils of the eyes. Some types of flip-up telescopes have vertical adjustment mechanisms incorporated into the ocular suspension to allow for independent raising or lowering of the oculars to deal with this issue.

The best way to detect chromatic aberrations in magnification systems is to look through the lenses at a black-and-white image, preferably one with sharp lines of demarcation. An Amsler grid (white lines on a black background, as in Figure 8) is an ideal target for detecting chromatic aberrations.

Noncoaxial alignment of telescope oculars and sight lines can also cause another problem: diffractive viewing effect. This phenomenon is detected by passing a pencil from the nonmagnified peripheral field directly into the center of the magnified field. If there is good coaxial alignment of the telescopes, the pencil will pass directly to the center of the magnified field. If it crosses the field above or below the center, the oculars are not coaxial.

Noncoaxial telescope oculars can also create enlarged scotomas.

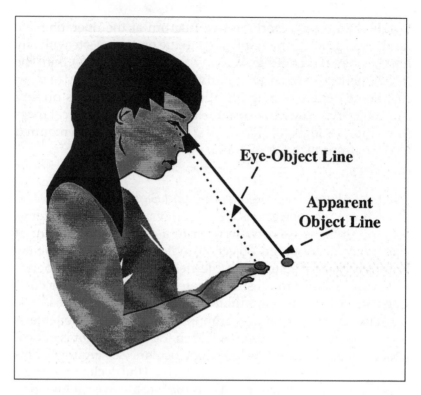

Eye-Object Line

Apparent Object Line

FIGURE 7.—Chromatic aberrations and diffractive veiwing effects may result when the line of sight is not coaxial to the cylinder of the telescope oculars.

"Flip-up" Capability

How does an operator decide between adjustable "flip-up" and through-the-lens custom-made telescopes (see Figure 9)? The decision is a challenging one. The factors affecting the decision and the advantages and disadvantages of each type of surgical telescope are not as obvious as first meets the eye!

Flip-up advantages are as follows:

- Flip-up telescopes can be flipped up for unmagnified appraisals of field of view.
- The declination angle can be adjusted for multiple users.
- Delivery and replacement are faster than with custom systems.
- Clinicians who alter their practice ergonomics can adjust the declination angle as needed.

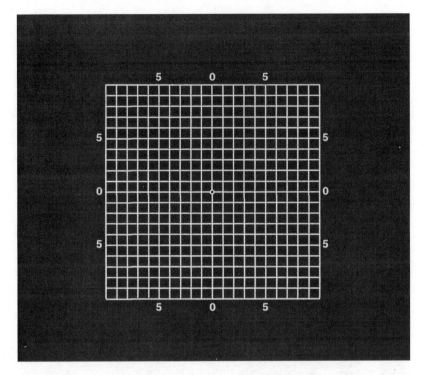

Figure 8.—An Amsler grid is an ideal target for detecting chromatic aberrations.

Flip-up disadvantages are as follows:
- Flip-up telescopes invite contamination (during adjustment), even with flip-tabs.
- They are usually associated with larger scotoma because of the suspension mechanism (recent designs have avoided this problem).
- They are heavier and bulkier than fixed systems.
- There is a greater risk of distortion for astigmatic users with greater than +2.0 correction and a larger declination angle.

Through-the-lens system advantages are as follows:
- The telescope is always in the correct position for viewing the surgical field (if properly customized to working distance and declination angle).
- Mechanical maintenance requirements are low (no flip-up mechanism to require attention).

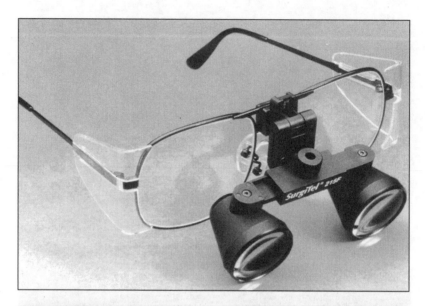

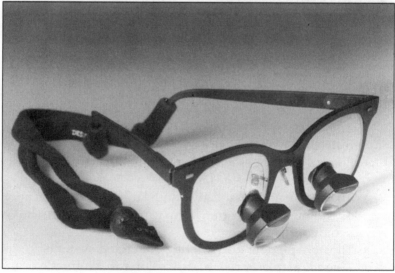

FIGURE 9.—Adjustable "flip-up" (top) and through-the-lens custom-made telescopes (bottom).

- Through-the-lens telescopes are lighter in weight.
  Through-the-lens system disadvantages are as follows:
- Through-the-lens systems are not adjustable for extraordinary surgical procedures (thereby requiring postural compromise for those situations).

- Optical maintenance costs are higher.
- A change of prescription or other adjustment currently requires return shipment to the manufacturer.
- Frames which are strong enough to support proper optical alignment of through-the-lens systems are heavier and less esthetic than the frames required for flip-ups.

Many clinicians choose to have both types of telescopes available. This arrangement also provides a back-up magnification system for times when one system is being repaired, when prescriptions are being changed, or when one system has been misplaced. Use of surgical magnification quickly becomes a dependency. It is a dependency built on excellence, but it is nonetheless a dependency. It's always best to be ready for breakdowns in equipment!

Contact/Cross-Contamination Potential

Telescopes can be cleaned, but even with those that boast sealed oculars there is no reliable way to satisfactorily disinfect the equipment. Some flip-up surgical telescopes have sterilizable flip-tabs intended to allow manipulation and adjustment without cross-contamination. Unfortunately, in practice a clinician is unable to reliably grasp a flip-up control tab on the forehead without inadvertently touching a nonsterile surface (the body of the telescope, hair, cap, or the skin of the operator's forehead), resulting in a high likelihood of contamination. The process of adjustment is almost certain to require overgloving or regloving.

Need for Adequate Light

Many operatories already have too much light (or too little), or have too much (or too little) contrast between background lighting and lighting of the oral cavity.[13,14] Although lighting in operatories is an ergonomic issue unto itself, it is closely interwoven with surgical magnification. Dental and medical equipment manufacturers are turning much attention to the development of low-profile, light-weight light sources whose purpose is to provide ideal lighting for dental and surgical needs (see Figure 10).

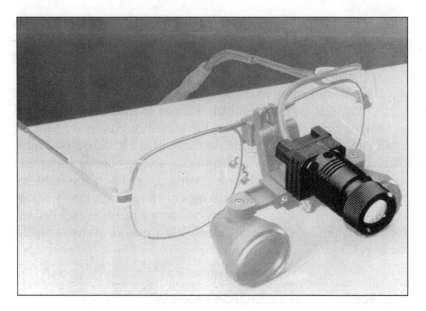

FIGURE 10.—A lightweight light source.

A few observations about lighting follow:
- Magnification increases the need for adequate lighting. The higher the magnification is, the more light is required.
- Fiber-optic light sources decrease in brightness over time as a result of fiber breakdown caused by bending of the bundles.
- Light coaxial to the line of sight is the most shadow free.[15]
- Head-mounted light units may temporarily blind assistants who are working in the operatory when the beam of light is flashed in their eyes.

Subjective Concerns

Weight distribution and resultant forces exerted may vary according to the facial anatomy of the operator and the manner in which lenses and telescopes are used. Furthermore, a broad range of weights is associated with surgical magnifiers (approximately 60g to 135g).[16] Some operators prefer headband mountings, and others prefer spectacles mountings. For the former, consideration must still be given to the issue of simple eye protection. Usually the weight on the nose pads is increased when flip-up scopes are in their raised positions.

Magnifiers need to be stable throughout the range of head tipping normally used to view the operating field and in positions used to see around the magnified field. Stability for spectacles-mounted systems can be enhanced with various retaining bands, Velcro straps, cords, cloth tubes, and so forth, some of which offer added safety against inadvertent damage to the oculars when the magnifiers are removed (see Figure 1b). Headband-mounted systems usually have built-in stability adjustments. Nose pieces should be carefully adjusted, and some systems allow lateral bending adjustments of the temple pieces. Care must be exercised not to inadvertently alter the declination or convergence angles when such improvements in the system stability are being made.

Overall physical comfort of the magnifiers is very important for an instrument that will likely be worn many hours of every working day. Some manufacturers offer frames designed to increase comfort by the addition of multiple nose pads and padded straps for the temple pieces. If the magnifiers aren't comfortable, they won't be worn!

Learning Curve for Use of Surgical Magnification

As with any new piece of dental equipment, fluent use of a surgical magnification system requires definite techniques that must be learned and practiced. The higher the magnification of the system is, the more difficult the transition. Specific challenges include all phases of instrument passes, manipulations of biomaterials in the operatory, the determination of planes and larger intraoral and extraoral landmarks, gauging parallelism of nonadjacent tooth preparations of prosthodontic abutments, and assessment of radiographs. Most clinicians report that they achieve a basic familiarity and comfort with magnification after about 10 days of use, but that real fluency may require as much as 2 months of full-time clinical use.

Summary

Guidelines for better ergonomics with surgical magnification are as follows:

- The depth of field of your surgical telescopes should accommodate your working distance, *not* vice versa.
- The choice between flip-up and fixed (through-the-lens) telescopes depends primarily on individual preference and intended usage.
- Poorly fitted or incorrectly used surgical magnification equipment is more likely to *cause* ergonomic problems than to *solve* them.
- Choose the lowest level of magnification required for surgical control to maximize the depth of field and to minimize the blind-zone scotoma.
- Ensure coaxial alignment of telescopes and sight lines.

Features required for a good surgical magnification system are as follows:

- The *working distance* of system must match the balanced musculoskeletal working distance of the operator.
- The *declination angle* must be adjusted to match the declination angle of the operator.
- The *depth of field* must allow for the full range of visual needs, from the nearest magnified object to be observed to the farthest.
- The system should provide the *minimum degree of magnification* required.
- *Field size* is adequate for visual clarity.
- The *scotoma* (blind zone) must be as small as possible.
- *Protection for the operators' eyes* is adequate.

Disadvantages of using surgical magnification for clinical treatment include:

- cost of equipment and
- a learning curve for optimal use, including movement of instruments onto field of operation and peripheral orientation.

Advantages of using properly selected and adjusted surgical magnification for clinical treatment include:

- better, clearer vision,
- supported optimal ergonomic balance,
- decreased fatigue,

- improved eye protection, and
- a higher level of clinical professional accountability.

The arguments for including surgical magnification in the oral health armamentarium are similar to the arguments made four decades ago for having air turbine high-speed hand piece technology available in regular dental practice. The nearly universal response of clinicians who have made this transition is that they would never again choose to practice without the availability of surgical magnification.

REFERENCES

1. Kanca J, Jordan PG. Magnification systems in clinical dentistry. *J Can Dent Assn.* 1995;61(10):851–856.
2. Magnification. C.R.A. Newsletter. 1995;19(10):3.
3. Burton JF, Rucker LM. The use of magnification devices in dentistry: a survey of dental practitioners. *Proceedings of IADR*; Singapore; 1993.
4. Leknius C, Geissberger M. The effect of magnification on the performance of fixed prosthodontic procedures. *J Calif Dent Assn.* 1995;23(12):66–70.
5. Lunn R, Sunell S. Posture, position, and surgical telescopes in dental hygiene. *J Dent Ed.* 1996;60(2):122.
6. Coburn DG. Vision, posture, and productivity. *Practice Management.* 1984:74:13–15.
7. Rucker LM, Richter W, Beattie C. Fine visual acuity and the performance simulation setting. *J Dent Ed.* 1985;49(1):86.
8. Rucker L, McGregor C, Woo G, Leong YM. Effects of low-magnification surgical telescopes on preclinical operative dental performance. *J Dent Ed.* 1992;56(1):34.
9. Rucker L, McGregor C. Surgical magnification in clinical simulation: enhanced visual control of performance. *J Dent Ed.* 1996;60(2):122.
10. Bridgman GF, Burton JF. A new multifocal spectacle lens for presbyopic dentists. *J Dent Res.* 1992; 71:985.
11. Burton JF, Bridgman GF. Spectacles to maintain the flexibility of vision for the older dentist: the Otago Dental Lookover. *Quintessence Intl.* 1991;22:879–883.
12. Burton JF, Bridgman GF. Presbyopia and the dentist: the effect of age on clinical vision. *Intl Dent J.* 1990;40:303–312.
13. Mayyasi AM, Beals RP, Templeton AE, Hale PN Jr. The effects of ambient illumination and contrast on dynamic visual acuity. *A J Optom.* 1971;48(10):844–848.

14. Lit A, Finn JP, Vicars WM. Effect of target-background luminance contrast on binocular depth discrimination at photopic levels of illumination. *Vision Res.* 1972:12(7):1241–1251.
15. Rucker L. Let there be light—but where should it be? *Bull Coll of Dent Surg.* 1996;14:13.
16. Rucker, LM, ed. Surgical Magnification Web Site. Surgical Telescope Evaluation Program. http://www.interchg.ubc.ca/lrucker/step/welcome.htm; 1996.

Chapter 9

Posture for Dental Hygiene Practice

Patricia J. Nunn, RDH, MS

Abstract

This chapter is designed to help dental hygienists develop a greater understanding of the cumulative trauma disorders (CTDs) which have been noted as frequently occurring occupational hazards of dental hygiene practice. The purpose of this section is to create as awareness of cumulative trauma injuries and to provide practical suggestions for improving faulty postural habits associated with CTDs to help prevent or reduce the incidence of work related musculoskeletal disorders in indivduals who provide peridonal debridement.

Introduction

Dental hygiene practice frequently requires maintaining the same working postures and using repetitive actions involving the shoulder, forearm, wrist, and hand for extended periods of time. The human body was not designed to engage in repetitive motions for extended periods of time, especially while maintaining the same body position, and most particularly if not in an ideal postural stance. Two broad categories of posture-related musculoskeletal problems arise from patient treatment requirements: back and neck pain and cumulative trauma disorders of the hand and wrist. Hygienists must begin to pay as close attention to their own physical needs as they do to the needs of the patients they serve.

Oberg and Oberg studied dental hygienists in Sweden and found 80% of dental hygienists complained of pain in the upper body and back.[1] A 1980 study of Hawaiian dental hygienists showed that 44% experienced back pain, 33% encountered nonspecific muscle aches, and 28% complained of neck

217

aches.[2] In a 1984 study of 841 dental hygienists who graduated in 1982 by Boyer, Elton, and Preston, it was noted that
the most frequently experienced health problems were primarily associated with the back and neck, followed by the
hand and wrist.[2] The cost of cumulative trauma disorders is
tremendous both for the injured dental hygienist and for the
employer. The average annual treatment cost for on-the-job
disabling back injuries is about $27,000 per injured person.[3]
The costs cited do not include money lost by decreased productivity, by lack of ability to generate income, and by myriad
other factors associated with the inability to work.

Most of what we are learning about prevention of cumulative trauma disorders in dental hygiene practice is only now
beginning to be addressed in dental hygiene literature. Previously, few texts addressed the problem of preventing cumulative trauma disorder in dental hygiene practice. Some texts
have addressed preventing cumulative trauma disorder to a
minimal degree and have provided a few practical approaches
to prevention. The topic has been addressed thoroughly in
medical literature, however, and some facts are known about
the ways to treat and prevent cumulative trauma disorders.
Cumulative trauma disorders are often associated with dental hygiene practice habits and many can be prevented by good
postural practices. Many hygienists educated several or many
years ago often have to think hard about instrumentation habits because the ways they were taught to carry out dental hygiene procedures were not always what is best for posture.
The goal now is to incorporate what is known to satisfy two
basic requirements:
1. patient therapy objectives will be accomplished, and
2. the accomplishment of treatment objectives will not hurt
   either patient or operator.[4]
The Occupational Safety and Health Administration
(OSHA) enumerates four signal risk factors for ergonomics-
related injury:
1. repetitive motion for more than 2 hours at a time;
2. awkward postures for longer than 2 hours at a time;
3. unassisted frequent manual handling; and
4. unassisted forceful manual handling.[3]
Dental hygiene practice routinely meets at least three of
the four factors (numbers 1, 2, and 4). For example, providing

therapeutic periodontal debridement, the clinician must assume postures that will allow access to the area of treatment. These positions may cause the dental hygienist to compromise his or her own posture for the sake of visualization or access to the treatment site (signal risk factor 2). Additionally, the use of hand instruments in areas of significant calculus or for root planing require numerous repetitive (signal risk factor 1) and often forceful motions (signal risk factor 4) to render the patient treatment site biologically acceptable. Therefore it becomes necessary for both the dental hygienist and the dentist employer to determine and carry out ways to offset the potential for injury.

Dental hygienists must make a commitment to acquire education on basic ergonomic information and proper medical management if affected. Fragala stated in "Prevention of Back Injuries: New Directions for Training" that sitting causes more disc "loading" (application of weight or force along the long axis of the body) than either standing or walking.[5] It is no wonder that the hygienist is exhausted from a day of sitting to do his or her work, especially if sitting on an improperly designed stool at a poorly planned work station. It is critical that the dental hygienist understand the theoretical principles of good ergonomic practice. Once one grasps the principles, ways to implement the theory into each person's own dental hygiene practice can be determined. Job redesign and job rotation are two very concrete ways that the hygienist can have an impact on his or her health and comfort. Ergonomically sound engineering controls, including provision of adjustable work stations, may provide another way to relieve some of the problems associated with practice.

Operator Posture

One of the key factors in maintaining musculoskeletal health is maintaining the body's neutral position. Neutral position can be defined as the position of an appendage which is neither moved away from nor directed toward the body's midline, nor laterally turned or twisted.[6] One can determine individual neutral position (comfort zone) of the back through the following steps:

1. Sit tall in a chair with weight evenly distributed; legs should be separated with feet flat on floor.
2. Tighten stomach muscles to flatten back against the chair back.
3. Let the hips slide slightly forward on the stool as you rotate the topmost portion of your pelvis in a backward motion (like a cat arching its back).
4. Let the topmost portion of the pelvis rotate forward until the abdomen is pushing out; allow the back to lift away from the chair back.
5. About midway between the two positions is the location that is most comfortable—the neutral position (see Figure 1).

Neutral position should be maintained as much as possible throughout daily activities. A good way to remember is to pretend that there is a steel pole going from one hip through to the other with each end bolted to the chair. This will only allow rotation of the pelvis forward and backward from the hips. Think of vertebrae as neatly stacked into neutral position and make every effort to avoid bending or twisting to see. To get closer to the area of operation, rotate closer or further away while maintaining the neutral position. Do not forget the steel rod connecting the hips, and allow muscles to work to hold the pelvis in neutral position.

A few "rules" that will help the practitioner maintain optimum position when seated on an operator stool include body position on the stool, having the stool at the correct height for the operator, securing lumbar support, and being aware of and using engineering controls to enhance posture.[7]

Center body weight on the stool with the back in neutral position and the shoulders relaxed. Do not perch precipitously on the front edge of the stool. Many clinicians have had the stool shoot out from behind and suddenly found themselves seated securely—on the floor.

The stool should be at the correct height for the individual operator. You can determine the correct height by sitting with the buttocks as far back in the chair as possible with the knees even with or very slightly below the level of the hips. This allows weight to be evenly distributed over the back of the thighs. Legs should be abducted (drawn away from the axis

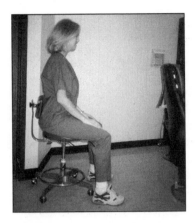

FIGURE 1.—Neutral wrist posture.

or median plane) and slightly rotated in an outward direction, enough so that the legs are to the sides of the stool and forming a tripod (Figure 2). Feet should be firmly on the ground, although not necessarily always flat on the ground. Foot position can and should be varied to give different back muscles a rest every so often. One foot can be placed on the rung of the stool or propped on the rheostat or even a foot rest. After a while, alternate by putting up the opposite foot and placing the "rested" foot solidly on the floor. Then alternate yet again by having both feet flat on the floor. The process could be repeated throughout the appointment and throughout the work day. One foot should always be flat on the floor, though, to maintain stability (see Figure 2).

It is acceptable and often best not to keep one's legs underneath the patient's chair. Many chair backs and/or operators are simply not built to accommodate one another. When the chair back is raised enough to get the legs under the chair, the operator is often forced to elevate the shoulders to be in an effective position for the desired procedure. Elevated shoulders put strain not only on the shoulder muscles and joints, but also on the arms, back, and neck.

Adjust the stool's back rest to provide lumbar support. Lumbar support assists back muscles by maintaining the spine in its normal, natural position.[7] If a stool cannot furnish the necessary support, a pillow, cushion, back rest, or even a rolled-up

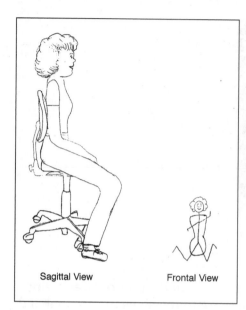

FIGURE 2.—Neutral sitting position.

Sagittal View   Frontal View

towel, can be used to fit the natural lordotic curve ("small of the back"). It may be a wise investment for a clinician to purchase his or her own stool if the one available is not the best for the individual body type. Manufacturers are becoming more aware of ergonomic concerns, and as time progresses, more engineering controls, such as armrests, stools that are more easily adjustable for height, lumbar and arm support, and other elements of a well-designed work station should become more readily available. Clinicians and their employers should watch for and consider these new advances as they come onto the market.

While you are at work, your shoulders should be consciously relaxed any time tension can be felt. It is important that the clinician pay attention to the body. It is ever so easy to become so engrossed in the procedures at hand that the twinges and other messages from the muscles are ignored until true pain is experienced. The elevated shoulder is possibly one of the most common posture errors dental hygienists make while providing patient care. To help maintain the shoulders in a relaxed position, the elbows should be approximately even with the occlusal plane of the instrumentation area.[7] The patient chair height for work on the maxillary posterior teeth may be slightly different from that needed for work on the mandibular. Also, working on a large, tall adult generally requires a different patient chair height than would be indicated for a small, short person.

The clinician should have the patient in proper position so that visualization can be attained without having to bend the neck. This will be discussed further in the section on patient positioning; the point here is that one must be able to see adequately in order to provide patient care. The ideal distance between patient and operator's eyes is 14 to 16 inches. At this distance, with normal vision, the operator should be easily able to visualize the area of operation by asking the patient to appropriately vary his or her head position. The clinician should have routine eye examinations and make sure that the eye care professional is aware of occupational needs. The area in which most dental hygiene procedures are carried out is considered to be "middle distance," so it may be necessary for vision correction to be adjusted accordingly. An option for enhancing vision may be the use of magnification systems. Surgical magnification systems provide the capability of seeing detail without getting physically closer to the treatment field and thus decrease the possibility of compromised posture.

Some other operator considerations in improving postural comfort include placing the cart or bracket tray and light to allow easy access from the operator's position with a minimum of turning, bending, and reaching. Remember to maintain shoulders in a neutral, relaxed position at all times. Remain conscious of optimum operator-patient positioning throughout a procedure. Do not cross the legs. Take a break every 30 to 60 minutes by standing up and doing gentle back bends, stretching, and walking around a little. It is probably a good idea not to work in the same position for longer than 1 hour. Remember the patient's back, too, by allowing the patient 5-minute breaks following each 60 minutes of active treatment—even lying down can be posturally stressful.

Patient Positioning

The operator's posture is critical in maintaining his or her musculoskeletal well-being, but equally important is the position of the patient while clinical procedures are accomplished. With the patient position incorrectly established, such as the chin up instead of down, or the head being turned away from the clinician when it should be turned toward the clinician, the clinician, who is focusing intently on the area of concern, inadvertently adjusts his or her own posture to support visualization of the field. That inadvertent posture adjustment may then place the clinician in a position that can be detrimental.

Mandibular instrumentation can generally best be accomplished by lowering the patient's chair back into the semisupine position (somewhat upright from a true supine position). The chair base should be lowered or raised until the patient's mandibular occlusal plane is parallel to the operator's elbows. The chair should not be raised to allow placement of legs under chair back if they do not fit with the patient at the appropriate height for operator. Be certain shoulders are relaxed when checking elbow height. The patient should be asked to lower the chin, and/or to turn to the appropriate side for optimum visualization. Generally, for posterior instrumentation of the buccal in quadrants 1 and 4, or the lingual surfaces of quadrants 2 and 3, the patient's head should be turned away from the operator to the degree where visualization is possible. For posterior instrumentation of the lingual of quadrants 1 and 4 or the buccals of quadrants 2 and 3, the patient's head generally should be turned toward the operator. The light should be directed straight down over area of instrumentation and adjusted directionally to optimally illuminate the instrumentation area. The light may come from the patient's left, right, or in the center, but regardless of the direction it emanates from, it is aimed straight down onto the mandible. The chin and light are down for the bottom (mandibular) arch.

For maxillary instrumentation, the patient should be lowered into true supine position (a more horizontal position than for mandibular). The chair base is lowered or raised until the patient's maxillary occlusal plane is parallel to operator's elbows with shoulders relaxed. Again, one should not attempt to raise the chair to allow placement of legs under chair back if they do not fit when the patient is at an appropriate height for operator. The patient should be asked to *raise* the chin and/or to turn to the appropriate side for optimum visualization. The light is directed down over the patient's chest, then up toward the area of instrumentation, and adjusted to optimally illuminate the area (from the patient's left, right, or center). The chin and light are down for the top (maxillary) arch.

Regardless of which arch the area of instrumentation is in, optimum operator positioning should be maintained throughout the procedure. The neutral spine position should be determined and maintained throughout patient treatment. When it is necessary, moving forward should be done by rotating from the hip. One should absolutely *not* bend or arch the spine, and *not* twist the torso or lean laterally. The patient's head usually is capable of turning toward one side or the other, and most patients can lift the chin up and down. The clinician should not hesitate to ask the patient to make head position adjustments.

Hand and Wrist Posture

Carpal tunnel syndrome and other cumulative trauma disorders are more frequently being mentioned as occupational hazards of dental hygiene practice. Carpal tunnel syndrome seems to be the most common neuropathy, but other repetitive stress disorders associated with dental hygiene practice may be associated with practice habits and may be prevented by good wrist posture practices. Ganglionic cyst, trigger finger, trigger thumb, tendonitis, tennis or golfers elbow, and several other conditions[9] (see Table 1) are just some examples that testify to the fact that ergonomic principles *must* be applied to the practice of dental hygiene and to dentistry.

Wrist-related occupational disorders are predisposed by many factors. The most important of these factors is ergonomically related to forceful and repetitive small movements. Most of what has been discovered about dental hygiene and repetitive stress, like other postural issues, is only now gaining attention in dental hygiene literature.[10-19] This topic, however, has been addressed thoroughly in medical literature, and some facts known about the process and about ways to treat and prevent carpal tunnel syndrome[6, 20-25] can be extrapolated to dental hygiene practice. Dental hygienists should learn the basics of safe wrist posture and evaluate their instrumentation habits.

The wrist joint between the hand and the arm contains many tendons that connect forearm muscles to fingers and thumb. The extensor tendons that straighten the fingers are on the dorsal side (back) of the wrist. The flexor tendons decrease the angle between two adjoining bones (e.g., bending the elbow decreases the angle between the humerus and the ulna) and which are used to bend the fingers are on the volar (palmer or front side) of the wrist. These tendons pass under ligaments to prevent them from springing away from wrist. The gap between the ligaments at the front of the wrist is known as the carpal tunnel. Passing through the carpal tunnel are the arteries and nerves supplying the hand and wrist. The median nerve, which innervates the palm and radial sides of the hand (thumb side) is the most important nerve that passes through the tunnel (see Figure 3).

A predominant cause of repetitive strain injuries is constant flexion and extension motions of the wrist. Chronic, repetitive movements of the hand or wrist, especially with the hand in "pinch" position, seem to be the most detrimental. The "pinch" position is attained as the thumb, index, and middle fingers are tensed together creating tension in the hypothenar eminence (the fleshy elevation on the ulnar side of the palm). Poor wrist positioning and incorrect hand posture in the performance of instrumentation techniques compound the problem. Poor wrist posture can cause compression of the median nerve. Other common contributors to repetitive strain injuries include movements in which the wrist is caused to digress from the neutral, straight position (e.g., lateral deviation from neutral); working for too long a period without allowing respite for the wrist; frequent repetitive wrist and forearm motion, including "pulling" motions; use of the wrist and hand in awkward positions; mechanical stresses to digital nerves from sustained grasps or serrated handles and contact with the handle on the radial aspect of the index finger; and use of vibratory instruments, especially small hand tools such as ultrasonic or sonic scalers.[6,21-24] Some of the contributory factors, while effective for dental hygienist tasks, can constrict

Table 1.—Cumulative Trauma Disorders or Injuries That May Be Triggered or Aggravated by Poor Dental Hygiene Postural Practice Habits

Condition	Possible Cause
Biceptal Tenovitis	working with the elbow too high in relation to the shoulder
Carpal Tunnel Syndrome	repeated wrist flexion, especially with fingers in pinch position
Cubital Tunnel Syndrome, aka: Ulnar Neuropathy	using an excessive amount of wrist action, especially using repetitive motions of lower arm
DeQuervain's Disease, aka: DeQuervain's Tenosynovitis	deviation of the wrist involving radial or inward hand motion and firm grips
Raynaud's Syndrome, aka: Vibration White Finger Disease	one cause is use of vibratory tools
Rotary Cuff Irritation	working with the elbow too high in relation to the shoulder
Tendonitis	repeated abduction of a body member (movement away from midline or the member to which it is attached—one of the more common shoulder joint diseases
Tennis Elbow, aka: Golfer's Elbow, aka: Lateral Epicondylitis	tendonitis in elbow region following effort requiring palm-upward hand motion against resistance, especially with an inward twist of the forearm
Tenosynovitis of the wrist	extreme wrist deviation from side to side (lateral deviation)

Table 1.—*Continued*

Thoracic Outlet Syndrome	nerve compression disorder resulting from working with the elbow higher than the shoulder
Trigger Finger, aka: Tenosynovitis of the Finger	any finger, except the thumb, is frequently flexed against resistance

References: "Cumulative Trauma Disorders," *National Safety News*, March 1994. Dr. Ghazi Ryan, Board Certified Orthopedics and Hand, Fall 1995.

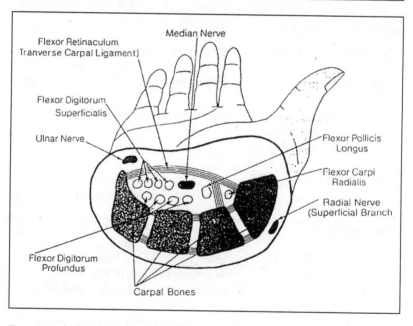

FIGURE 3.—The carpal tunnel.

the median nerve and the entire musculoskeletal components of the hand, wrist, and forearm for long periods of time.

Carpal tunnel syndrome in particular seems to be more common in the following individuals:

1. pregnant women;
2. women who have just begun to take birth control pills;

3. women who have premenstrual syndrome;
4. middle-aged women; and
5. men and women who suffer from rheumatoid arthritis, myxedema (advanced hypothyroidism), or acromegaly (abnormal enlargement of extremities of the skeleton caused by hypersecretion of growth hormone [GH] from the pituitary gland).

Anything basically that can cause an increase in the contents of the carpal tunnel (e.g., generalized edema resulting from fluid retention) puts one at risk. Also, in a study reported in the *American Journal of Physical Medicine and Rehabilitation,* Patrick Radecki states that carpal tunnel syndrome also seems to be related to a gender specific wrist ratio. He found that women whose wrist ratio (the proportion between wrist depth and width) is high are more likely to experience carpal tunnel syndrome.[23] The American Dental Hygienists' Association reports that in 1994–1995, females comprised a total of 98.1% of all program graduates. Since most dental hygienists are women, this may be a relevant risk factor.

Evidence is available that points to a strong relationship between wrist positioning during work and the onset of cumulative trauma injury—caused singly in combination by three factors:

1. Poor wrist posture while working or just plain swelling that involves the wrist can result in an inability of the median nerve to get oxygen and nutrients from its blood supply. Lack of blood supply results from constriction of the tendons and muscles where they pass into the hand via a gap (the carpal tunnel) under a ligament at front of the wrist. The contents of the carpal tunnel, the median nerve and blood vessels, can be thought of like a water hose that is bent and compressed together to stop the water flow. The same basic effect occurs when the carpal tunnel is bent and compressed onto the median nerve and blood vessels passing through the tunnel. Isometric contractions of the musculature *around* and *in* the tunnel cause increased pressure within the tunnel itself. Sustained isometric contractions of these muscles will not allow normal venous pumping to occur; thus, local edema of low oxygen and nutrient value occurs.

2. Working with the instruments with poor wrist positioning and executing repetitive motions can cause blows or tendon friction that bruise a nerve.

3. A small space in the carpal tunnel (the wrist ratio) is a factor in cumulative trauma injury.

While nothing can be done about skeletal size or sex, if risk factors fit, one needs to be especially aware of things that *can* be controlled and do what can be done to lessen the possibility of cumulative trauma disorders. Just because the hygienist has a smaller wrist ratio does not mean that he or she is immune from carpal tunnel syndrome. The bad news is that all dental hygiene practitioners are at risk just because of the type of wrist usage necessary to perform the tasks of dental hygiene. The good news is that, regardless of the demands of the profession, steps can be taken to minimize the risk of cumulative wrist trauma.

Periodontal treatment modalities create a need for repetitive motions during therapy in order for patient treatment goals to be met. After the dental hygienist becomes aware that what is done to the wrist during a workday can have a direct impact on how healthy a wrist or hand will be, he or she should make every effort to adapt work techniques to a more wrist-safe method. Just paying attention and watching what is done and making adjustments when one realizes that ergonomic principles are not being followed can go a long way toward working comfortably and safely.

Some basic and simple procedures can be incorporated into the normal periodontal debridement procedures. Maintain the wrist in normal, neutral position as much and as often as possible to keep the carpal tunnel open so nerves and blood vessels have open access. Wrist motion should not exceed a functional optimum of 10 degrees flexion to 35 degrees extension, measured from the radius to the second metacarpal just below the index finger (see Figure 4). Rest the forearms whenever possible. Never bend the wrist severely forward, flex it backward, or use ulnar or radial deviation (side-to-side motion). Avoid long periods of flexed or extended positions.

It is probably in the best interests of wrist and hand health to extremely limit use of digital motions. The best motion for hand instrument activation seems to be a rotating motion using a secure, hard-tissue fulcrum and moving the entire hand, wrist, and forearm as a unit to supply the necessary movement. Use the little finger extensor on the back side of the hand to balance the hand. When the instrument is held with the little finger down against the ring finger and in against the rest of the hand, the hypothenar eminence is tight, which helps to stabilize the hand by contracting all the little muscles under the little finger. Unfortunately, having the little finger in this position raises the pressure in the palm and carpal tunnel by isometric contraction. By tightening up the extensor instead of the hypothenar eminence, we also stabilize that side of the hand, but since this muscle runs along the back of the hand and not through the palm, it will *not* increase pressure in the palm or carpal tunnel. So let that little finger go!

Leverage is crucial! The greater the leverage is, the less force is needed to do the job effectively. Use a stable, hard-tissue fulcrum as close to the resistance (the instrument cutting edge) as possible.

Use a slow, deliberate, applied force in a directed manner, allowing relaxation between strokes rather than a rapid series

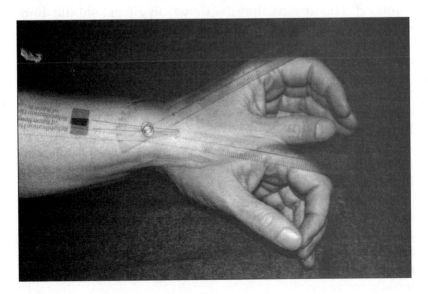

FIGURE 4.—Flexion range for optimum wrist function.

of strokes with increasingly more pinch force. Instrumentation techniques have been developed to reduce the need for quick repetitive motions. Fast motion can be thought of as mobility whereas, the ability to maintain control over a motion can be thought of as stability. In order to have increasing levels of mobility, one must have increasing levels of stability to maintain control. If one simply keeps on going faster and faster and faster, control of that sharp instrument becomes more difficult. This means that while the hand is moving quickly, it is also necessary to tense the arm and hand to maintain the stability necessary to control motion Just a 10% increase in speed at which a person is working causes a 32% increase in the pinch force (isometric contraction) necessary to maintain control.[20]

Sharp instruments are probably one of the wisest time investments that the dental hygienist can make for effecting adequate instrumentation without the need for repetitive motions. With sharp instruments, one needs fewer, less forceful, less tension-producing motions to be effective.

Use definitive, deliberate, directed instrumentation techniques. A study by Atwood and Michalak noted that human tendons can take relatively few finger manipulations per minute.[10] This means that the dental hygienist should find some ways to allow the affected muscles to relax regularly. This can very easily be accomplished by only tensing muscles during a working stroke that actually removes a deposit.

The acronym PAARR is a good way to remember the steps that will allow those minuscule breaks for the muscles by providing intermittent contraction and relaxation of the muscles. Place the curette subgingivally using only light pressure; Angulate the instrument to the appropriate angle; Adapt the toe third of the cutting edge to the tooth; Remove by tightening the fulcrum (on a hard-tissue surface), pressing the adapted cutting edge against the tooth surface, and activating the working stroke; and, as soon as the stroke is completed, immediately Relax the grasp. Only the removal portion of instrumentation requires tightened muscle tension. It is critical to relax the grasp between each working stroke to allow a degree of muscle recovery.

To provide additional muscular rest, the dental hygienist should get into the habit of taking periodic breaks, alternating tasks, and stopping at times during instrumentation to exercise the hands and fingers. Mix tasks by alternating appointments for patients with more difficult treatment needs with those who have less rigorous needs, and by alternating treatment procedures. Flexing the hand and stretching the fingers are easy and unobtrusive ways to exercise while working. Stretching can be accomplished by simply opening the fingers wide. This finger stretching can even be done as the hygienist reaches for the next instrument. Another beneficial exercise is to gently rotate the wrist in small circles. A caution should be noted: the hand(s) should be kept above the level of the heart. Often, one's first instinct is to shake the hands or exercise the hands in a downward position; however, the need is for excess of blood to temporarily leave the vessels in the carpal tunnel and go back to the heart, not for more blood to come to the wrist.

Mechanical devices should be used with care to prevent wrist trauma. The use of sonic and ultrasonic scalers and use of slow speed handpieces have be rethought from functional standpoints. Ultrasonic and sonic instrumentation seem to be the new standard of care for most periodontal patients. These types of instrumentation can be a curse and a blessing in relation to cumulative wrist trauma. The best way to optimize performance and minimize risk when using vibratory instruments, scalers, or handpieces, is to remember to maintain the neutral wrist and light grasp and to pinch less during use.

Ergonomic instrument design may help in the quest to reduce cumulative trauma disorders in two basic ways. Less muscle tension is required to place, angulate and adapt, or just to hold lighter instruments. The biggest area for improvement in instrument design may be instrument handles; handles with the largest possible diameters will allow application of force through different joints of the same finger. Instruments are becoming available that allow both these principles to be applied to some degree, but further adaptation requires additional research. The instrument of tomorrow may only vaguely resemble the instrument of today.

Gloves also can contribute to cumulative trauma disorders. Most literature pertaining to glove use states that gloves should fit well. Unfortunately, what constitutes a good fit is often left to the reader. Fortunately, the best way to tell whether gloves do fit well is fairly simple. The gloves should fit the hand and fingers snugly. They should *not*, however, fit tightly across the wrist or the forearm nearest the wrist, especially on the palmer aspect of the hand (see Figure 5). A tight fit squeezes the carpal tunnel and the nerve inside it. There should be enough glove at the wrist that the latex wrinkles at the wrist. Some gloves are advertised as wrist friendly, but the best way to provide a wrist-safe fit is just to try on different brands.

There is a good possibility that some dental hygienists leave the practice of their profession because of musculoskeletal pain and injury that could have possibly been avoided by sound ergonomic practice. One way for members of the oral health care team to increased the likelihood of having long and comfortable careers is through education and sound work practices that may help reduce or even eliminate musculoskeletal pain. The practitioner should make every effort to use good ergonomic principles, to control the work environment, to avoid

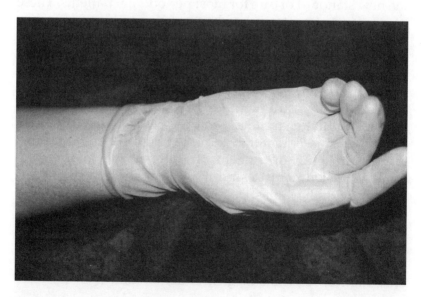

FIGURE 5.—A correctly fitting glove.

repetitive stressful motions of all parts of the musculoskeletal system, and to change poor habits as they are noticed.

REFERENCES

1. Oberg T, Oberg U. Musculoskeletal complaints in dental hygiene: a survey study from a Swedish country. *Journal of Dental Hygiene*. 1993:67.
2. Boyer EM, Elton J, Preston K. Precautionary procedures: use in dental hygiene practice. *Dental Hygiene*. 1986;60:516–523.
3. Ergonomics—is OSHAs blueprint too hot to handle? *Occupational Hazards*. 1995;57(4):35–38.
4. Nunn PJ, Nunn TD. Perfect posture. *RDH*. 1993;13(9).
5. Fragala G. Prevention of back injuries: new directions for training. *Occupational Hazards*. 1993;56(12).
6. Armstrong TJ. *Ergonomics Guides*. American Industrial Hygiene Association; 1983.
7. Nield-Gehrig JS, Houseman, GA. *Fundamentals of Periodontal Instrumentation*, 3rd ed. Baltimore: Williams & Wilkins; 1996.
8. Wilkins EM. *Clinical Practice of the Dental Hygienist*, 7th ed. Baltimore: Williams & Wilkins; 1994.
9. Montante WM. Cumulative trauma disorders. *National Safety News*. 1983;November/December:46.
10. Atwood MJ, Michalak C. The occurance of cumulative trauma in dental hygienists. *Work: A Journal of Prevention, Assessment, and Rehabilitation*. 1992;2(4);17–31.
11. Bauer ME. Carpal tunnel syndrome: an occupational risk to the dental hygienist. *Dental Hygiene*. 1985;59;218–221.
12. Conrad JC, Conrad KJ, Jetzer TC. Peripheral nerve dysfunction in practicing dental hygienists. *Journal of Dental Hygiene*. 1990;October:382–387.
13. Conrad JC, Conrad KJ, Osborn JS. A short-term epidemiologic study of median nerve dysfunction in practicing dental hygienists. *Journal of Dental Hygiene*. 1992;February:76–80.
14. Conrad JC, Conrad KJ, Osborn JS. Median nerve dysfunction evaluated during dental hygiene education and practice (1986–1989). *Journal of Dental Hygiene*. 1991;July–August:283–288.
15. Gerwatowski LJ, McFall DB, Stach DJ. Carpal tunnel syndrome: risk factors and preventive strategies for the dental hygienist. *Journal of Dental Hygiene*. 1992;February:89–94.
16. MacDonald G, Robertson MM, Erickson JA. Carpal tunnel syndrome among California dental hygienists. *Dental Hygiene*. 1988;July/August:322–329.

17. MacDonald G. Hazards in the dental workplace. *Dental Hygiene.* 1987;May:212–218.
18. Nunn P, Hart C, Gaulden F. 'Perfect' instrumentation can be hazardous to your health, or ergonomic applications for the prevention of carpal tunnel syndrome. *Access, American Dental Hygienists' Association.* 1995;9(1):37–43.
19. Osborn JB, Newell KJ, Rudney JD, Stoltenberg JL. Carpal tunnel syndrome among Minnesota dental hygienists. *Journal of Dental Hygiene.* 1990;64(2):79–85.
20. Arndt R. Work pace, stress and cumulative trauma disorder. *Journal of Hand Surgery.* 1987:12A.
21. Beaton-Starr M. Carpal tunnel syndrome and the workplace. *Work: A Journal of Prevention, Assessment, and Rehabilitation.* 1992;2(4):61–66.
22. Brumfield RH, Chapoux JA. A biomechanical study of normal functional wrist motion. *Journal of Hand Surgery* (British and European Volume). 1984;43(3).
23. Radecki P. A gender specific wrist ratio and the likelihood of median nerve abnormality at the carpal tunnel. *American Journal of Physical Medicine and Rehabilitation.* 1994;73(3).
24. Schneck RR. Keep in touch with pain. *Safety and Health, National Safety Council.* 1988;December:39–42.
25. Su J. Industrial rehabilitation of individuals with carpal tunnel syndrome. *Work: A Journal of Prevention, Assessment, and Rehabilitation.* 1992;2(4).

Chapter 10

The Musculoskeletal Health of the Dental Care Worker

Ellen A. Kolber, MS, MA, OTR, CHT

Abstract

This chapter focuses on the primary prevention of musculoskeletal injuries specific to dental work. There is significant evidence that the practice of dentistry includes exposure to numerous risk factors associated with injury. Limiting exposure through ergonomic intervention offers considerable reduction of these factors. Issues related to the physical status and work style of the individual are also likely to have a major effect on the health of the dental care worker. Although research has not yet provided insight related to specific attributes of these variables, it is believed that physical conditioning and overall activity level play a role in maintaining the health of soft-tissue structures. It is also accepted that the use of various postures increases risk and that implementation of neutral and aligned postures reduces risk. Postures employed during dental tasks relate both to the configuration of the office and to basic movement habits learned by the dental worker. Modifying these patterns requires consideration of specific structural components of the body, as well as analysis of the specific motions employed during work tasks and activities of daily living. This chapter focuses on theoretical and practical issues related to the physical condition, postural components, and work style issues relevant to the dental office.

Introduction

Primary prevention measures in the dental office address the reduction of prepathogenic disease conditions; the objective is to avoid the occurrence of symptoms associated with musculoskeletal injury. Ergonomic interventions such as the acquisition of adjustable dental chairs and the initiation of regular rest breaks are examples of commonly used primary prevention strategies for reducing the risk factors associated with musculoskeletal pain. Optimum function of the body's soft-tissue structures and normal physiologic activity are maintained by not exceeding the structural limitations of the muscles, tendons, nerves, and joint structures. Once the individual begins to experience clinical symptoms, microscopic structural changes have already occurred and some degree of clinical musculoskeletal disease is present. Prognosis for recovery of musculoskeletal overuse injuries is generally considered inversely proportional to severity and length of time for which the injury has been present.[1] Therefore, the longer an individual has sustained a cycle of pain, indicative of inflammation and alteration of the normal structural components of soft tissues, the greater the degree of tissue damage and impaired physiological function. This makes a very strong case for the implementation of both primary and secondary prevention (early intervention) strategies in addressing the onset of pain and discomfort.

Given the failure to avoid prepathogenic clinical disease, secondary prevention strategies are key in limiting further structural changes and the effects of tissue damage.[2] An example of a secondary intervention measure is the attempt to modify poor postural alignment in order to improve the body's ability to deal with external forces. Early intervention efforts are aimed at the avoidance of further inflammatory tissue response and the healing and remodeling of scar tissue so that it more closely mimics the structure and function of the surrounding, uninjured tissue.[3] The healing process of the affected tissue, stated simply, includes the resolution of inflammation and a laying down of viable collagen fibers, sometimes referred to as scar tissue or adhesion formation. Unless healing occurs in the acute and subacute stages (less than 3 months) and further reinjury is avoided, a progression of the condition often ensues. Chronic disease involves an unfortunate cyclic pattern of further inflammation and reinjury. Events include the ongoing occurrence of microruptures, inflammatory tissue response, and the continuous formation of painful adhesions that leave the individual more vulnerable to reinjury.[4,5]

Once consistent and moderate pain is present, significant tissue changes are likely to have already occurred. In addition to a decline in the dental worker's feeling of general health and wellness, subsequent decreases in productivity levels may occur. Tertiary prevention strategies are implemented to avoid an ongoing disease process. Chronic disease consists of continued progression of the disease and reinjury and further deterioration of the individual's functional status within the dental environment and in the performance of activities of daily living. Rehabilitation goals addressed by physical and occupational therapists include scar and tissue remodeling and maintenance of functional and productivity levels. Table 1 outlines the levels of prevention according to the stage of the injury and recommended interventions for dealing with the disease in the various stages.

The etiology of musculoskeletal overuse injuries is multifactorial, meaning that the presence of more than one risk factor and perhaps the interaction of several factors greatly enhances risk of injury. Preventive approaches are aimed at reducing exposure to risk factors associated with musculoskeletal pain and are specific to the individual and the individual's environment. Risk factors associated with work-related musculoskeletal injuries include the use of repetitive motions, forceful exertions, awkward and extreme positions, confined and static postures, vibration, cold temperatures, mechanical stresses imposed by an external object, and an imbalance between work and rest.[7-9] A number of these factors are clearly operative in the workplace of dental care practitioners.

In addition to environmental and postural factors, numerous personal attributes have been associated with the onset of musculoskeletal pain. These include insufficient strength, physical deconditioning, the presence of fixed postural malalignment, relative inexperience on the job, inefficient work habits and techniques, vitamin deficiencies, inadequate wrist size and shape, other anthropometric (size) dimensions of the worker, history of previous injury, presence of systemic disease, congenital abnormalities, heredity, and gender.[7,10-12] This chapter will discuss primary prevention strategies relevant to fitness, posture, work style, and lifestyle of the dental care worker. This information is offered as an adjunct to the implementation of an ergonomic program, not as an alternative.

Table 1.— Levels of Prevention and Stages of Musculoskeletal Injury*

Level of Prevention	Symptoms	Symptom Relief	Recommendations
Primary	Fatigue or mild discomfort in one site following performance of dental tasks.	Following rest and time away from work.	Include breaks & stretches. Work in neutral postures. Seek ergonomic advice. Pace yourself. Pay attention to pain and fatigue. Limit & alternate activity.
Secondary first stage of injury	Pain, feeling of stiffness, or mild sensory symptoms in one site during or following the performance of dental tasks.	Following rest, stretches, & focused effort. Responsive to OT and PT & ergonomic changes.	See above recommendations. Increase frequency of breaks & stretches. Seek medical attention. Consider avocational hand use.

Table 1.— *Continued*

Level of Prevention	Symptoms	Symptom Relief	Recommendations
Tertiary			
second stage of injury	Symptoms in several sites during or following performance of dental tasks.	Only after consistent rest & modified activity; easily reinjured.	See above recommendations. Seek OT & PT & intervention. Seek alternate means of performing activities of daily living. Consider judicious use of splints.
third stage of injury	Symptoms described above & loss of function, during or following performance of dental tasks and after rest. May affect sleep.	May occur infrequently. Surgery may be required.	May need to significantly curtail hand-intensive work & leisure activities.
fourth stage of injury	Symptoms from even minor manual activity, may have signs of tenderness, weakness & loss of control.		
fifth stage of injury	Loss of capacity for use as a result of continuous pain, sensory symptoms, numbness and weakness.		

*Based on Fry's levels of injury derived from clinical symptoms[6]

The dental care worker who has consistent pain and discomfort should seek the advise of a physician.

Physical Conditioning of the Dental Care Worker

Physical conditioning objectives for the dental care worker involve a consideration of the specific physical requirements of this work, as well as the needs and goals of the individual dental care worker. A job analysis of dental work reveals the presence of a number of physical factors that increase the risk of sustaining a musculoskeletal injury. Training programs for athletes frequently match training activities with specific performance needs. Creating a conditioning program that includes components of the job, however, would likely further expose the dental worker to known risk factors and would therefore be counterproductive. It is recommended that the dental worker's conditioning program address issues inherent in the physical demands of dental work from the perspective of minimizing certain imbalances that are present in dental work. For example, there is a significant muscle activity imbalance between the large muscle groups, which are relatively inactive, and the smaller muscles of the arms and hands, which are engaged in constant and often repetitive motions. The larger muscle groups are responsible for cardiorespiratory health and overall endurance. Because they are relatively inactive, except to perform static holding contractions, the overall effect of the work is sedentary. Simultaneously, extreme metabolic and functional demands are placed on the smaller muscles of the arms and hands. If the largely sedentary activity of dental work is not balanced by less sedentary activity, over time the individual is likely to incur levels of deconditioning and poor physical fitness which will not support healthy, pain-free function of the forearms, hands, and fingers.

There is evidence in the literature that poor physical conditioning increases the risk of injury. An association between poor physical condition and the development of musculoskeletal pain has been suggested in Australian literature studying computer keyboard users. No direct causal relationship, however, has been demonstrated between levels of deconditioning and incidence of work-related musculoskeletal injuries.[11] Research as to whether exercise can actually decrease risk of injury in workers is inconclusive. Recommendations for specific exercises and exercise levels specific to the prevention of work-related musculoskeletal pain remain similarly unclear. Silverstein cites several studies in which on-the-job exercise programs were found to be effective in reducing fatigue and absenteeism, reducing hand and wrist disorders, and increasing blood flow.[13] However, the results of her study reveal that after 1 year of worker involvement in an on-job exercise program, which included stretches and strengthening and relaxation exercises, there were no statistically significant differences in discomfort levels based on participation. Possible explanations suggested by the authors include study length inadequate to realize the benefits of the exercise; increasing work productivity demands which may have overshadowed the benefits of exercise; and length, variety, and type of exercise that did not adequately address the physical demands of the job. It is notable that no cardiorespiratory exercises were included as part of this program.

The Components of Fitness
The four components of physical fitness are
- cardiorespiratory endurance,
- muscular fitness,
- flexibility, and
- body mass index.

Acceptable levels in all areas are seen as necessary for the individual to be considered physically fit and able to tolerate the stresses and demands of a long work day as well as daily life activities.[14]

The American College of Sports Medicine (ACSM) recommends that before beginning any exercise program, men over 40 and women over 50 years of age, as well as anyone who is considered to be at high risk for coronary artery disease, should have a full medical examination.[15,16] ACSM guidelines state that a medical examination might not be necessary if moderate (as opposed to strenuous) exercise is undertaken gradually.[16] *The American College of Sports Medicine Fitness Book,* edited by W. Larry Kenney, is an excellent basic reference for the beginner, providing specific information on methods of evaluating yourself and exercises in all areas of fitness.[17]

Cardiorespiratory fitness is the sustained ability of the heart and blood vessels to transport oxygen from the lungs to the body's tissues. Efficient cardiac muscle function facilitates transport of blood flow to all organs and systems of the body. Blood flow assists with oxygen transport, nutrient supply, and removal of the by-products of muscle metabolism. Cardiovascular exercise is widely used in the treatment of soft-tissue injuries for its enhancing effect on glycogen (energy) storage and oxygen consumption.[5,18] Poole cites tissue biopsy research that reveals a relationship between excess lactic acid (which is a muscle metabolite), and glycogen depletion, and incidence of tendinitis. It is a reasonable assumption that good cardiorespiratory fitness may help maintain a more optimal environment in which muscles can perform and recover.

Muscular fitness refers to the strength and power that a muscle can generate. Although "strength" and "power" are often used interchangeably, strength is more precisely defined as the capacity of a muscle to generate maximum muscle contraction. Power is the amount of work performed, therefore associated with endurance of the muscle.[19] Strength training causes an increase in the size of myofibrils, which are the components of the muscle fiber that are responsible for the contractile properties of muscle. This process is known as muscle hypertrophy. A hypertrophied muscle can contract more efficiently and generate more force over more time and is not as susceptible to tears and fatigue. Power training produces an increase in muscle mitochondria (a source of energy) and an increase in the number of capillaries per muscle fiber, thereby increasing blood flow. In animal studies, exercise was found to have a beneficial effect on increasing the tensile strength of tendons.[20] Greater tensile strength allows more tension to be generated before the occurrence of tissue microfailure and cellular degradation. Physical activity plays a role in reducing vulnerability to tears in muscles and in tendons by increasing the ability of muscles and tendons to tolerate greater loads and to contract against external forces.

Flexibility/range of motion can be compromised as a result of functional shortening of soft-tissue structures. It can result from injury, as a response to the deposition of scar tissue and adhesion formation, which form within and between the soft-tissue structures surrounding the joints. Noninjured structures may shorten as a result of poor postures and movement patterns which place muscles and tendons in shortened positions and use only limited arcs of motion. Shortened muscles have reduced numbers of sarcomeres, the contractile portion of the muscle. This results in altered, abnormal patterns of fiber recruitment (patterns of contraction) that are less efficient and out of balance with other muscles. The outcome leads to inefficiency in terms of the generation of contractile force and ultimately changes the intricate biomechanics of the joints over which the muscles act.[21] Therefore, seemingly benign decreases in flexibility and range of motion resulting from altered biomechanics and structural changes to soft tissue may increase dental workers' predisposition to injury and pain over time.

Body mass index refers to the amount of lean mass (muscle and bone) in the body relative to the amount of adipose tissue (fat). In Green's study on computer users, there was a tendency for females who weighed more and had higher body mass indexes to suffer from musculoskeletal pain.[11] It is not known, however, whether excessive weight in dental care workers would reveal a similar trend. Nor are specific causal factors related to this finding known. In any case, increased body mass index is a significant indicator of fitness level and should be considered as part of an individual's overall physical health and status. Cardiovascular exercise is recommended when weight loss is desirable.

General Exercise Principles

A number of factors should be considered in the development of an exercise program designed to address the fitness needs and physical demands of the dental care worker. Current thinking has relaxed guidelines for how much exercise the average person needs to stay healthy. Exercise specialists suggest that moderate physical exercise be performed at a level between 70% and 85% of maximum heart rate, for session of 20 to 30 minutes, three to four times per week.[16,22] Significant evidence indicates, however, that engaging in moderate physical activity for at least 30 consecutive minutes during performance of daily activities on most days also offers significant health benefits.[15] In general, moderate exercise is now emphasized over vigorous, exhausting, painful exercise. In fact, studies show that the most common cause of injury during exercise is exercising too aggressively. Engaging in even a light exercise program is believed to have significant benefits.

In general, choice of specific exercises and programs should be geared toward general fitness goals and needs of the individual. For example, because optimal seated posture requires good function and strength of the abdominal muscles and sufficient hamstring length and flexibility, these particular muscle groups should be addressed by the dental care worker, who tends to sit for extended periods of time. As previously discussed, hand-strengthening exercises, which impose forces to the finger flexors, may be contraindicated, because they add to the cumulative exposures from dental-work tasks. Providing sufficient rest and recovery time to fatigued muscles is probably of greater overall benefit than attempting to fortify these muscles against injury by performing vigorous strengthening exercises. Exercising muscles that are fatigued from excessive work demands is not recommended. Programs should be tailored to meet the needs of each individual.

WARM-UP ACTIVITIES AND STRETCHES

Exercise sessions should begin with warm-up activities. An adequate warm-up reduces muscle and joint soreness during the early stages of an exercise program and may decrease the risk of injury.[16] Two types of warm-ups can be performed. A 5- to 10-minute full-body warm-up, such as jogging in place, raises deep-muscle temperature and should be performed before stretching and weight training to prevent injury. A second type of warm-up focuses on specific body segments that will be used in the performance of the physical activity to follow. Specific warm-ups are effective in preparing the individual physically and psychologically for activities involving skill and coordination, but are less effective in raising the temperature of postural muscles. It is recommended that the dental care worker perform a full-body warm-up prior to exercise activities and that specific warm-ups be performed prior to certain sports and work activities. The physiological effects on various soft-tissue structures, incurred as a result of the physical tasks of dental work, are likely to be similar to those that occur following exercise. It is therefore believed that performing warm-up activities before dental activities is beneficial. The performance of segmental warm-ups of the upper extremity are more feasible in the office setting than performance of full-body warm-ups. Hand warm-ups, which promote the diffusion of synovial fluid (the tendon lubricant in the hand and fingers) are shown in Figure 1.

The overall benefits of stretching and flexibility exercises are documented in the fitness and exercise physiology literature.[16,20,23] It is recommended that the dental care worker stretch before work and periodically throughout the day. Performing a full program of sustained stretches to all muscle groups in the manner suggested above may not be possible. Stretching the distal forearm; the hand and finger muscles; and the muscles of the shoulder girdle, neck, and back will increase blood flow and maintain an optimal physiological environment for function and health. It has been suggested that one criteria for the selection of exercises is whether they can be done in an inconspicuous manner in the office environment and cause minimal disruption of work performance.[24] Several methods of stretching the forearm muscles (both hands together and hands separately) are shown in

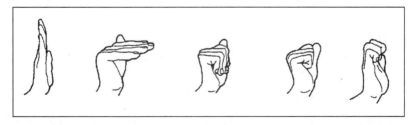

FIGURE 1.—Hand warm-ups, also called "tendon-gliding" exercises, assist in the diffusion of synovial fluid, which helps to decrease friction between tendons.

Figure 2 (a and b). The finger extensor muscle muscles are stretched when a fist is made and the wrist brought into flexion as shown in Figure 2c. The lateral neck muscles can be stretched as shown in Figure 3. The short periods of time between patient treatments can provide adequate breaks in which stretches can be performed in the office setting, throughout the day.

Holding a stretch for 30 to 60 seconds is believed to be most effective in increasing the length of soft-tissue structures. Stretches of short duration benefit muscular performance by allowing the muscles to contract more efficiently and by preparing them better to take on loads. A momentary stretch performed immediately before exercise or activity is known as a prestretch and has been demonstrated to be effective in increasing the amount of force that the contraction can produce. This phenomenon is attributed to the energy that is stored in various contractile and noncontractile components of the muscle and that can be used during the muscle contraction following the stretch. This is relevant for the dental care worker both in the performance of exercise and in the physical demands of dental work.

The benefits of performing periodic stretches throughout the day are apparent. They should be performed gently, with-

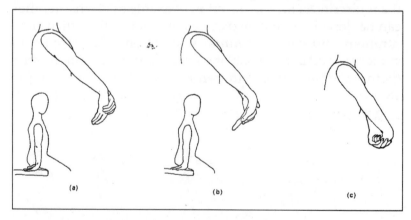

FIGURE 2.—Stretches for the forearm muscles, including two ways of stretching the wrist extensor muscles (a), two ways of stretching the wrist and finger flexor muscles (b), and one way of stretching the finger extensor muscles. The more closed the fist is in the latter stretch, the greater the stretch.

FIGURE 3.—A stretch for the lateral neck muscles. While one hand stabilizes the trunk by holding onto the seat, the other hand gently assists the stretch by pulling the head down toward the shoulder.

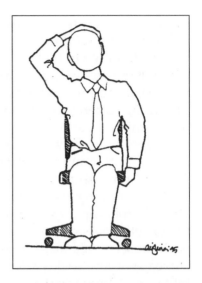

out bouncing, and should not cause pain. Pain indicates that the structural limit of the muscle tendon unit is being exceeded. Overstretching can cause tears in the restraining soft tissue and can lead to injury. Stretches of the upper extremities and neck should be performed intermittently, three to four times per day. It is recommended that sustained stretches not be performed to structures that already overstretched.[13,21] The individual who has lax or loose ligaments that allow joints to hyperextend, or attenuated muscle-tendon units, should avoid stretches that may cause further joint instability or postural imbalances. For example, an individual who has rounded, forward shoulders as shown in Figure 8 should avoid a sustained stretch to the upper back. The stretch may further exaggerate the imbalances responsible for this posture.

CARDIORESPIRATORY/ENDURANCE TRAINING AND MUSCULAR/RESISTANCE TRAINING

Resistance/power training and endurance training consisting of aerobic exercise is usually performed on alternate days. It is recommended that aerobic exercise such as running, bicycling, or swimming be the cornerstone of a fitness program. Aerobic exercise enhances cardiorespiratory endurance, the aspect of fitness that provides the greatest overall health benefits. Since dental work makes relatively little use of the musculature responsible for cardiorespiratory health, implementing aerobic exercise may be of particular benefit in the conditioning of the dental worker.

ACSM has recently included resistance (strength) training in its recommendations for a general health and fitness program.[16] Strength and power training are important for maintaining muscle mass and may help an individual function more efficiently.[15,23] The effectiveness of using strength and power training as a method of decreasing susceptibility to injury remains unclear. Although it is not known whether strength training reduces musculoskeletal vulnerability to strain in the upper extremities, a number of studies point to the effectiveness of exercise for improving endurance of the back muscles as a factor that may prevent the first-time occurrence of low back pain.[26] Literature addressing the rehabilitation of individuals recovering from injury does correlate increases in strength with diminishing risk of reinjury. Occupational therapists and physical therapists regularly include strength and power training in their rehabilitation programs for patients with overuse injuries following the acute stage of injury.[5,18]

Although findingsin the experimental research literature are scarce, there is a strong theoretical argument that supports the use of strength and power training to reduce the risk of injury and reinjury. Training yields a physiologic response within the contractile portion of the muscle that allows the muscles to generate greater contractile forces and maintain longer contractions. This stronger muscle will not have to work so hard to generate and maintain contractile force. A further rationale supporting the use of exercise as a preventive measure is that exercise increases blood flow through a stressed area.[13,27] Blood flow brings needed nutrition and oxygen and helps clear away the byproducts of muscle metabolism such as lactic acid. This creates a favorable physiologic environment in which mucles and tendons can function efficiently.

Resistance or weight-training programs often emphasize strengthening of the proximal, postural muscles of the trunk and shoulder girdle prior to strengthening of the distal extremities of the arms and legs. These proximal muscles are responsible for providing a stable foundation and base from which the hands can be efficiently engaged.[21] A limitation in strength and endurance of the upper back and shoulder muscles will limit the strength, endurance, and the function of the distal muscles, including the forearm, wrist, hand, and fingers.

Endurance and strength of the trunk muscles are particularly significant in terms of their influence on the ability to maintain upright, erect posture. When the trunk muscles are fatigued, they no longer function well to maintain upright, erect posture during standing and sitting. The result is often a tendency to slouch, causing a forward shift in body mass. This new posture is termed "kyphotic" and is characterized by backward rotation of the pelvis, reversal of the lumbar curve in a backward direction, a significant increase in the forward curvature of the thoracic midback, and subsequent forward positioning the shoulders.

This slouched posture places very high forces on the discs of the low back, as well as on restraining ligamentous structures. When fatigued muscles or poor postural habits do not support upright posture, the spinal ligaments are relied upon for this purpose. If these ligaments, which are nonelastic and unforgiving, are strained, pain is likely to result. Thus, the relationship between fitness, posture, and pain is evident.

It is recommended that neither strength nor power training be attempted when muscles or tendons are painful or moderately fatigued. It is known that even in cases of normal but sustained physiological muscular effort, evidence of early microfailure occurs in soft-tissue structures.[25] It is possible that at the end of a day of working with patients, the dental workers' hands, for example, may undergo the initial physiological effects of overuse, manifesting a feeling of fatigue or discomfort. If the tissues are allowed to rest, any cellular damage or inflammatory reaction is likely to fully resolve. However, continued exposure to the forceful activity of strenuous exercise may actually inhibit the normal tissue recovery process. It is therefore suggested that the dental care worker not perform strenuous exercise such as wrist curls or squeeze a gripper on a day when he or she has seen many patients or experiences signs of overuse in the upper extremity (discomfort, swelling, or fatigue). However, other muscles, such as those of the lower-extremity and postural muscles of the trunk, may not be as fatigued. If this is the case, then these other muscle groups can be safely engaged in a strengthening program.

There are a number of types of strengthening programs, each imposing different performance demands upon muscles, tendons, and joints. Choice of exercise method is based on the consideration of several factors. All methods are based on the overload principle which states that exercise must be of sufficient intensity, duration, and frequency to develop maximum tension and cause muscle fatigue. Muscles are hypertrophied in response to increased resistance (loads), resulting in greater strength.[18,28] Resistive concentric isotonic exercise is the most widely used method of increasing strength and can conveniently be performed at the home or office. In this type of exercise, the muscle shortens as it contracts against the force of a weight, such as a dumbbell. Progressive resistive exercises (PREs) are resistive concentric exercise in which the individual performs a total of three sets of 10 repetitions, each set with a progressively heavier weight, with each muscle group exercised. The first set (the first 10 repetitions) is performed with 50% of the maximum weight tolerated, the second set (the second 10) is performed with 75%, and the third set (the third 10) is performed at maximum resistance tolerated. In other words, the individual starts with a relatively low weight and systematically increases as the sets progress. Determining maximum resistance is a trial-and-error process. Maximum resistance must be determined at the beginning of the program and upgraded as strength gains are made. The use of cuff weights that can be fastened to extremities by straps eliminates the need to activate the muscles of the hands and forearms when further contraction of these muscle groups is not desired.

Another effective approach, known as a regressive resistive exercise (RRE), is similar to PRE but in reverse. The individual begins with 100% of the maximum resistance tolerated, then decreases to 75%, and then 50% (10 repetitions at each level, 30 repetitions total for each muscle group).[29]

Cool-Down and Stretching Activities and Flexibility Training

In addition to a warm-up performed before strengthening exercise, it is suggested that the individual also include 5 to 10 minutes of cool down, by slowly reducing the intensity of the endurance activity at the end of the workout session. This helps prevent an abrupt drop in blood pressure, which can result when blood pools in the extremities. This can cause dizziness or fainting. Cooling down also decreases risk of fatal heart arrhythmias during the immediate recovery period.

Flexibility training includes additional stretches that are intended to address specific deficits in flexibility or range of motion. Target structures may include muscels, tendons, or tight structures around a joint. It is recommended that flexibility excercises performed to elongate structures be performed after endurance training. Muscles, tendons, and ligaments are more responsive to flexibility exercises performed after training.[16] Flexibility deficits that affect the ability to assume good aligned posture will be discussed in the next section.

In summary, an effective program of daily activity includes increasing one's overall activity level; focusing on conditioning muscles that are deconditioned and not extensively used in the course of a normal day; and performance of warm-up, stretching, and cool-down activities. Maintaining motivation to sustain participation in the program is important. During the first 6 to 8 weeks of training, increased strength and power performance are mainly due to neuromuscular adaptation involving more efficient recruitment of muscle fibers during contraction. After that time, gains are attributed to the actual structural changes in muscle fibers that cause muscle hypertrophy.[20] Cross-training, in which a number of different types of physical activity are performed, has the benefits of reducing boredom and providing a variety of demands on the body. This facilitates the physiological adaptation required for cardiorespiratory and muscular fitness, flexibility, and optimal body mass composition.

Posture and Movement

Posture is a complex term used to refer to a number of movement and positioning concepts. Although poor posture is frequently cited as a significant risk factor in musculoskeletal pain, a clear definition cannot readily be found in the ergonomics literature,[30] and is not consistently used to refer to the same concept in the rehabilitation literature. Posture has been defined in a number of ways: a position or attitude of the body, the relative arrangements of body parts for a specific activity, and a characteristic manner of bearing one's body.[31] This section will define the various types of posture, describe components of optimal posture, and offer recommendations for improving postural alignment and postural habits.

Posture can be classified, in terms of the effect that a muscle contraction has on a joint or body segment, as either static or dynamic.[32] A posture is static if there is no movement, either because all the muscles around the joint are relaxed or because the antagonist muscles that oppose the action of the active muscle group are contracting with equal force and magnitude and therefore counter the forces produced by each other. Examples of static posture include standing, lying still, and attempting to squeeze a hard object. Muscles that maintain the static position are described as performing a static or isometric muscle contraction. Tasks involving static posture held for long periods of time are known to be risk factors for musculoskeletal pain.[30] In dentistry, as in other precision tasks, static muscle contraction is performed at the joints closer to the trunk (the proximal segments), so that segments farther from the trunk (the distal segments), such as the wrist and fingers, have a stable base from which to move and perform precision-oriented motions. Static posture is also present in the neck, the lower and upper back muscles, and the shoulder muscles. An example of excessive static loading of the upper trapezius muscle in a shortened position is shown in Figure 4. Varying degrees of cervical flexion are often maintained by the dental care worker[26] to achieve optimal visual access to patients' mouths. This poor postured alignment performed concurrently with excessive sustained static muscle contraction is believed to account for musculoskeletal pain found in neck, shoulders, and back in dental care workers.[33,34]

Dynamic posture refers to positions of the body assumed while the segments are engaged in movement. This term is often employed to indicate motion. Dynamic posture or movement is the result of a change in muscle length, as the body segment moves through an arc or motion around a joint. Isotonic contraction is the general term used to denote a muscle contraction involving any type of change in muscle length causing movement. More specifically, concentric, isotonic muscle contraction is used to refer to a muscle that shortens as it moves the segment. This type of contraction is used most frequently in most movements and activities of daily living. An example of a concentric, isotonic muscle contraction occurs in the elbow flexors when a glass of water is raised to the mouth. In an eccentric, isotonic muscle contraction, a muscle lengthens as it moves a segment. Examples occur in the elbow flexors when the glass of water is slowly placed back down and in the quadriceps when the body is being lowered to sit. Eccentric contractions slow down body segments and are performed when a muscle actively resists motion created by an external force such as gravity.[35]

In general, optimal static and optimal dynamic posture are defined by alignment in which there is symmetrical loading of the body or body parts and in which the mechanical advantage of the muscular and skeletal systems is most efficient. Poor trunk posture characterized by slouching not only requires the back muscles to work harder, but also places greater systemic demands on the cardiac system as a result of the heart's role in meeting the increased demands of the disadvantaged muscles. Posture should be evaluated and considered in the context of the specific task performed and in light of the physical requirements of the task.

FIGURE 4.—Static loading of the neck and shoulder girdle muscles. The effect is exaggerated when the shoulder girdle is elevated because of poor postural habits or lack of height adjustablility in the worksite.

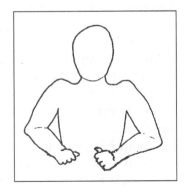

A poorly designed, nonadjustable dental office may make the performance of stooped or asymmetric postures unavoidable. Configuration of the dental office that requires the dental care worker to bend or stoop increases forces to the spine. Bending poorly distributes stresses on certain restraining ligaments and on portions of the intervertebral disks, thereby increasing the loads to delicate spinal structures. In a forward bending position, additional contraction of the back muscles results from the center of mass moving forward. The forces from this additional contraction are transmitted to other structures of the spine. Twisting or rotating the trunk while seated or standing, rather than rotating the seat in a swivel chair or pivoting the feet while standing, also places potentially harmful forces on the spine. It is therefore recommended that the dental care worker rotate the seat while sitting and pivot the feet while standing, to avoid twisting. Elevating the shoulder and hand in an unsupported manner, a position that is frequently exaggerated in nonadjustable or poorly designed offices, increases forces on the shoulder, as well as on the back. Maintaining reaches below shoulder height by lowering the instrument trays and the patient reduces these forces.

Seated posture is affected by the position of the pelvis. Optimal pelvic positioning is within what is termed, the middle range. A moderate lumbar curve is maintained. In this neutral posture, fatigue is minimized, especially if a back support from the chair is available, because the back and abdominal muscles do not have to work as hard. A supportive and correctly adjusted chair will assist in preserving a desirable low back curve, thus minimizing the need for muscle activity and strain to the ligaments of the spine. To benefit from the back support of the chair, however, the individual needs to use the chair back by positioning the pelvis all the way back in the seat and allowing his/her back to rest against the chair back. The dental care worker is often observed to lean or bend forward, thereby necessitating greater muscle contraction particularly from the back muscles and imposing greater forces on vulnerable structures of the spine. Having the dental worker's chair as close to the patient's as possible, may help minimize the tendency to lean or slouch forward. Sitting backward on a chair so that the dental worker is leaning forward against the chair back may be helpful. There are chairs that are commercially available that are designed to be used in this way.

When one or both arms are elevated, a posture frequently used in dentistry, forces on the spine increase. Proper height adjustment of the dental worker's chair relative to the patient and the floor provides pelvic stabilization to the spine through solid foot contact and support from the floor. It can also minimize reaches, a factor known to reduce the rate of fatigue in the upper back, neck and shoulder muscles.[36]

Optimal posture is characterized by joint position in which the segments are positioned and used in the middle or neutral ranges of joint motion. The use of awkward and extreme postures is frequently cited as a risk factor for musculoskeletal pain.[8,30,37] In addition to reducing compression and shearing forces within a joint, neutral postures have the effect of placing muscles at their resting lengths. Muscles contract most efficiently positioned at (or actually just beyond) resting length. In addition, frictional forces to soft tissues are minimized when the joints are in neutral. In ulnar deviation of the wrist, for example, when the hand is bent to the side in the direction of the little finger, frictional forces between tendons are greater than when the wrist is straight. The risk for DeQuervains disease, a tendinitis condition of two thumb muscles in the wrist, is increased when the wrist is in ulnar deviation. This occurs from shearing forces of the these tendons against the widest part of the wrist from the radius bone of the forearm.

Dynamic movement performed within normal, physiologic ranges enhances the health and nutritional environment in which muscles and tendons function. However, excessive dynamic motion, also termed repetitive motion, is a notable risk factor for injury. Specific parameters outlining safe amounts of motion are not currently available. The injury mechanism in tendons is attributed to excessive motion of a tendon over an adjacent structure such as bone, fibrous tissue, or another tendon, causing cumulative increases in frictional forces. This often results in cellular and tissue degradation and a localized inflammatory response.

Muscle and tendon lengths, which result from dynamic and static postures and long-term postural habits, are major determinants in the ability to generate force and maintain posture.[21,38] Dynamic and static posture influence length adaptations that occur to structures over time. For example, if the abdominal muscles are weak and easily fatigued during seated posture, ability to maintain a mid-range lordosis is limited. As previously stated, the upper back and shoulders will tend to collapse forward in response to pelvic positioning. The rhomboids and middle trapezius muscles of the middle and upper back, which stabilize the shoulder girdle and help maintain erect upper back posture, will be placed in a stretched, elongated position. If this forward-shoulder and rounded-back posture is subsequently adopted and used, these muscles are likely to become overstretched and may actually increase in length. Overstretched muscles must work harder than muscles of the appropriate length to accomplish the same movement and stabilizing functions. Such a structural change may progress to affect other soft-tissue components, as a compensatory response, causing a further worsening of postural alignment. The next progression in this scenario is frequently a shortening of opposing muscles, the pectoralis muscles of the chest. A situation that may have begun as a functional limitation caused by muscle weakness or poor postural habits may progress to become a muscle imbalance or fixed limitation. Ligaments responsible for stabilizing joints that are constantly subject to excessive tension as a result of poor posture will also eventually attenuate or stretch, thereby decreasing their effectiveness as joint stabilizers. Postures voluntarily assumed for the performance of everyday activities, over time, profoundly influence soft-tissue length, balance, and efficiency. Functional deficits may become structural limitations. This may result in increased muscle fatigue and pain caused by the straining of overused, over-stretched muscles and ligaments, and compensatory patterns of movement.[38]

Of further consideration, is the role of the central nervous system in regulating posture and balance mechanisms, muscle tone, and movement and reflex patterns. It has been suggested that the risk of musculoskeletal pain may be increased as a result of conflicting demands on the central nervous system.

These conflicting demands occur when dynamic motion of the distal extremities is superimposed on the static muscles of the trunk. This phenomenon has been identified and addressed as a significant issue inherent in the tasks of computer keyboard users and musicians.[39,40]

Cocontraction is a term used to describe the situation that arises when one group of muscles works inefficiently against the contraction of the opposing group, a function mediated in the central nervous system. The prime movers, the major muscles used to perform the motion, therefore have to work that much harder to overcome the opposing muscle contraction. To some extent, this is a normal occurrence similar to isometric or static contraction, in which several different muscle groups contract simultaneously, to stabilize a joint. However, cocontraction, as an involuntary phenomenon, involves nonpurposeful contraction of the opposing muscle group resulting in a loss of energy. The outcome is excessive energy expenditure, which is inherently inefficient.

Other inefficient movement patterns include unintentional jerky motions and uncoordinated movement patterns.[41] In contrast are the gracefulness and posture of a dancer, for example, whose movements are smooth and appear to flow in a natural, effortless, way. The dancer's movements are aesthetically pleasing, in part, precisely because they are efficient, balanced, and well-timed. The complexity of events occurring in the central nervous system are also influenced by the function of the sensory system and the arousal mechanisms in the brain associated with sensory and psychological processing. Both affect muscle tone and the quality of motor output. The competing intellectual and performance demands of dentistry may further contribute to challenges of the central nervous system in regulation movement.

Methods for Improving Posture

Modifying postural habits and movement patterns is difficult. Change may require addressing musculoskeletal issues such as insufficient range of motion, muscle strength, and endurance. It is also likely to involve modifying motor programs, which are the brain's means for storing and retrieving commonly used patterns of movement. Motor programs are processed automatically within the central nervous system. It is possible to change postural alignment and movement habits, with significant motivation and training. It is diffcult because when attention is drawn away from the postural performance components, to engage in the other physical and mental activity required for task performance, efforts to control movement patterns are generally short-lived.[31] For the dental worker, this problem is illustrated in the attempt to maintain a neutral wrist position while performing a highly skilled, precision-oriented procedure. Only when the new posture or method is integrated and organized into the normal movement repertoire of the dental worker is the posture truly learned and performed without the need for additional cognitive focus.

GENERAL APPROACHES, TO IMPROVE POSTURE

There are a number of methods that are used in attempt to improve posture and movement patterns. Exercise systems such as yoga and martial art forms help in developing physical and movement skills that can be carried over into the postures and movement patterns of daily activities and have been shown to reduce stress. It is highly recommended that individuals participate in activities like yoga, martial arts, dance, and sports. These activities offer opportunities for movement experiences that facilitate adaptive responses by the musculoskeletal and nervous systems. Besides enhancing overall strength and endurance, these experiences facilitate body awareness and provide occasions to move in ways that are novel. Individuals who use their bodies in very restricted ways tend to be less effective and efficient in their motor responses. The quality of a motor response is in part, a result of information provided by sensory receptors in joints and tendons and those of the inner ears which control balance reactions. The type of sensory input from these receptors influences the resultant movement. By modifying the quality of sensory input, one can alter motor output.

Responding to the body's signals of discomfort or fatigue to alternate posture is fundamental in improving postural habits. Body awareness is the ability to sense and accommodate to sensory signals sent to the brain from the peripheral nervous system. It improves in response to attention, practice, and motivation. Developing a habit of "checking" the body for discomfort or tension and finding strategies to move more efficiently may be difficult if an individual is not "in tune" with those types of physical sensations and able to make subtle adaptations.

Practice is believed to be an important factor in acquiring new motor skills. Consistent, conscious focus on the desired performance promotes the relearning of habits and skills. It is believed that new movement patterns are learned and integrated when they are carried over from practice into performance. At this stage, they no longer require focused conscious attention. It has been found that focusing for short periods of time on improved posture that helps to create new, more efficient motor habits that are carried over into performance between these practice sessions. Short periods of practice time performed relatively frequently are known to be more effective in enhancing learning than longer periods performed less frequently.

A number of mental imagery techniques have been effective in assisting people to change their posture.[42] It has been found that the use of visualization can facilitate learning and integration of skills. An example of using an image to improve erect standing or sitting is to envision a long, vertical spine. An example of a way to improve the quality of movement is to feel the movement of the trunk, arms, and legs coming from the body's center (of mass). This is suggested by the image of the dog wagging the tail as opposed to the tail wagging the dog.

Specific Methods for Particular Problems

Excessive muscle tension in reaction to stress or acquired habits may produce static contractions that lead to pain. Movements that break tension may be helpful, if performed regularly and integrated into one's work habits. Nodding the head up and down (as if to say "yes"), rotating the head from side to side (as if to say "no"), and rolling the shoulder girdle in a backward circular pattern are relaxation exercises that the dental worker can implement while working to reduce tension in the neck, upper back, and shoulders. The forearms and fingers are most relaxed when positioned in the dental worker's lap or relaxed down at the side. When the hands are not in use, it is recommended that they be allowed to rest down in a comfortable position without holding onto instruments or being positioned in anticipation of the next task.

As stated previously, is recommended that the dental care worker sit back in the chair when possible with the buttocks back in the seat, and using the chair back for support whenever feasible. Positioning oneself as close as possible to the patient and the tools and instruments lessens the necessity of bending forward or maintaining a forward stooped, unsupported position in the chair. It also decreases reaches. "Finding" the curve in the low back (the lumbar region), which is "lost" when one is seated for long periods of time is also helpful in improving alignment and decreasing loads on the spinal ligaments. This is done by rotating the pelvis anteriorly in either standing or sitting (see Figure 5). Readjusting the dental worker's chair (and tool tray) relative to each patient is important in maintaining optimal height positioning.

People who sit for long periods of time are at great risk of low back pain caused by the flexed or posteriorly tilted

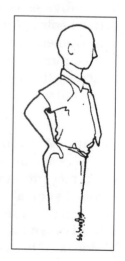

FIGURE 5.—Reversing the curve in the low back. During seated activity, the normal lordotic curve is lost. To reverse the curve, momentarily arch the back by sticking out the chest and abdomen. This stretch can be performed standing, as illustrated, or sitting.

position of the pelvis. Dental care workers frequently change their posture from sitting to standing and therefore do not generally sit for extended periods of time, relative to other professions. However, the concept of dynamic sitting may have relevance and application in regard to lengthy dental procedures. In dynamic sitting, the individual is encouraged to perform frequent, subtle weight shifts and readjustments. Movement is encouraged because it aids in increasing nutrition to relatively avascular spinal structures. In addition, changing spinal and pelvic positions lessens forces on certain soft-tissue structures and redistributes the demands every time a postural readjustment is made. A fatigued structure can therefore rest and recover while other soft tissue components assume the workload.

Recommended postures for the upper quadrant, consisting of the upper back, neck, shoulders, arms, and wrists, have been briefly discussed in this chapter and described in greater depth by other authors. Therefore, only suggestions regarding optimal thumb and finger positioning will be addressed here. The position of the thumb is significant in terms of the function it serves as a stable post for the other fingers to pinch against. Because the thumb is used intensely during almost all grasp patterns, the joint structures are subject to constant forces. It is therefoie at greater risk for soft tissue and arthritic changes. Therefore, using the thumb in ways that minimize exposure to forces is especially significant. Long-term use of the thumb with the distal joint in hyperextension increases compression and shearing stresses to the joint at the base of the thumb (see Figure 6). Stability of the tip and middle joints of the thumb is compromised by the cumulative forces which elongate ligaments over time. If the force requirement of a manual task is so great that the strength of the finger and thumb muscles is insufficient to contract against the external force that are causing the distal joint hyperextension, then the task cannot be safely performed. Either the tools or the task should be modified. The fingers and thumb should not pinch or be used with the tip joints bent backward but should instead be used with the tips slightly flexed to avoid strain to the ligaments (see Figure 7). To diminish the effect of forces transferred to the base of the thumb, the thumb should be positioned in abduction (away from the plane of the palm).

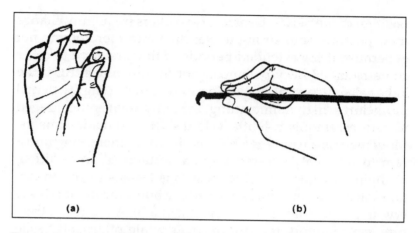

FIGURE 6.—Potentially harmful positioning of the thumb and fingers: the thumb performing a pinch with the tip joint positioned in extreme hypertension (a) and tool use with the thumb and fingers in moderate hyperextension (b).

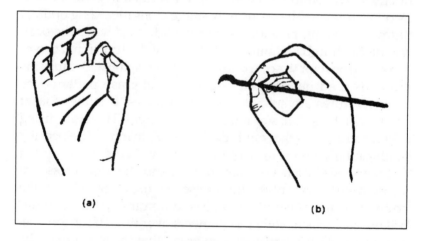

FIGURE 7.—Recommended positioning of the thumb and fingers: the thumb performing a pinch with the tip joints of the thumb and index fingers positioned in moderate flexion (a) and tool use with the thumb and fingers in gentle flexion.

STRUCTURAL POSTURAL PROBLEMS

Some structural (or fixed) postural problems are very obvious and can be observed in the poor alignment of an individual from side view. A number of patterns are frequently seen. A forward head position, described as "bird-watching posture," indicates a shortening and loss of balance of the neck musculature. This may accompany a forward shoulder and a rounded back posture and is considered fixed, if the individual cannot easily assume a position of aligned neutral head, neck, shoulder, and upper back alignment (with the ears essentially in line with the shoulders). Fixed forward shoulder and a rounded back posture indicates a shortening of the pectoralis minor (a chest muscle) and overstretching of the middle trapezius and rhomboid muscles (two middle back muscles) (see Figure 8). When the muscles of the head, neck and shoulders are of optimal relative lengths and no weakness is present, the shoulder girdle can effectively position the head for manual use.

Adequately engaging the back extensor and abdominal muscles will improve the ability to maintain erect, upright posture. Weak muscles and those not adequately used because of poor motor habits, place body structures, even at distances to these muscles, in jeopardy. For example, poor abdominal strength contributes to poor spinal alignment, which may cause poor shoulder girdle posture, affecting distal structures in the arms and fingers. The goal of improving postural habits and movement patterns while addressing strength and

FIGURE 8.—Forward head and shoulder posture. When an individual assumes this positioning over a long period, soft-tissue structures will eventually accommodate, making it difficult to assume and maintain erect alignment.

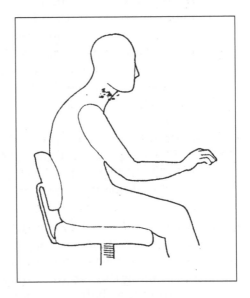

muscle/tendon length limitations, is recommended for some individuals.

ALTERNATIVE METHODS OF POSTURAL RE-EDUCATION

Alternative methods of postural training and re-education have only recently gained credibility among mainstream professionals and consumers. Practitioners who perform these techniques are known generally as body workers. They may apply methods of a specific school or philosophy, or be eclectic in their approach, drawing on several techniques. Movement and posture, from the point of view of the bodyworker, are often addressed in the larger context of health and wellness. Information in this section will highlight a number of the specific methods developed to improve posture and movement. There are many other effective systems of postural re-education. An excellent source that lists and describes various alternative methods is a book by Mirka Knaster.[43] Much of the information on the approaches described below, comes from this book.

1. *The Feldenkrais Method: Functional Integration and Awareness Through Movement* is a well-known, highly regarded method of improving ease of movement by presenting the brain with modified, more effective input from the joints, muscles, and tendons and thereby establishing new patterns of motor responses. The Feldenkrais method attempts to "rewire" or re-educate the nervous system. Instructors use a gentle hands-on method of manual cues to re-establish new movement patterns and teach structured movement experiences to improve these skills.

   For more information contact
   The Feldenkrais Guild, PO Box 489, Albany, OR 97321-0143, (800) 775-2118, (503) 926-0981.
   Feldenkrais Resources, 830 Bancroft Way, Suite 112, Berkeley, CA 94710, (800) 765-1907, (510) 540-7600 .

2. *The Alexander Technique* addresses postural habits by focusing on balance in the head/neck relationship. The Alexander teacher gently guides the head into proper positioning during gross movement tasks such as rising from the chair. This gives the student the opportu-

nity to experience movement that enhances the lengthening of the spine. Attention is also focused on reducing the use of unnecessary muscle tension.

For more information contact

North American Society of Teachers of the Alexander Technique, PO Box 517, Urbana, IL 61801, (800) 473-0620.

Alexander Technique International, Inc., 1692 Massachusetts Ave., Cambridge, MA 02138, (617) 497-2242.

3. *Rolfing,* also known as *Structural Integration,* uses superficial- and deep-tissue hands-on techniques and educational movement sequences with the intention of reducing strain in the body's fascia (connective tissue), to eliminate impediments to unrestricted movement. The individual receives a series of sessions focused an developing awareness of alignment and habitual movement patterns. Exercises are geared toward deepening breathing and toward improving ease of movement, muscle tone, coordination, and flexibility.

For more information contact

The Rolf Institute of Structural Integration, PO Box 1868, Boulder, CO 80302-1868, (800) 530-8875 or (303) 449-5903.

Guild for Structural Integration PO Box 1559, Boulder, CO 80306-1559, (800) 447-0150 or (303) 447-0122.

4. *Pilates and the Physical Mind Method,* both originating from the work of Joseph Pilates, use a system of exercises and a variety of equipment invented by the late Pilates. Correct use of the equipment makes the user aware of how to move in balanced ways. Although this is a strength-oriented approach, it also addresses flexibility. The premise is that through strengthening, increasing flexibility, and learning balanced muscle techniques, the individual is able to use more efficient posture and movement patterns and to prevent injuries.

For more information contact

Physical Mind Institute, 1807 Second St., #28129 Santa Fe, NM 87505, (800) 505-1990 or (505) 988-1990.

Center for Sports Medicine, St. Francis Hospital, 900 Hyde Street, San Francisco, CA 94109, (415) 353-6410.

5. *Biofeedback Training* is a method used to gain conscious control over various physiologic functions of the body such as heart rate, muscle activity, and skin temperature. Sometimes known as surface electromyography (EMG), biofeedback can help an individual decrease muscle activity such as that implicated in headaches and pain and that deriving from postures that require excessive muscle contraction. Conversely, biofeedback also can be used to increase active recruitment of muscle fibers in weak or unused muscles. For example, biofeedback may be effectively employed to improve posture that positions the shoulders in an abnormally protracted (forward) position because the back muscles lack strength or are not being used adequately to maintain the shoulders in a normal, erect posture. Biofeedback training is often used as an adjunctive technique by health care professionals such as massage therapists, psychologists, and physical and occupational therapy.

6. *Massage Therapy* is a collective term for numerous soft-tissue approaches used to relieve discomfort in soft tissue. Swedish massage techniques are probably the best known among these. However numerous schools have been developed based on alternative theories of health, such as Shiatsu, which is based on Eastern traditions. Shiatsu is founded on principles similar to those underlying the theory of acupuncture. Individuals who perform work or activities which tend to cause soft tissue strain, often find relief from periodic massage sessions. No matter what type of massage approach is utilized, receiving treatment from a state-licensed practitioner is recommended. A license is required by law in many states.

Work Style and Work Pace

Work style and work pace are believed to play a significant role in the onset of pain. Many health care professionals are currently under pressure to increase revenues by treating more patients. Working faster and treating more patients greatly increases the physical demands of the dental office. Greater pressures to keep treatment numbers high increases repetitions and speed of task performance. Increasing rates of task performance have been shown to increase the use of awkward and extreme postures of other manual tasks.[44] This is likely to be true in dental care, as well. Pressures to work quickly may be contrary to the dental worker's need to take time to properly adjust the components of the work site. Psychological stress has also been found to play a role in the onset of work-related musculoskeletal pain. It is likely that the role played by psychological stress is due to increased tension in muscles.

The need for break time to allow soft tissues to rest and recuperate is frequently referred to in the research literature. Even very brief rest breaks allow important metabolic activity to occur to maintain a healthy environment in which muscles and tendons can work. Not a great deal is known in terms of recommended work-rest cycles for repetitive activity of the upper exttremity. Much is not known in this area, information quantifying critical levels of rest required for specific levels of activity. It is suggested, however, that the more intense the activity being performed, the more rest tissues require in order to recuperate. Sustained use of an awkward posture and use of static muscle contraction, as well as greater demands on muscle forces increase rest requirements.

Lee et al offer a definition for breaks for computer operators.[24] These include microbreaks, minibreaks, and major breaks. A microbreak is a very short break of less than 10 to 15 seconds, necessitating no significant interruption of work. It is a initiation of a very brief pause that is integrated into the style of the worker. The brief rest breaks provide significant and opportune recovery time between activities. An example would be allowing the arm and shoulder to rest down during moments when elevation required for hand use is not needed. Another example would be putting a tool down while it is not in use, instead of continuing to grasp it.

A minibreak is defined as a short rest period of less than 1 to 2 minutes, in which interruption of the worker's activity may or may not be necessary. For dental care workers, these breaks might fit in well between patients. A generally accepted rule applied to the rest requirements of computer keyboard users is to not work more than 30 to 45 minutes without a minibreak. It may be necessary for the dental care worker to take more frequent minibreaks, performing no more then 20 to 30 minutes of dental work, depending on the intensity and requirements of the task. It is recommended that these breaks be interspersed throughout the work day. A minibreak can be used as a time to perform an activity that has different physical requirements than the tasks that the dental care worker has been performing, such as standing to make a telephone call or performing stretches or relaxation exercises.

A major break is an unspecified amount of time that lasts more than the few minutes allotted for minibreaks. This is an excellent time to perform gentle, full-body stretches as well as specific neck and upper-extremity stretches.

Attempting to pace and balance physical demands throughout the day will help to provide natural pauses and time for recuperation. Viewing the effect of physical activity on the body in a larger context of several days or a week will assist in anticipating especially demanding periods that may require planning. The performance of stretches and relaxation exercises should be performed throughout the workday. A work environment that supports and fosters safety among the entire office staff is ideal in terms of fostering follow-through among all office staff. An important aspect intrinsic to the creation and maintenance of this safe work culture, is advocacy and support from office management.

Summary and Conclusions

Reducing risk factors associated with incidence of musculoskeletal pain and injury in dental work is facilitated through ergonomic assessment and modification. Significant factors associated with habits of the individual worker are amenable to change, including fitness level, posture, and various aspects of work style. It is recommended that dental care workers employ preventive solutions for environmental issues, as well as for factors related to personal attributes. Primary prevention is clearly the most cost-effective, humane, and energy efficient approach to addressing safety issues in the dental office.

The relationship between specific components of fitness and musculoskeletal injuries in high-risk work has not been clearly established. However there is empirical evidence that physical condition and quality of movement have profound effects on musculoskeletal health. Good vertical alignment of the head, neck, spine, and pelvis during seated activity promotes endurance and muscular efficiency and perpetuates the use good alignment. Poor vertical alignment has the opposite outcome; the interrelationship of these factors is believed to be significant. Awareness of the effect of optimal posture and patterns of muscle use and their contribution to states of fatigue and discomfort may foster motivation for correcting problem areas.

The integration of 30 minutes of moderate physical activity into the daily activity of the dental worker may help to address the inactivity of the larger muscle groups of the legs and trunk and static muscle activity of the back, neck, and shoulders in the dental worker's day. More intensive stretching, strengthening, and cardiorespiratory exercise to have additional health benefits. It is not known whether the exercise is truly effective in preventing musculoskeletal injuries. It is likely that there is a direct dose-response relationship that at its most excessive, cannot be overcome by optimal ergonomics, postural retraining, or conditioning exercises.

There are many approaches to improving fitness and posture. Work and physical activity that place varying demands on the body will address a number of fitness needs and help maintain motivation. Fitness, alignment and use of efficient movement patterns can be thought of as ideal physical states that can be continually challenged to improve. Balance in activity and rest and work style are important components in the prevention of musculoskeletal injuries of the dental care worker.

ACKNOWLEDGMENT

The author would like to thank Cristina Burwell for her assistance with the illustrations used in this chapter.

REFERENCES

1. Ranney D. Work-related chronic injuries of the forearm and hand: their specific diagnosis and management. *Ergonomics.* 1993;36(8):871–880.
2. Mausner JS, Kramer S. *Epidemiology, an Introductory Text.* 2nd ed. Philadelphia: WB Saunders; 1985.
3. Hardy MA. The biology of scar formation. *J of Phys Ther.* 1989;69(12):1012–1024.
4. Powell SG, Burke AL. Surgical and therapeutic management of tennis elbow: An update. *J of Hand Ther.* 1991; April:4(2):64–68.
5. Poole BC. Cumulative trauma disorder of the upper extremity from occupational stress. *J of Hand Ther.* 1988; July:1(4):172–180.
6. Dennet X. Fry HJH. Overuse syndrome: a muscle biopsy study. *Lancet.* 1988;(April):905–908.
7. Stock SR. Workplace ergonomic factors and the development of musculoskeletal disorders of the neck and upper limbs. *Am J of Industrial Med.* 1991;19:87–107.
8. Armstrong TJ. Ergonomics in cumulative trauma disorders. *Hand Clinics.* 1986;2(3):553–565.
9. Kroemer KHE. Avoiding cumulative trauma disorders in shops and offices. *J Am Ind Hyg Assoc.* 1992;53(Sept):596–604.
10. Armstrong TJ. Chaffin DB. Carpal tunnel syndrome and selected personal attributes. *J Occup Med.* 1979;21(7):481–485.
11. Green RA. Briggs CA. Anthropometric dimensions and overuse injury among Australian keyboard operators. *J Occup Med.* 1989;31(9):747–750.
12. Arndt R. Working posture and musculoskeletal problems of video display terminal operators—review and reappraisal. *J Am Ind Hyg Assoc.* 1983; June:44(6):487–446.
13. Silverstein BA, Armstrong TJ, Longmate A, Woody D. Can in-plant exercise control musculoskeletal symtoms? *J of Occup Med.* 1988;30(12):922–927.
14. Dickey T, ed. The elements of fitness. In: *The New Wellness Encyclopedia.* New York: Houghton Mifflin; 1995.
15. Howley ET, Franks BD. Evaluation of health status. In: *Health Fitness Instructor's Handbook.* 2nd ed. Illinois: Human Kinetics. 1992; 15–25.
16. Wilmore JH, Costill DL. Prescription of exercise for health and fitness. In: *Physiology of Sport and Exercise.* Illinois: Human Kinetics; 1994:513–530.
17. Kenney WL. *The American College of Sports Medicine Fitness Book.* Illinois: Leisure Press; 1992.

18. Lowe C. Treatment of tendinitis, tenosynovitis, and other cumulative trauma disorders of musicians' forearms, wrists, and hands . . . restoring function with hand therapy. *J of Hand Ther.* 1992;April:84–90.

19. Knowles JM, Calibey TC. Prevention, treatment and rehabilitation of sports injuries. In: Rothman J, Levine R, eds. *Prevention Practice: Strategies for Physical and Occupational Therapy.* Philadelphia: WB Saunders; 1992:132–144.

20. Kannus P, Jozsa L, Renström P, Järvinen M, Kvist M, Lehto M, Oja P, Vuori I. The effects of training and immobilization, and remobilization on musculoskeletal tissue. *Scand J Med Sci Sports.* 1992;(2):100–118.

21. White SG, Sahrmann SA. A movement system balance approach to management of musculoskeletal pain. In: Grant R, ed. *Physical Therapy of the Cervical and Thoracic Spine.* 2nd ed. New York: Churchill Livingstone;1994;339–357.

22. Mount J. Designing exercise programs for the elderly. In: Rothman J, Levine R, eds. *Prevention Practice: Strategies for Physical and Occupational Therapy.* Philadelphia: WB Saunders; 1992:218–223

23. Liemohn W, Sharpe G. Muscular strength and endurance, flexibility, and low-back function. In: Howley ET, Franks BD, eds. *Health Fitness Instructor's Handbook.* 2nd ed. Illinois: Human Kinetic Books; 1992:179–207.

24. Lee K, Swanson N, Sauter S, Wickstrom R, Waikar A, Mangum M. A review of physical exercises recommended for vdt operators. *Applied Ergonomics.* 1992;23(6):387–408.

25. Nordin M, Frankel VH. *Basic Biomechanics of the Musculoskeletal System.* Philadelphia: Lea and Febiger; 1989.

26. Hagberg M, Hagberg C. Risks and prevention of musculoskeletal disorders among dentists. In: *Occupational Hazards in the Health Professions.* Boca Raton, Florida: CRC Press; 1989:324–330.

27. Hansford T, Blood H, Kent B, Lutz G. Blood flow changes at the wrist in manual workers after preventive interventions. *J Hand Surg.* 1986;11A(4):503–508.

28. Zemke R. Remediation biomechanical and physiologic impairments of motor performance. In: Trombly CA, ed. *Occupational Therapy for Physical Dysfunction.* 4th ed. Baltimore: Williams and Wilkins; 1995.

29. Pedretti LW, Wade IE. Therapeutic modalities. In: Pedretti LW, ed. *Occupational Therapy: Practice Skills for Physical Dysfunction.* 4th ed. New York: Mosby; 1996.

30. Haslegrave CM. What do we mean by a "working posture"? *Ergonomics.* 1994;37:781–799.

31. Smith LK, Weiss EL, Lehmkuhl LD. Standing and walking. In: *Brunnstrom's Clinical Kinesiology*. 5th ed. Philadelphia: FA Davis; 1996:401–435.

32. Norkin CC, Levangie PK. Posture. In: *Joint Structure and Function*. 2nd ed. Philadelphia: FA Davis; 1992:419–447.

33. Shugars D, Miller D, Fishburne C, Strickland D. Musculoskeletal pain among general dentists. *General Dentistry*. 1987; July:272–276.

34. Kajland A, Lindvall T, Nilsson T. Occupational medical aspects of the dental profession. *Work Environ Hlth*. 1974;11:100–107.

35. Norkin CC, Levangie PK. Muscle structure and function. In: *Joint Structure and Function*. 2nd ed. Philadelphia: FA Davis; 1992:92–124.

36. Chaffin DB, Andersson GB. Biomechanical considerations in machine control and workplace design. In: *Occupational Biomechancis*. 2nd ed. New York: John Wiley & Sons; 1991:376–410.

37. Putz-Anderson V. *Cumulative Trauma Disorder: A Manual for the Musculoskeletal Diseases of the Upper Limbs*. New York: Taylor and Francis; 1988.

38. Hansford T. Corrective exercise for postural and biomechanical dysfunction. In: Program Guide for Seminar: Upper Extremity Cumulative Trauma Disorders: Evaluation, Management, Problems and Solutions, Feb 25–27. San Diego: American Society of Hand Therapists, 1994.

39. Grandjean E. *Ergonomics in Computerized Offices*. New York: Taylor and Francis; 1987.

40. Edwards RHT. Hypothesis of peripheral and central mechanisms underlying occupational muscle spasm. *Eur J Applied Physiology*. 1988;57:275–281.

41. Winter DA. *Biomechanics and Motor Control of Human Movement*. New York: John Wiley & Sons; 1990.

42. Sage GH. *Motor Learning and Control: A Neurophysiological Approach*. Iowa: William C. Brown; 1984.

43. Knaster M. *Discovering the Body's Wisdom*. New York: Bantam Books; 1996.

44. Arndt R. Work pace, stress, and cumulative trauma disorders. *J Hand Surg*. 1987;12A(5):866–869.

Chapter 11

Human-Centered Ergonomics: Proprioceptive Pathway to Occupational Health and Peak Performance in Dental Practice

Michael M. Belenky, DDS, MPH, FACD, FPFA

Abstract

Ergonomics offers dentists, dental hygienists, and other members of the oral health team the opportunity to realize their peak performance potential without compromise of themselves, their work, or their patients. Through the use of human-factors engineering, they can easily determine the changes in posture, process, and practice environment that will prevent or reduce repetitive stress injuries, physical and mental fatigue, musculoskeletal disorders, and impaired care delivery. These beneficial changes can be achieved in both traditional and newer practice settings, leading to increased efficiency, greater productivity, superior care, and an improved quality of life for providers of dental services to the patient community. Ergonomic optimization of practitioner posture, patient positioning, treatment process, operatory equipment, and facility design affords the dental profession a direct and practical route to peak performance in the 21st century.

Human Priorities for Human Endeavor

Concern for the occupational health of workers, the manner in which they perform, and the quality of their product prompts many in academia, industry, and government to place a high priority on human-centered factors in the workplace and on changing the "way we work."

Ergonomics—the scientific study of human beings and their relationship to a work environment—commands the attention of today's industrial managers. Contemporary government standards for occupational safety and health require those in management to conduct exhaustive risk analyses and to prescribe and monitor "safe" modes of human performance whenever workers may be at risk of injury from conditions of their employment.[1] The rising incidence of work-related injuries, in the United States and elsewhere, is further reason for concern and action.[2] The human and financial costs of medical care, rehabilitation, and disability that follow such injuries are no longer acceptable to employees, employers, or society at large. Industries now commit substantial fiscal and personnel resources to the investigation and optimization of work settings through human-factors engineering. They must establish and maintain performance standards and settings that do not compromise worker health. To attain these objectives, they recognize the many commonalities among humans, their tendency to perform similar tasks in similar ways, and their inclination to respect and respond to the body's proprioceptive senses; for to ignore nature is to invite failure in the highly competitive world of modern business. Management today knows how to sustain a happy, healthy, efficient, and effective workforce, and to operate profitably. Their secret is respect for human factors in the design and operation of the work environment. Whenever possible, they adapt machines and work stations to the needs of human beings, rather than adapt humans to the requirements of machine as in traditional work settings. They have discovered human-centered ergonomics and rejected machine-centered ergonomics. A similar opportunity awaits dentistry. We have only to identify a need and call for action. Industry's ergonomic revolution has shown us the way.

Human Factors in Dentistry: An Occupational Profile

Dentists and the profession at large are generally held in high regard by the patient population.[3] But beyond this shared accolade, many of our occupational attributes are dissimilar. Many of us are engaged in "independent" practice and are proud of our "individualism." For the same oral condition we may propose differing treatments. For the same treatment we may select different instruments. We work in as many different ways as there are dental care workers in practice, each of us certain that "my way is the best way." However, there is one "reward" of dental practice that we all share to some degree and to which we can all attest—the high incidence of back, neck, shoulder, arm, and hand ailments, which impair both our health and our potential for peak performance.

Surveys conducted by Murtomaa, Hope-Ross and Corcoran, Rundcratz, and Shugars et al reinforce this observation and lend objective substance to what is subjectively apparent to all who are engaged in active dental practice.[4-6] Data from their investigations suggest that a substantial number (38 to 72%) of dental professionals incur occupationally related pain and discomfort. In a 1987 survey of 2000 members of the American Dental Association, Shugars found that musculoskeletal pain is an occupational ailment for 60% of general dentists. Those experiencing pain reported that it occurred from 65 to 125 days per year and led to absence from work, increased breaks from practice activity, income loss, and altered practice procedures. It is likely that musculoskeletal stress and fatigue lessen practitioner control of finite intraoral performance and increase the potential for technical compromise. Nearly a third of those responding to the survey reported that musculoskeletal pain arising from practice interrupted physical and leisure activities, and a fourth reported that the pain interfered with sleep.

Dentists and dental hygienists seek varied treatments to obtain relief from these problems, but few realize more than a limited degree of permanent relief. The numerous individual work styles in dentistry today vary widely and are likely contributors to the postural stress, muscle fatigue, and tension in the upper back, neck, and shoulder complex. Physicians, physical therapists, chiropractors, and others who treat such occupational maladies respond alike when asked "what do dentists and dental hygienists tell you when you suggest that they alter the way they work?" Dentists and dental hygienists commonly respond that there is little they can do to eliminate or reduce the distortion of natural posture and the ensuing discomfort and pain. They find the distorted postures necessary to see and to perform dental procedures in the varied treatment sites of the oral cavity. They see no alternative but to seek continuous palliative therapy so that they can sustain their practices. Those who are conscious of opportunities at hand today would suggest other options, especially in view of the dramatic ergonomic alternatives now being applied to other areas of human endeavor.

In any examination of dentistry's occupational profile over the centuries, it is quite evident that the manner in which practitioners of dentistry work has changed very little, except for advances in technology and materials. Whether in ancient times or today, one observes a common physical profile, an unnatural body form reflecting degrees of contortion and distortion which range from the moderate to the extreme. A great deal has changed and improved in the art and science of dentistry over the centuries, but little has changed in the manner of work.[8] If dentistry is to offer the best and brightest of today's youth only this prospect for their future, many may seek the lucrative alternatives that now compete with the profession.

In part, the way we work is the product of the way we teach students in the more than 600 dental schools of the globe. Educators are challenged to prepare students for the realities of practice today and possibilities yet to come in the practice of the future. The scientific and technologic advances that have come to dentistry in the last half of this century are many and are indicative of future potential for yet greater progress en route to oral health for all. They include fluoridation for the prevention of dental caries; high-speed handpieces; restorative materials that bond to enamel, dentin, and metals; ultrasonic scaling of teeth; chemicals that preclude or reduce the formation of plaque and the onset of dental and periodontal disease; soft-tissue regeneration and replacement; telescopic loupes for greater visual control of intraoral performance; computer-assisted design and manufacturing of fixed prostheses; osseo-integrated implants; lasers for surgery of soft and hard tissues; radiovisiography and computer imaging; computer-based information and practice management; electronic patient records; and equipment and facility design tailored to specific concepts of care delivery, enhanced by computer technology. Today's young dentists enter a profession of great achievement and endless promise for the future. Some are the product of extraordinary advances in dental education: instructional methods enhanced by computer-based interactive self-learning exercises; modern classrooms and laboratories; multimedia audiovisual projection devices for classroom and laboratory illustration; realistic simulation settings for the pre-clinical acquisition and perfection of psychomotor skills, including such enhancements as lifelike phantom heads and virtual-reality technology; and state-of-the-art clinical facilities for patient care. However, in the majority of dental schools, students prepare for patient care in traditional laboratories that bear no relationship to the realities of the treatment settings in which they will later practice. They perform bench-top technical exercises, where the priority concern of attending faculty is the quality of the outcome product—i.e., a cavity preparation or a finished restoration. The process of achievement is too often left to a student's own devices. Through intuition, experimentation, and repetitive practice, students perfect their skills in ways as different and many as their numbers. They acquire less-than-optimal work habits, repetitive-stress injuries, and cumulative trauma disorders that too often compromise their physical and mental well-being, preclude peak performance, and impair their potential for excellence in dental practice. They learn in ways that few industries could afford or permit; for efficiency, effectiveness, and a consistent quality of product depend on maximizing the potential of the human performer, leaving nothing to chance. The same opportunity resides in academia. Dental educators can define simple, direct, and consistent ergonomic processes for the performance of common tasks by students and produce a new generation of dentists for the future. There is but one obstacle to overcome—the human reluctance to change. This obstacle is formidable in academia, but of minor consequence for the dentist who experiences musculoskeletal ailments as a result of daily practice and seeks an alternative. It is virtually absent in the new dental student who enters the profession with an open mind, free of experiential bias, anticipating both health and success in dental practice.

Ergonomics, or human engineering, has been a part of dentistry for several decades. We would be remiss were we not to recognize and honor the great contributions of Kimmel, Walker, Kilpatrick, and the many others who sought to improve the condition of dental practice through research, innovation, and pioneering initiative.[8,9] Their focus on work simplification, increased productivity, the use of dental assistants, four-handed dentistry, TEAM dentistry, operatory and facility design, equipment and instrument design, and so forth changed the practice of dentistry forever. They are owed a debt of gratitude for more than the changes they brought to the profession. They opened the path to the future and challenged others to continue the march. Dentistry must accept the challenge.

Dentistry and its educational community have reason to be proud of past achievement. The many professional attributes previously cited support this conclusion. However, the past alone need not be a limiting prologue for the future. Many colleagues suggest that if dentistry is to be prepared for the challenge and opportunity of the 21st century, the profession must never remain static with respect to any issue; for the future belongs to those who will assume a dynamic stance and search for the infinity of opportunity. The world is in a state of constant change, at a meteoric pace. Dentistry's choice is progression or regression; to stand fast on the past is to remain in the past.

Dr Dominic DePaola, Dean of the Baylor College of Dentistry, wrote in an issue of the *Journal of Dental Education,*

We have limited resources and our primary obligation is to educate students . . . .When resources are limited, we must revise or reinvent and explore new and perhaps even better ways to teach students, and not simply try to do the same things we have done in the past with fewer resources.

He goes on to add, "Certainly there should not be any university or system of higher education that will tolerate a dental school that continues to disseminate data that will be obsolete in a short period of time."[10] Many dental educators will point to examples of progressive change in dental education, but they will also point to the fact that many of the methods and means now used are the very same as those used at the beginning of the 20th century.

Ergonomic Strategy for the Future: From Zero to Infinity

Change can be a matter of simply building upon experience of the past or exploring the infinity of opportunity from a starting point free of past bias. In this way, one is not bound to what has been, but is free to seek what might be, what could be, and, perhaps, what should be. For many experienced practitioners of dentistry, it is often difficult to put aside the experience and expertise of past years and to explore and discover new options for the future of human performance. We may come to conclusions like those of the past, or we may come to conclusions unlike those of the past. It is essential that dentistry remain conscious of opportunity and accept both the burden and the benefit of discovery.

Human engineering in dentistry has been carried to a new level of opportunity in part through the efforts of Dr Daryl Beach of the Human Performance and Informatics Institute (HPI) and the Global LAN Center, in collaboration with the World Health Organization (WHO), academic institutions, professional organizations, dental industry, and individual dental professionals. Years of study and refinement have yielded a new logic for human performance. Through extensive observation and the comparison of various options, an optimal human-centered concept of ergonomics has been identified and applied to dental education and practice for more than three decades. It is called *performance logic;* for it allows an individual to logically derive the most natural method for the practice of dentistry. Following the principles of performance logic one can use proprioceptive self-awareness to determine the most efficient, stress-free process for performing dental procedures; design an optimal human-centered setting for dental practice; provide the highest quality of oral care; and increase productivity and profitability.[11]

In 1987, the World Health Organization cited the importance of performance logic in a report on the proceedings of an expert committee, stating that "oral health can be improved and the cost of equipment reduced, if the workplaces are designed to ensure optimum performance . . . The Performance Logic approach may be considered as a pointer to the future."

One of the fundamental precepts of performance logic is to begin with basic conditions and add to them only as needed. Every decision related to this concept of human-centered ergonomics is based on a philosophy called "zero concept for health and health care."[12]

Human-Centered Priorities: Reordering Dentistry's Focuses of Concern

Unlike past initiatives, human-centered ergonomics focuses first, and accords first priority to the task or patient (F-1), the reason for the profession's existence; secondly to the performer (dentist, dental hygienist) (F-2), and third and last to the environment or treatment setting (F-3). It is only after establishing the correct performer-to-patient relationship (F2-F1) that it is possible to develop a treatment setting to accommodate the requirements of practitioner and patient. While the practice environment is a substantial focus of concern, it should neither dictate nor influence the practitioner-to-patient relationship.

Proprioceptive Self-Derivation (pd): A Natural Basis for Decision

The determination of practitioner posture, patient positioning, the performance process, and the treatment setting is the product of proprioceptive self-derivation (pd) in human-centered ergonomics. The individual arrives at his or her conclusions by responding to the body's internal sensors through pertinent derivation protocols. These conclusions are never the product of mentor prescription, but are instead individually derived. The practitioner is neither directly told nor directly shown how to sit, how to position the patient, or how to maintain these relations in the performance process; for he or she may forget. Rather, the practitioner is personally and primarily involved in the decision making that leads to these conclusions, through pd, and fully understands and remembers the product of such derivations.[13] The proprioceptive pathway to occupational health and peak performance in dental practice requires practitioner attention to five simple steps.

Five Steps to Occupational Health and Peak Performance

These steps are as follows:

1. derivation of a natural, comfortable posture for the practitioner;
2. positioning the patient to accommodate the practitioner;
3. positioning operatory equipment to accommodate the practitioner;
4. positioning the operating light to illuminate the patient's oral cavity; and
5. maintaining established relationships among the practitioner, patient, equipment, and operating light by use of five movements and a 10-step protocol that ensure optimal performance without compromise of self, patient, or task.

Posture for Practitioner Health and Peak Performance

Given a task to be performed—a patient in need of oral care—the dentist or dental hygienist must first establish a natural and comfortable posture for optimal perception and control of a finite procedure. Inasmuch as one must overcome the influence of gravity to perform any act in earth's atmosphere, gravity is the zero point for the derivation of a posture. Furthermore, when the task to be performed demands a high order of consistent precision and accountability, it is necessary to do even more than simply overcome the force of gravity. The practitioner must establish a posture that also ensures stability and control of performance. This is accomplished through proprioceptive self-derivation that uses a standard protocol. It may be done with an operating stool, a sophisticated measurement frame such as the one in the Center for the Study of Human Performance in Dentistry at the Dental School of the University of Maryland or any device that can elevate and lower a small seating platform. The seating platform used for this purpose must be no larger than required to support the ischial tuberosities of the pelvis, and it must be free of any contoured padding or other design features that could influence the way in which one sits. The seat must not impose a bias in this determination. With eyes closed, the practitioner first determines a seating height for the lower half of the body, then an upper-body posture, followed by head position, and then an arm and hand position for the control of a precise and finite act. Without distorting the natural posture established at this point, the practitioner opens his or her eyes and attempts to view the task point or working point set by the thumbs and the forefingers of the dominant operating hand. If the practitioner can see the proprioceptively determined working point, the derivation of an optimal posture is complete. If not, then a slight adjustment of the head, the hands, or both will permit viewing the working point, and the derivation is completed. This self-derived posture contradicts the postures traditionally prescribed for contemporary dental practice. Traditional prescriptions for posture would have one sit with knees higher than buttocks, rotating the pelvis to the posterior, undoing the natural lordotic curvature of the spinal column, and leaving the upper surface of the thighs parallel to the plane of the floor. They further prescribe that one should place the forearms parallel to the plane of the floor. The working point so established would force the prospective patient's head into the lap of the practitioner, requiring the practitioner to drop his or her head to see the oral cavity. Such posture is, in fact, a prescription for musculoskeletal discomfort or pain and compromise of performance. In marked contrast to this prescription, a proprioceptively derived posture does not distort the body's natural form. The knees and buttocks are at a common level, the thighs slope downward from posterior to anterior, the spinal column is essentially erect, the lordotic curvature of the spine is maintained, the forearms are elevated above the horizontal, and the working point is significantly elevated (see Figure 1).[14]

Several thousand students and practitioners of dentistry and dental hygiene have derived their postures proprioceptively in the manner described. They now practice while maintaining their natural postures. In one of many studies conducted to determine the most natural and comfortable posture for dental practice, 100 unbiased physical therapy students were asked to

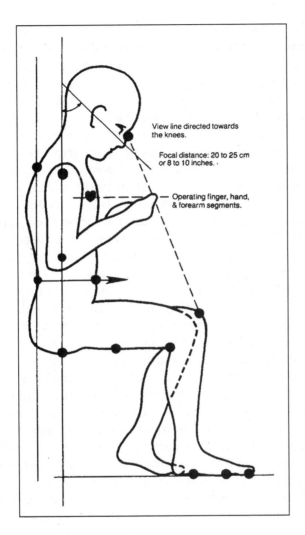

View line directed towards the knees.

Focal distance: 20 to 25 cm or 8 to 10 inches. ·

Operating finger, hand, & forearm segments.

FIGURE 1.—The balanced operator.

proprioceptively derive postures they would use to perform a finite act of precision, such as threading a needle or winding a watch. Each subject responded to a standard protocol three times. The results of the 300 observations confirmed the reliability and validity of the derivation process and clearly identified a preference for a posture unlike that seen among most practitioners, past and present.[15]

Positioning the Patient

The working point of a proprioceptively derived posture is the zero point for subsequent derivations. Having determined a point in space at which one prefers to consistently perform a finite task, it is possible to fix and stabilize the location of a patient, the practitioner, the dental assistant, and the armamentaria of the treatment setting. Setting everything to and from this point makes it possible to perform most dental procedures without compromise of posture. Without the initial determination of this consistent performance point, it is impossible to consistently fix and stabilize anything, and the practitioner is forced to continually reset and reposition the location of the patient, the treatment team, and the equipment. The correct fixation and stabilization of all elements of the practice environment minimizes the need for physical contact, reduces the chance of contamination, and improves the prospect for asepsis (see Chapter 13, "Ergonomically Correct Design Concepts of a Functioning Dental Office").

The practitioner is able to maintain a natural posture when the patient is placed in a supine, natural, full-rest position, with priority accorded head location, so that the patient's maxillary incisors contact the dentist's operating fingers at the preferred working point (see Figure 2). This can be achieved with most patient supports, including dental beds and dental chairs. Research indicates patient acceptance and preference for this supinated body position.[16,17] Any initial patient reluctance to accept nontraditional positioning is quickly alleviated when the patient realizes that this enables peak performance on the part of the dentist or dental hygienist.

Resetting the Practice Environment

To accommodate the practitioner-to-patient relationship and minimize the need for resetting and repositioning elements of the practice environment, the dental assistant, dental operating light, dental instruments, and the adjacent cabinetry are placed in a proprioceptively correct relationship to the working point. These relationships are optimized in treatment settings specifically designed for human-centered ergonomics (see Figure 3).[18] Reasonable alternatives to the ideal

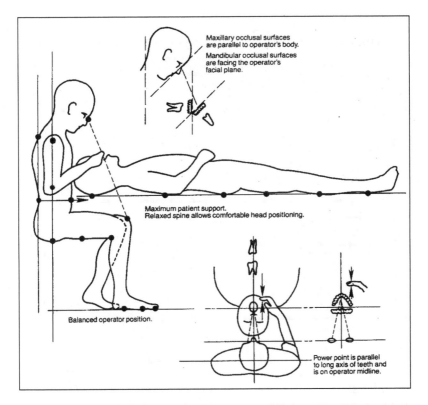

FIGURE 2.—Ideal patient positioning in relation to equipment.

can be achieved in traditional dental operatories, with varying degrees of compromise. The principles of human-centered ergonomics can be applied in existing treatment settings to reduce occupational ailments and improve prospects for peak performance.

Instrument Control

Zero-based decision logic, when applied to instrument control in intraoral performance, minimizes the number of instruments and the hand parts used to grasp them, and maximizes the manner of their application to optimize their intended effect upon performance. Only those instruments required for a particular procedure should be included in the preset sterilized trays or packs commonly used in aseptic

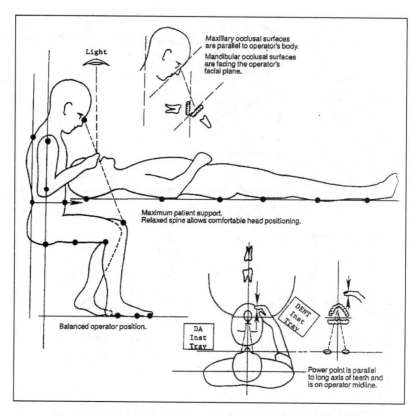

FIGURE 3.—Ideal patient positioning in relation to operator position.

practice. The hand grips by which they are held, placed, and stabilized in the oral cavity should be limited to the first three digits of the operating hand, unless instrument design requires greater control. Instruments should be applied so that their functional movement occurs in the mid-saggital plane and their controlled movement is a product of flexion rather than extension whenever possible. Intraoral stabilization is maximized by placing the third digit (middle finger) on the tooth or site of performance whenever possible and otherwise as close as possible to the procedural site (see Figure 4).[19]

Visual Perception

Whenever possible, direct viewing of procedural sites is preferred. However, when direct viewing compromises a

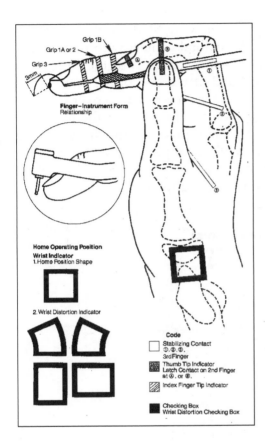

Figure 4.—Finger grips for intraoral treatment.

practitioner's proprioceptive posture, indirect viewing with a dental mirror is the necessary alternative. The use of mirrors in dentistry is too often the default option, when direct viewing of all aspects of a procedure is impossible. In part, this is the result of inadequate familiarization with the ease and benefit of mirror use in dental education. The dental mirror may be the most underused and beneficial instrument for the preservation of practitioner health, and yet it is too seldom the viewing medium of choice when circumstances logically call for its use.

The mirror that satisfies principles of human-centered ergonomics is much smaller than that in common use. This allows for correct placement and maximum viewing in the limited spaces of the oral cavity. The angular relationship between the extended axis of the handle and the reflective surface is set at 45 degrees to facilitate viewing by the seated practitioner. Its minimal bulk permits total contact with finger parts holding the mirror. It should be held lightly by the thumb and forefinger of the mirror hand at the end of the handle and introduced into the oral cavity by a wrist drop over the midface, between the cuspid points. For viewing the maxillary arch, the mirror is placed as far as possible from the site being viewed and is moved in a elliptical pattern that permits the practitioner to see all points of a tooth or procedural site without compromising posture (see Figure 5).[19]

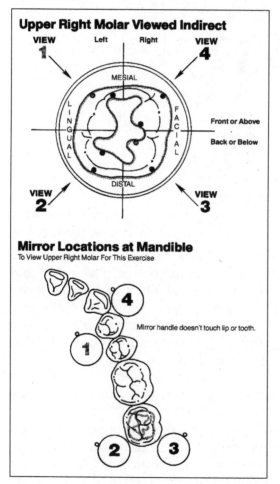

FIGURE 5.—Correct use of the dental mirror.

Five Movements That Maintain Practitioner Posture

Use of the following five movements enable the practitioner to maintain a natural and comfortable posture during the performance of dental procedures (see Figure 6):

1. operator movement about head of the patient, clockwise or counter-clockwise;
2. patient head movement by rotation, left or right;
3. patient head tilt, up or down;
4. patient mandible movement, minimally or maximally, for preferred mouth opening; and
5. elevation of the patient support, up or down.

Ten-Step Protocol for Optimal Perception and Control of Performance Without Compromise of Practitioner, Task, or Patient

Following is a 10-step decision process by which a dentist or dental hygienist can proprioceptively derive the performer-to-task spatial relations that assure achievement of performance outcome without compromise of self, task, or patient. It applies to the majority of treatment procedures in all disciplines of dentistry. When exception presents, it should be accommodated exceptionally (see Table 1).[19]

Key to this and any decision process is a consistent starting point. The starting point from which this protocol begins is the practitioner seated in a stable, natural posture, at the 12 o'clock position, directly behind the patient's head. The patient's head is centered, and the maxillary occlusal plane is offset from the vertical axis by 5 to 10 degrees. The patient's maxillary incisors are in contact with the forefinger of the practitioner's dominant operating hand, which is at the dentist's preferred working point. To begin from any other starting point would compromise the decision process and the practitioner's posture.

1. Establish appropriate intermaxillary opening.
2. Grasp instrument or item to be used with thumb and forefinger.
3. Place instrument or item in correct relationship to task site.

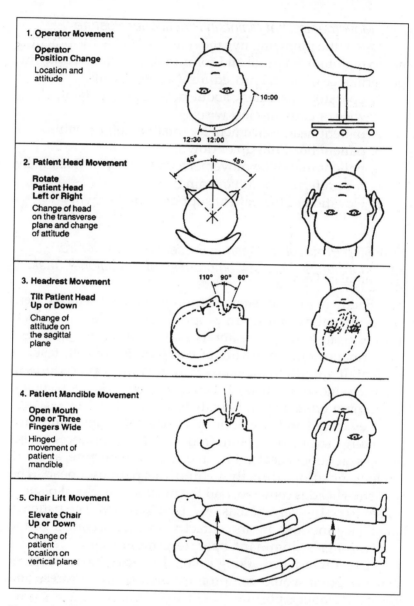

1. Operator Movement

**Operator
Position Change**

Location and
attitude

10:00

12:30 12:00

2. Patient Head Movement

**Rotate
Patient Head
Left or Right**

Change of head
on the transverse
plane and change
of attitude

45°   45°

3. Headrest Movement

**Tilt Patient Head
Up or Down**

Change of
attitude on
the sagittal
plane

110° 90° 60°

4. Patient Mandible Movement

**Open Mouth
One or Three
Fingers Wide**

Hinged
movement of
patient
mandible

5. Chair Lift Movement

**Elevate Chair
Up or Down**

Change of
patient
location on
vertical plane

FIGURE 6.—Five movements to maintain operator balance.

4. Stabilize instrument or item with middle finger on task
   site or as proximally as possible.
5. Check posture to determine whether steps 1 through 4
   have compromised posture. If not, then proceed directly
   to Step 6. If posture is compromised, correct posture by

Table 1.—Ten Steps to Optimal Perception and Control Without Compromise of Practitioner, Patient, or Task

1. Establish Appropriate Intermaxillary Opening
2. Grasp Instrument or Item with Thumb and Forefinger
3. Place Instrument or Item to Place at Task Site
4. Stabilize Instrument or Item with Middle Finger on Task Site or as Proximal as Possible
5. Check Posture and Correct if Compromised
6. Check Vector or Force Application to Assure Alignment with Mid-Saggital Plane
7. Plan to Move Instrument or Item from Distant Point to Near Point
8. Establish Eye-to-Task Sightline with Direct or Indirect Viewing
9. Simulate Performance
10. Perform Act

---

rotation of patient's head right or left and by practitioner movement clockwise or counter-clockwise.

6. Check vector of force (axis of instrument or item action) to ensure alignment with mid-saggital plane. If adjustment is necessary, correct by patient head rotation or practitioner movement.
7. Plan to move instrument or item from distant point to near point on task site.
8. Establish eye-to-task sight line, using direct or indirect viewing as appropriate.
9. Simulate performance to ensure optimal perception and control.
10. Perform act to achieve the planned outcome.

This 10-step protocol applies to procedures and intraoral sites common to the practice of general dentistry and many specialty disciplines. If used correctly, it will consistently provide the dentist and dental hygienist with correct postural and positional relations that preserve practitioner health and enable peak performance. One may encounter tasks to which the principles of human-centered ergonomics will not apply—they are few. When they present, they are accommodated in an exceptional manner. It is unlikely that any practice concept will satisfy each and every task encountered in dentistry. The intent of human-centered ergonomics is to focus on those challenges that are common and that predominate in dental practice.

Diverse Applications in Dentistry

Human-centered ergonomics has been applied success-fully to dental hygiene and periodontics, operative dentistry, pediatric dentistry, fixed prosthodontics, removable pros-thodontics, endodontics, exodontia, and orthodontics. Ex-amples may be found in both dental education and private practice. Human-centered ergonomics has been taught for more than three decades to students and experienced prac-titioners alike.

Achieving the Optimal in Nonoptimal Practice Settings

The realities of dental practice require that most practitioners use traditional equipment and work settings for the trial of a new concept. Few students and practitioners can expect to begin in an optimal environment designed for human-centered ergono-mics. Some may be able to change their work environment at the outset. Some may do so at a later date. Most will have to be content with the present circumstances of their practice.

A five-step protocol has been developed for the applica-tion of human-centered ergonomics to traditional dental prac-tices. It assumes an operatory equipped with a dental chair, dental operating light, stools for the dentist and assistant, in-strument delivery systems, and cabinets, all of which may be placed in a variety of positions. The degree of positioning flex-ibility will determine the degree to which a practitioner can satisfy the principles of this ergonomic concept.

In step 1, the practitioner adjusts the height of the operat-ing stool to accommodate a natural, comfortable, and proprioceptively derived posture. Once seated, the practitio-ner reconfirms this posture and prepares to set the rest of the practice setting to satisfy the preferred working point for opti-mal perception and control of finite performance. In step 2, the practitioner positions the patient in the dental chair, places the patient in a supine position, and locates the patient's head so that the patient's maxillary central incisors contact his or her preferred working point. In step 3, the practitioner sets and stabilizes the instrument delivery systems of the dentist and dental assistant proximally, to facilitate ease of access. In step 4, the dental operating light is set and stabilized directly above the oral cavity and slightly to the rear, so as to illuminate most operating sites from one position. This eliminates the need for frequent repositioning of the light. In step 5, the practitioner employs the Five Movements to Control Practitioner Posture and the 10-Step Protocol for Optimal Perception and Control to determine the postural and positional relations necessary to perform a dental procedure without compromise of self, task, or patient (see Table 2).[19]

Accepting the Challenge in Academia

At the Dental School of the University of Maryland and the Faculty of Dentistry at the University of British Columbia,

---

Table 2.—Five Steps to Human-Centered Ergonomics in Traditional Dental Practice Settings

1. **Establish Your Optimal and Comfortable Posture** for the Control of Finite Performance by Proprioceptive Self-Derivation.
2. **Position the Patient** to Maximize Your Physical and Visual Access to the Oral Cavity and to Assure Control of Performance without Compromise of Posture.
3. **Place and Stabilize Your Instrument Delivery Modalities** of in Proprioceptively Correct Proximal Locations.
4. **Place and Stabilize the Dental Operating Light** to Provide Adequate Illumination from One Position.
5. **Use the 5 Movements to Maintain Operator Balance and the 10-Step Critical Path to Optimal Perception and Control of Performance without Compromise of Practitioner, Patient, or Task** to determine the correct postural and positional relations for practitioner, patient, and assistant.

human-centered ergonomics (performance logic) has been the basis for preclinical psychomotor education and clinical practice in most disciplines of dentistry in the 4-year undergraduate curriculum. On the first day of their dental education, students are acquainted with fundamentals of performance logic. This initial inquiry into the principles of human-centered ergonomics continues for several months, and students begin to apply concept principles in early technique laboratory courses preceding subsequent simulation exercises. Students individually derive their postures proprioceptively and make impressions on their student partners, in a clinical setting, within the first months of their dental education. They advance to realistic patient simulations of periodontic and operative dentistry technique in sophisticated simulation facilities. The realism of such learning environments prepares and eases their transition to patient care in later years. To facilitate learning, these programs employ certain lead-up exercises to prepare students for psychomotor performance.[18]

In the second year, students acquire clinical skills in the disciplines of pediatric dentistry, endodontics, prosthodontics, exodontia, and dental auxiliary utilization in simulation facilities, prior to beginning patient care in the general practice clinics. In the third and fourth years, students apply principles of human-centered ergonomics to comprehensive patient care. Although these dental school experiences are conducted in ideal settings, students are also shown how to apply human-centered ergonomics to practice settings like those they will encounter in the "real world" of dentistry.[18]

The Dental School and the Faculty of Dentistry offer courses in human-centered ergonomics to the practice community several times each year. These courses are presented by a consortium of North American educators and are conducted in school settings, at major professional meetings, and in private offices. *The high incidence of work-related repetitive stress injuries and cumulative trauma disorders among dental workers prompts many dentists and dental hygienists to attend these courses.*

Both institutions are WHO Collaborating Centers for the Development of New and Advanced Methods for Training Dental Personnel. They have conducted international symposia on performance logic and performance simulation, welcomed faculty from nearly 40 nations and more than 70 educational institutions to select courses in human-centered ergonomics, and hosted several overseas colleagues on sabbatical leave to study this new priority in dental education.[20]

Human Priorities for Dentistry in the 21st Century

To change or not to change, that is dentistry's ever present choice. The profession may elect to rest upon past laurels, justifiably proud of its heritage and record of achievement in service to the patient community. Its priority can remain with the many new and exciting advances in the science and technology of dentistry, postponing change in the way we work. However, most in dentistry are acutely aware of the impact of occupational demands upon their well-being, the quality of practice life, and their potential for peak performance. It is now time for dentistry to recognize and act upon the high incidence of work-related ailments in the profession at large. If human beings can go from early flight to space exploration in less than a century, dentistry can reject its historic adaptation to the presumed requirements of equipment and settings considered "state-of-the-art" and accord like or greater priority to the real and human-centered requirements of those who provide oral health care in the near term. The transition from machine-centered ergonomics to human-centered ergonomics is a major focus of concern and action in many industries seeking to optimize the quality of employee performance while reducing the risk of occupational injury. The objectives for dentistry now, and in the years to come, should be no less.

REFERENCES

1. Silverstein B, et al. Draft, Ergonomic Protection Standard: Summary of Key Provisions. Washington, DC: Occupational Safety and Health Administration; June 1994.
2. Dainoff MJ, Dainoff MH. *People and Productivity: A Manager's Guide to the Electronic Office.* Toronto, Canada: Holt, Rinehart and Company; 1986.

3. Gallup poll rates dentists in top three groups in public confidence. *ADA News.* November 7, 1994; 29.
4. Murtomaa H. Work-related complaints of dentists and dental assistants. *International Archives of Occupational Health.* 1982; 50:231–236.
5. Hope-Ross K, Corcoran D. A survey of dentists' working posture. *Journal of the Irish Dental Association.* 1985;32(3):13–18.
6. Shugars D, Miller D, Williams D, Fishburne C, Strickland D. Musculoskeletal pain among dentists. *General Dentistry.* 1987; 35(4):272–276.
7. Belenky M. Human performance and clinical simulation: the integration of human-centered ergonomics and psychomotor education in dental education. *Proceedings, 2nd International Symposium on Simulation in Dental Education: State of the Art.* Köln, Germany, 6–7 April, 1992.
8. Kimmel K, Walker R. *Practising Dentistry: Ergonomic Guidelines for the Future.* Berlin and Chicago: Buch-und Zeitschriften-Verlag "Die Quintessenz"; 1972.
9. Kilpatrick H. *Work Simplification in Dental Practice: Applied Time and Motion Studies.* 3rd ed. Philadelphia: WB Saunders Company; 1974.
10. DePaola DP. Dental schools are members of the academy: survival demands a primary focus on scholarship. *Journal of Dental Education.* 1994;58(1):7–11.
11. Morganstein W. Performance logic: the ultimate application. *Journal of Dental Practice Administration.* 1983;1(1):31–__.
12. Beach D. Zero concept for health and health care, report of a conference on the health of the dental professional, Chicago. *Journal of the American Dental Association.* 1987;114(4):515–518.
13. Moffitt W. Performance logic in periodontics. Presented at the Annual Meeting of the American Association of Dental Schools, Washington, DC, 1986.
14. Belenky M, Manski R, Terashita M. Human performance in dentistry: student self-derivation of optimal posture and position for the application and control of finite psychomotor skills. Abstract, *Journal of Dental Education.* 1989;53(1):60–61.
15. Colangelo G, Hobart D, Belenky M, Bechtel R. Elbow angle during a simulated task requiring fine psychomotor control. *Journal of Dental Education.* 1991;55(12):785–788.
16. Schoen D, Belenky M, Grace E, Cohen L. A comparison of patient satisfaction using two different support systems. *Journal of Dental Practice Administration.* 1989;6(2):61–64.

17. Grace E, Schoen D, Cohen L. Chair inclination and patient comfort. *Journal of Dental Practice Administration.* 1990;6 (2):__–__.
18. Wittenstrom J. *A Human-Centered Base for Office Design,* Chapter 6 in: *Successful Office Design* Practice Management Series. Chicago: American Dental Association; 1994:55–66.
19. Belenky M. Performance Logic in Clinical Dentistry: A Teaching Syllabus of the Center for the Study of Human Performance in Dentistry. Dental School, University of Maryland at Baltimore; 1994.
20. Belenky M. Human performance in dental education: the Maryland model. *Journal of the Japanese Association for Dental Education.* 1991;17(12):103–116.

Optimizing Dental Operatory Working Environments

Lance M. Rucker, DDS, and
Marcia A. Boyd, DDS, MA

Abstract

It is a sufficient challenge for any dental professional to understand and practice the principles of good surgical ergonomics, even in an *ideal* working environment. Although the worker must combat the effects of prior habits that may conspire against postural health, a truly ideal work setting supports and promotes balanced working postures rather than eccentric, imbalanced postures. However, it is quite another level of challenge for a worker to be confronted with a less-than-ideal equipment setting, complicated by poorly designed and poorly arranged operatory hardware, cabinetry, and pathways for the movement of dental personnel and patients to and from the operating site.

Compromised dental operatory environments can be made to work effectively to support good postural balance if specific guidelines are followed to ensure that the basic principles of good surgical ergonomics are not unwittingly undermined because of the operatory setting.

Introduction

In 1987, more than 300 Swedish dentists were surveyed, and intervention regimens were devised for their wide-ranging back, neck, and shoulder pains.[1-6] Half were given ergonomic instruction, and the other half were given physical therapy in addition to their instruction. In a 1990 follow-up survey, the researchers found that both approaches were equally futile in dealing with the dentists' problems. A most interesting observation from their study, however, was that "significantly more dentists without symptoms of pain [had] applied a wedge cushion under the upper part of the back of a patient to get an optimum view into the oral cavity." This observation may not have been so trivial as the researchers assumed.

The nuts and bolts of surgical ergonomics have been laid out in previous chapters. The real challenge is to apply those principles to equipment and settings that are less than ideal. When the operatory furniture will not allow optimal patient and operator positioning, which parameters of the postures and positions are most critical to good surgical ergonomics? Are there ways in which equipment might be easily modified or adjusted, or used so as to minimize the compromise and optimize the ergonomics?

Surgical Ergonomics in Compromised Settings

Every setting involves a certain degree of compromise, although some are more obviously compromising than others. Therefore, as a rule, one should assume that *all* equipment is potentially compromising equipment. However, what is probably more detrimental to the postural balance of the operator than the hardware configuration of the operating setting (i.e., the physical layout of the operatory equipment) is the way in which the operator *uses* the settings available.

The good news is that very few hardware settings actually preclude balanced use. Admittedly, some settings may challenge the orienting of the participants (operator, patient, and assistant) so that optimal balance may be achieved by all during the psychomotor performances. However, for most hardware settings, a surprisingly low level of awareness and/or postural accommodation is required to allow complete balance during all critical phases of a clinical procedure.

Five Criteria for Using Any Operatory Equipment

There are five criteria for balanced use of any operatory setting. Only when these criteria are met can there be any chance of applying the concepts of good surgical ergonomics:

1. operator stabilization with proper seating height;

2. patient support that places the oral cavity at the optimal control operating point;
3. control of the maxillary plane;
4. clearance around patient's head to allow unimpeded operator access from the 10 o'clock position to the 12:30 position; and
5. positioning of the light.

OPERATOR STABILIZATION WITH PROPER SEATING HEIGHT

For a seated operator, the single most crucial prerequisite for balanced intraoral operation is an operating stool (or chair) that can be adjusted to the proper height for each operator as shown in Figure 1 (see Chapter 11, "Human-Centered Ergonomics").

In a multiuser setting, it is especially important that this operator stool be height-adjustable to serve the range of leg-

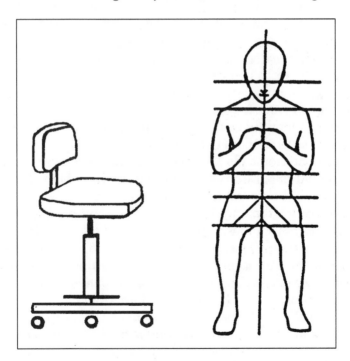

FIGURE 1.—For a seated operator, the most crucial prerequisite for balanced intraoral operation is a stool or chair that can be adjusted to the proper height.

lengths and variations in footwear. High-heeled shoes or thick soles demand a higher seating base. Most secretarial or clinic stools with standard gas-cylinder adjustability will serve most operators. If the stool is a one-touch height-adjustable stool, it can easily be adjusted so that the several clinical operators who use it during a day can maintain stable, balanced working bases.

Stools with a negative slant tip the user backward, requiring either back and thigh muscle isometrics or a static backrest pressure to keep the operator's torso upright. These stools should be avoided. If the operator is especially tall or the seat height is too short, this same backward tipping occurs. If the seat pan contour is too great, the operator may find the effect destabilizing.

In general, a simple one-touch height-adjustable stool will best serve all operators in maintaining a stable, balanced working base. It is a nice bonus if the seat is also comfortable for nonoperating interactions (e.g., when the operator is interviewing the patient or performing nonclinical functions).

Once the seated posture is balanced, the other criteria can be met.

PATIENT SUPPORT THAT PLACES THE ORAL CAVITY AT THE OPTIMAL CONTROL OPERATING POINT

This criterion calls for adjustment of the patient chair (or bed) so that the oral cavity is brought to the balanced operating point of the operator, not vice versa.

More often than not in ergonomically compromised practices, the dental chair is initially positioned so that the patient's oral cavity is only part of the way to the optimal operating position. Then the dentist is left to adapt around the patient's body and/or the equipment to access the patient's mouth. The assistant must then adapt to this adaptation!

Generally, most modern equipment allows the operator and assistant to work in surgical balance. The objective can be met with an articulating dental chair, as well as with a platform, dental bed, or dental chair that flattens entirely (see Figure 2).

The greater the angle of articulation of the chairback is, the greater the challenge is in achieving criteria 3 and 4. For

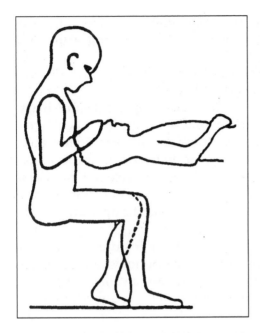

FIGURE 2.—Using a platform, a dental bed, or a dental chair that flattens entirely to provide surgical balance.

example, when the patient is semireclined in an articulating chair, the position of the patient's mouth no longer dominates the relationship to the dental chair. The patient's weight sliding down into the seat and the dimensions of the seat will determine the relationship to the dental chair. This automatically demands operator accommodation such as reaching around the chairback or reaching over the top of the extended chair or the headrest. Alternatively, the compromise forces the operator to move to the 7 to 9 o'clock range so as to gain access to the oral cavity *en face*. This accommodation invites, and usually forces, a twisting of the operator's torso with one or both elbows raised in adaptation.

Some patients may complain about movement of the dental chair backwards toward the horizontal position in spite of the fact that they are likely to recline to this position each night for sleeping. They are often even more restless about being tilted back and then maintained just beyond 45 degrees, at about the supine position of a partially reclined chair. There are strong negative psychological stimuli associated with being so positioned. The swallow reflex is encumbered and the base of the tongue is not fully at rest to safely occlude the oropharynx. Some practitioners are able to avoid these side effects by pre-positioning the patient chair horizontally and then inviting the patient to self-position, prior to treatment.

CONTROL OF THE MAXILLARY PLANE

Inadequate control of the angle of the patient's maxillary plane* can cause the operator to work out of balance. Even with the correct light position, the angle of the patient's maxillary plane can determine the working posture of the spinal column. The maxillary plane dictates (and usually parallels) the angle of the operator's spine, regardless of where the operator is sitting and regardless of whether the operating site is maxillary or mandibular.

You probably already know that your posture is controlled by the patient's head position. What you may *not* have realized is that the maxilla provides a readily available *gauge* by which you can make changes that will let you work in comfortable, balanced postures.

For most intraoral access sites, the maxillary plane should be extended approximately 7 degrees beyond the vertical (see Figure 3a). For treatment of most maxillary second and third molars, the maxillary plane may be extended to approximately 25 degrees beyond the vertical. For treatment of the anterior mandibular sextant, the head and neck may be flexed to bring the maxillary plane to approximately 8 degrees ahead of the vertical.

The goal should be the initial achievement of an essentially vertical maxillary plane. In practice, many operators miss this goal. It is not uncommon to see dentists attempting to treat supine patients with maxillary planes tipped forward more than 30 degrees ahead of the vertical. These dentists are easily recognized by out-of-balance torso postures such as that illustrated in Figure 3b.

Control of the maxillary plane is best achieved by adjustment of the angle of the patient's backrest, by articulation of the headrest, and/or by creative use of neck-pillows or mini-

---

*Although the maxilla is most accurately represented by a curved surface, we are for purposes of this discussion referring to its "occlusal plane," which is defined as the plane of most cusps tips and incisal edges from tooth 1.6 to tooth 2.6 (Federal Dentaire Internationale).

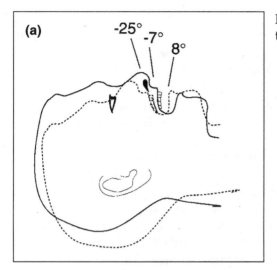

Figure 3.—Control of the maxillary plane.

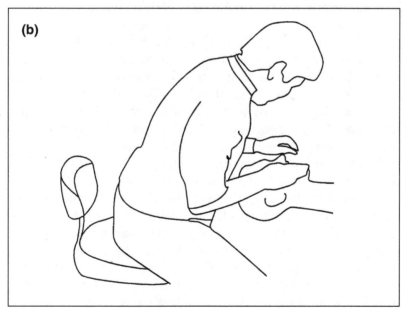

bolsters. Some patients may achieve the required access via voluntary head extension and flexion.

Once the goal is achieved, ask the patient for further extension as needed to treat distal maxillary molars, or invite flexion when treating mandibular anteriors. Most patients will appreciate (or even require) support from pillows or wedges in order to maintain such positions.

Sometimes facial anatomy can be deceiving: remember, it isn't the angle of the patient's forehead or the nose that is important for attaining uncompromised intraoral access. The true angle of the maxillary plane is most accurately and conveniently checked from the right side the patient's head, upper lip and cheek retracted, with your head tipped to the 9 o'clock position (or from 3 o'clock for assistants or left-handed operators).

In exceptional situations, the maxillary plane cannot be easily controlled. For example, the patient may be unable to lie supine without encountering breathing problems (e.g., with congestive heart problems). Such a patient may be able to hyperextend the head and neck to provide a vertical maxillary plane (in spite of the raised backrest). Occasionally, depending upon the nature of the intraoral procedure, it may even be preferable from an ergonomic perspective to raise the patient's backrest to near vertical and to operate in a stand-up position. In such stand-up strategies, it is the chairside assistant who is likely to suffer the most. If you are unwilling or unable to stand, you must be resigned to your own seated postural compromise during the treatment of such patients.

What about the patient with physical restrictions to the articulation of the head and neck? This patient may be able to tolerate a greater head-down incline of the backrest to provide a vertical maxillary plane. Otherwise, once again, the dentist and assistant will be forced to operate out of balance.

Conscientious control of the patient's maxillary plane does not guarantee good postural balance for the operator, *but lack of control of the patient's maxillary plane is certain to cause poor postures* for both the dentist and the dental assistant.

A poorly controlled maxillary plane places the dentist's torso (upper body) out of balance, which can drive the dentist to select a lighting position that further reinforces the postural dysfunction.

Articulating headrests are usually helpful, depending upon their design. If they do not adequately support the patient's head, they may be coupled with a wedge or bolster for the head or neck. Patient chairs without articulating headrests definitely require some means of helping the patient achieve and support the extended and flexed head positions required for the angles that allow balanced surgical access to all areas of the mouth.

CLEARANCE AROUND PATIENT'S HEAD TO ALLOW UNIMPEDED OPERATOR ACCESS FROM THE 10 O'CLOCK POSITION TO THE 12:30 POSITION

Most dentists and hygienists attempt to use a wider range. The range from 7 to 9 o'clock is fraught with twists, sways, and elbow "winging." Furthermore, as discussed in Chapter 11, virtually all sites in the mouth can be accessed using the more conservative range from 10 o'clock to 12:30 (see Figure 4).

It is important to ensure that access is truly unimpeded. If the patient's back and head supports are designed so that the operator's thighs cannot be freely turned beneath the patient chair, the operator will be forced to gain access to certain clock positions by spreading the knees and thighs widely apart and leaning forward, or by twisting with knees together on one side or the other. The latter accommodation is usually coupled with further twisting and leaning of the torso and/or "winging" of one or both elbows.

Because the height of the seating platform is usually greater for the dental assistant, who requires access through the 1 o'clock to 4 o'clock range, the assistant will usually experience a slight twist of the torso during intraoral work and during certain extraoral instrument manipulations.

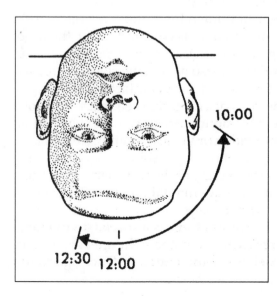

FIGURE 4.—Access to the patient's head from the 10 o'clock position to the 12:30 position should be unimpeded.

In some operatories, the patient chair base must be moved so that the operator can move freely throughout the range. Consideration must be given to the location of the delivery carts and trays so that they do not restrict proper working access for the operator and the assistant.[7] Ideally, the operator can retrieve, use, and return instruments with no Class V motions[8] and a minimum of Class III and Class IV motions. Fortunately, most modern delivery systems permit ergonomic balance in all phases of instrument management. However, it is more critical that the operator be in balance during the manipulation of instruments intraorally than during the retrieval and replacement of instruments. This rule applies whether the operator is working assisted or unassisted.

POSITIONING OF THE LIGHT

Many dental assistants and some dentists have been trained that the optimal location for the operatory light source for a supine patient is 1) directly above the patient's mouth for mandibular treatment sites and 2) directly above the patient's abdomen for maxillary treatment sites, so that it shines more directly on the maxilla. Unfortunately, when this second guideline is followed, *either* the maxillary sites are beset with shadowing *or* the operator must twist out of balance to see most operating sites clearly.

The issue is not one of human limitations or preferences; it is a problem of physics. In the case of *direct vision*, the need is to have the *light line as coaxial as possible to the sight line (as close to the same line as possible)* so as to have shadow-free intraoral operating sites. This fairly obvious fact implies a light line that just clears the head of the operator so that no shadow is cast on the oral field. A mouth mirror can also be used to reflect secondary illumination onto the operating sites. Head-mounted fiber-optic light sources are a solution for those who can tolerate the additional weight of these systems. They may also present a problem of unintentional blinding flashes into the assistant's and/or patient's eyes.

With *mirror vision*, however, there is a special dominating factor: the same mirror must carry the light onto the site as carries the view to the eye of the operator. Once again, for optimal illumination, the light line must be as coaxial as possible to the sight line. *The greater the deviation* of light line from eye line is, *the greater the shadowing.* As long as light line and eye line are within 15 degrees of each other (Figure 5a), the view will be essentially unshadowed and will be highly visible with use of standard mouth mirrors (up to size 5). What happens in most operatories is that dentists act like "fireflies drawn to the light." Rather than moving the light, the operator will tip or twist the body to bring the eye line closer to the light line "in order to see better" (Figure 5b).

The good news is that a single light source can provide a well-lit, unshadowed view to allow balanced operation on a supine patient. For both mandibular and maxillary treatment, the light source must be in the patient's mid-saggital plane directly above and slightly behind the patient's oral cavity, approximately 5 degrees toward the head of an operator in the 12 o'clock position. To confirm this location, test that your sight line to the maxillary central incisors is within 15 degrees of the light line throughout a full range of operator clock positions around the head of the patient.

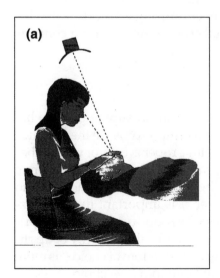
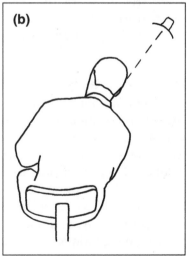

FIGURE 5.—Light line and eye line should be within 15 degrees of each other for an unshadowed view.

Because this positioning implies that there will be little need for anyone to move the light once the patient has been properly positioned, the light source can be as far above the heads of both operator and assistants as will *just* allow the assistant to reach it. It will be out of the way for both dentist and assistant but can still be moved for exceptional needs. The focal length of most modern operatory lights can be adjusted to work well at this range. (Consult your dental supplier for further details.)

The usual blocks to achievement of the fifth criterion are operating lights that are poorly mounted or that are restricted in their articulation so that they do not reach the designated location. These may be short-armed chair-based lights, or they may be fixed wall-mount or ceiling-mount lights. Most can be remounted to permit proper placement, to serve the operator's needs for surgical ergonomic balance.

The light line must be as coaxial as possible to the sight line, whether the operator view is direct or indirect (via a mouth mirror). The advantages of optimal light positioning are many, including

- superior intraoral illumination,
- support of balanced operating postures,
- the reduction of postural compromises, and
- the reduction of potential cross-contaminating contacts with light handles.

Default to Balance

When a patient is unable to present in supine posture because of medical restrictions or is unable to provide the operator with an adequate mouth opening for proper access, or when other exceptions conspire to compromise the operator's ergonomic balance, it is appropriate that the hardware can be adjusted to permit such exceptions. However, it is important that the flexibility that allows for such exceptions not undermine the primary promotion of ergonomic balance for the majority of applications. In ergonomics, the concept of "freedom of choice" is more often than not best replaced with "freedom *from* choice."

The working environment must support basic balanced operator-driven ergonomics, yet be flexible enough to accommodate multiple users and multiple patient requirements. Ideally, clinical settings should be arranged and used so that they *default to balance*. That is, the equipment should have as its default setting a configuration that supports balanced operation. Microchips can allow most simply for such default settings, but mechanical equivalents can also be used. Most important is the operator's awareness of counter-productive overadjustability (too much choice) and the promotion of simple, rapid adjustments. Dr Daryl Beach, one of the pioneers of dental ergonomic research, has claimed that if any setting requires more than 7 seconds to adjust, 50% of users will either not adjust it properly or will not adjust it at all (unless the job description includes specific responsibility for setup of equipment, as is the case in some operating room suites).[9] Compliance is reduced as the time requirement for proper setup increases to 15 seconds, at which point *no one* will adjust it properly, if at all. Observations in general clinical settings support these findings, but only when operators have good training in equipment adjustment. Otherwise, the compliance is even poorer.

Most measures of clinical success are based on visual parameters: how results should "look," rather than how the integrated process feels, sounds, or even smells. It is often assumed by the dentist, particularly the novice dentist, that it is more important to visually control an operation than to seek high *proprioceptive* and nonvisual *exteroceptive* control. Is the predominant emphasis on visual control in dentistry appropriate? One study has determined that a relatively small portion of an operator's dimensional accuracy in the use of the high-speed rotary handpiece for operative tooth preparation is attributable to visual control during the preparation.[10] This could imply that musculoskeletal postural balance should be compromised only with great circumspection for the sake of visual control.

During an operative procedure, a dentist is usually able to see the operating site before beginning an action. From time to time, the dentist is able to see where and how the instrument can be applied. The dentist may also stop the operation periodically to inspect visually the accuracy with which the desired end product is being achieved. However, because of the nature of rotary burs and their attendant water slurries, and the limitations imposed by subgingival sites, the dentist is often unable to maintain visual control of the instrument or bur tip throughout the entire procedure.

Trade-Offs

Sometimes operatory hardware must be rearranged to achieve the five basic criteria for balance. What happens if the rearrangement interferes with optimal access to instrument trays, egress paths from the operatory, and so forth? In the hierarchy of priorities for oral health care, what happens at the primary site of operation is more important than virtually everything else in the office protocol. If the operator must use a less-than-optimal stretch or twist to reach an instrument tray or dynamic instrument delivery system, or must step away from the operating position to wash or put on gloves, that is more acceptable than the persistence of conditions that mandate out-of-balance operation during the intraoral manipulation of dental instruments.

Barrier Issues

We live in an age of increasing awareness of contamination and cross-contamination. With these sensitivities has come a commensurate increase in barrier protection in all aspects of dental practice. The effects of increased use of barrier protection on surgical ergonomics are serious and often encumbering. Gloves reduce tactile feedback and may increase risks of carpal tunnel syndrome and other repetitive strain injuries.[11] Concerns about cross-contamination militate against intermittent manual contact with operatory adjustment buttons and knobs unless the contacted surfaces are barrier protected in a way that conveniently and safely allows such adjustments.

The concepts of balanced surgical ergonomics and default-for-balance hardware settings, as discussed above, minimize (and often eliminate) the need for adjustment during a procedure.[12–14] Specifically, once set, the light should *not* have to be adjusted, nor should the height and angle of the patient chair. Depending on the specific procedures planned, it may be necessary to adjust the articulating headrest to change the angle of the maxillary plane. This approach can reduce the costs of barrier protection as well as reduce the risks of cross-contamination.

Left-Handed or Right-Handed: Lateral Preferences and Optimal Operatories

Each of us has a preference, however slight, for the use of one hand over the other. Nearly 50% of North Americans are *anatomically* left-handed.[15] That is, they were born with distinctive differences in their corpus callosum, the part of the brain connecting the left and right cerebral hemispheres. Our society is dominated by the right-handed majority, and a wide range of cultural, historical, and societal pressures supports dominant use of the right hand. But for such pressures, all of those anatomically left-handed North Americans would probably use their left hand in preference to their right for most tasks.

However, only 14% of North Americans are *functionally* left-handed.[16] That is, a majority of the anatomically left-handed people *operate* right-handed. These people were converted to their right-handedness long before the origin of their conscious knowledge. Some researchers speculate that this may be important vis-à-vis reading and learning disorders. For some people it's a matter of custom; the percentage of functional left-handers is much less in certain societies. For other people it is a matter of convenience. Given that most of the world is set up for right-handed operation—instruments, machinery, workspaces—almost everything is designed for right-handed use.

There are certain times when being left-handed has its benefits. For example, left-handed women have a distinct advantage when buttoning their own clothes. The design for buttons and snaps on women's clothing is the reverse of that on men's clothing—a carry-over from times when ladies had right-handed servants to dress them. Of course, this also means that left-handed men are at a *dis*advantage in getting dressed and undressed.

Sometimes being left-handed confers very special status. Take baseball for example: a left-handed batter has considerable advantage, particularly against right-handed pitchers. A left-handed pitcher is highly valued in this game as well.

What about dentistry? Does it matter whether you are left-handed, right-handed, or ambidextrous? Of course it does. Most operatory equipment, cabinetry, and instruments are designed (by right-handers, usually) for the largest dental market: right-handed operators. Although "swing designs" are now available from some manufacturers, there are major implications for all other elements of the operatory, including fixed cabinetry, which dictate real compromises for even the cleverest convertible units on the market. This makes it difficult for left-handed dentists and dental hygienists to share operatories with right-handed practitioners. Therefore, from both economic and ergonomic perspectives, the ideal dental office would have left-handed chairside assistants paired with right-handed dentists and right-handed dental hygienists, all operating on right-handed equipment, or vice versa.

However, left-handed operators who do manage to find specialized equipment, who modify their operatories to properly serve their ergonomic needs, and who recruit matching hygienists to share their office spaces (unless they choose to relegate their hygienists to limited right-handed operatories only) are in for a real treat. *Right-handed chairside assistants find left-handed dentists especially easy to work with in four-handed dentistry.* Depending on the assistant's own degree of lateral manual preference, the right-handed assistant can work much more efficiently and smoothly with a left-handed dentist. *And* . . . more right-handed assistants are available than left-handed assistants. Certain problems may arise for expanded intraoral auxiliary duties, but if the delivery systems are ergonomically sound, a right-handed expanded-duties assistant should have no problem performing the usual range of expanded duties such as fissure sealants, impressions, and prophylaxes in a left-handed operatory.

The same observations apply for left-handed assistants working with right-handed dentists. In other words, higher demand for these assistants (from greater numbers of right-handed dentists, who are aware of the advantages) and less supply (because there are fewer left-handed assistants) spells BIG ADVANTAGE for left-handed dental assistants.

Well . . . there have to be *some* compensations to left-handers for living in a right-handed world, don't there?

Summary

Much can be done by dental personnel to optimize the ergonomics of operatory working environments. In particular, quick and easy modification of operatory hardware to accommodate the criteria explained in this chapter will allow for a more ergonomically balanced, efficiently operated working environment.

Remember the five criteria for using any operatory settings in balance:
1. operator stabilization with proper seating height,
2. patient support to place the oral cavity at the optimal control operating point,
3. control of the maxillary plane,
4. clearance around patient's head to allow unimpeded operator access from the 10 o'clock position to the 12:30 position, and
5. positioning of the light.

Only when these criteria are achieved can concepts of good surgical ergonomics be applied to optimize the quality of oral health care.

REFERENCES

1. Rundcrantz BL, Johnsson B, Moritz U. Occupational cervico-brachial disorders among dentists. *Swedish Dental J.* 1991;15:219–228.
2. Rundcrantz BL, Johnsson B, Moritz U. Occupational cervico-brachial disorders among dentists. Analysis of ergonomics and locomotor functions. *Swedish Dent J.* 1991;15(3):105–115.
3. Rundcrantz BL, Johnsson B, Moritz U, Roxendal G. Occupational cervico-brachial disorders among dentists: psychosocial work environment, personal harmony and life-satisfaction. *Scand J Soc Med.* 1991;19(3):174–180.
4. Rundcrantz BL, Johnsson B, Moritz U, Roxendal G. Cervico-brachial disorders in dentists. A comparison between two kinds of physiotherapeutic interventions. *Scand J Soc Med.* 1991;23(1):11–17.

5. Rundcrantz BL. Pain and discomfort in the musculoskeletal system among dentists. *Swedish Dent J Suppl.* 1991;76:1–102.
6. Rundcrantz BL, Johnsson B, Moritz U. Cervical pain and discomfort among dentists. Epidemiological, clinical and therapeutic aspects. Part 1. A survey of pain and discomfort. *Swedish Dent J.* 1990;14(2):71–80.
7. Panero J, Zelnik M. *Human Dimension and Interior Space.* New York: Watson-Guptill; 1979.
8. Kilpatrick HC. *Work Simplification in Dental Practice.* 3rd ed. Philadelphia: W.B. Saunders Co; 1974:672.
9. Beach D. Personal communication. 1984.
10. Rucker L, Gibson G, McGregor C. Getting the feel of it: the nonvisual component of psychomotor control in dentistry. *CDA J.* 1990;56(10):937–941.
11. Powell BJ, Winkley GP, Brown JO, Etersque S. Evaluating the fit of ambidextrous and fitted gloves: implications for hand discomfort. *JADA.* 1994;125:1235–1241.
12. Rucker LM. Performance simulation: the method. *J Res in Educ.* 1987;ED4:276–350.
13. Rucker L, Belenky M. Performance simulation training and its application to preclinical education: logic and methodology. *J Dent Ed.* 1986;50:1–21.
14. Belenky MM. Performance logic: the concept. *J Res in Educ.* 1987;ED4:232–275.
15. Cheek D. Were you originally left-handed? *Swedish J Clin Exp Hypn.* 1978;Sept:17–25.
16. Porac C, Coren S. *Lateral Preferences and Human Behavior.* New York: Springer-Verlag; 1977.

Chapter 13

Ergonomically Correct Design Concepts of a Functioning Dental Office

John C. Wittenstrom, DDS, and Sachiko Kawaguchi

Abstract

The organization and design of a dental office utilizing "performance logic" design concepts is described. The office environment is made up of well-defined stations grouped into area types. The area types are organized within the office according to a human-centered classification which emphasizes human-centered activities over machine-centered activities. The stations are designed according to preferred body conditions for each task. "Dental beds" are described, which are characterized by a stabilized head-rest which defines a zero point within the area. The benefits of this stabilized zero point are also described.

Introduction

Every dental care facility has room for ergonomic improvement. And every dental health care worker can improve the way he or she performs tasks—not just to work more efficiently and effectively, but to work more naturally and comfortably.

The design of the work environment itself, however, is often the reason the health care worker does not perform in the most natural and efficient way. A second reason for not working more naturally and efficiently is that most training programs worldwide still place more importance on what is done (the product) than on how it is done (the process). Fortunately, some training programs have begun to adopt a more process oriented approach.

This chapter describes the characteristics of a functioning dental office that was organized and designed using specific ergonomic concepts. These concepts are collectively referred to as "performance logic" concepts in this chapter to differentiate them from other ergonomic design and performance concepts. The term "performance logic," further described below, was coined by Daryl R. Beach, DMD.

The Performance Logic Approach

Performance logic is an approach for determining optimal human performance conditions for any specified act. These conditions include the details of the performer's body, the details of the person or object the performer is working on, and the details of the environmental objects, such as instruments and materials.

A basic tenet of performance logic is that for every step of every task there are preferred body conditions. These preferred conditions can further be defined as "reference" conditions, and the acceptable "reference range" of conditions. For example, a dentist's reference condition for lateral head balance is with no head tilt to the left or right. Most dentists, however, can accept tilting the head about 5 or 10 degrees to one side without adverse affects to the musculoskeletal system. The acceptable range of tilt is referred to as the reference range.

The details and application of the performance logic concepts are further described below.

Organization of the Office

The office is located in the center of downtown Minneapolis, Minnesota, which has a population of 370,000. The population of the seven-county surrounding metropolitan area is 2.4 million.

The size of the office is 2500 square feet. It is designed for optimum management and control by two dentists working together in a space- and expense-sharing arrangement. The office represents the minimum necessary space for two dentists in comprehensive general dental practice with well-defined and integrated stations, areas, and walkways.

The office is designed for the following staff:
- two dentists,
- one receptionist,
- one to two business personnel,
- two dental hygienists,
- two dental assistants, and
- up to two lab technicians.

Stations

A station is a three-dimensional unit of space that can be occupied by one person at any given time for a given purpose. The station can accommodate a given range of sizes of people as appropriate for actions associated with a given purpose.

CLASSIFICATION OF STATIONS

A station can be classified according to several factors, all of which are useful in the specification of ergonomically well-designed dental facilities.

Stations can be classified by function:
1. stations for information performance,
2. stations for motor performance,
3. stations for personal maintenance and development,
4. stations for environmental maintenance, and
5. mixed-function stations.

Stations can be classified by extent of rotation and side shift:
1. A *one-directional* station is characterized by the performer facing in one direction. This type of station may also include a side shift (side step) from left to right or from right to left to align the body with the appropriate task point, work surfaces, object, equipment or instrument(s).
2. A *multi-directional* (rotational) station can be of two types:
   - rotation around the task point (e.g., the patient's mouth); or
   - rotation around the vertical axis of the seated performer (e.g., to operate at two separate task points,

work surfaces, objects, pieces of equipment, or instrument(s).

Stations can be classified by the persons using the stations:

1. stations for a single person, such that a person with a given duty is assigned to a station (e.g., dental assistant); and
2. stations for multiple people, such that unspecified people use/share the station (e.g., reception area seats for patients).

Stations can be classified by relationship between the trunk and legs:

1. standing (e.g., the assistant using a model trimmer to trim a dental model);
2. sitting (e.g., the assistant assisting the dentist); and
3. supine (e.g., the patient being treated in the operatory).

Stations can be classified by relationship to walkways:

1. end-of-walkway station,
2. within-walkway station, and
3. beside-walkway station.

Areas

The stations that make up the dental office are grouped into different functional areas. An area is defined as a three-dimensional unit of space that consists of one or more stations for given acts and the space necessary between the stations for walkways.

Area Types

There are nine different area types. These area types are classified 0 to 9 according to a logic for human performance in which human-centered areas are given priority over machine-centered areas (Figure 1). There can be one or more of each of these different area types in a dental office.

Using the human-centered 0 to 9 classification results in facilities that have the potential for optimum management of information, therapy, and communications between people. This approach gives guidance for the successful incorporation of new technology while remaining focused on people. It

AREA TYPE		
	0	All areas (the total environmental setting)
	1	Information—reception, inlcuding walkways
Human-	2	Information—dentist & hygienist
Centered	3	Treatment
Areas	4	Laboratory
	5	Human maintenance
Machine-	6	Setting maintenance
Centered	7	Automated
Areas	8	Operator required
	9	Unaccountable space

FIGURE 1.—Area-type classification.

can also significantly save costs over the long term because it minimizes redesign projects within the office.

INFORMATION AREA—RECEPTION, INCLUDING PRIMARY WALKWAYS

This area includes the receptionist's station, which is the control center for office activity and the primary information area for patients.

The receptionist's station is purposely designed for only one person. Although this type of design requires nonreception activities to take place in other parts of the office, the advantages are significant. All people entering the office want to make eye contact with a receptionist on entering. This design helps people determine the location and position of the reception station relative to the front door. Having one receptionist also requires a skillful person who can handle multiple activities at a time. The computer network used in the office must be integrated into the receptionist's work station for optimum efficiency and effectiveness.

The information area also includes a "quick-check" area, which has a comfortable seat for patients and eliminates the need for an extra full-treatment area for emergency patients.

The quick-check area is located near the front of the office and is primarily for seeing emergency patients and patients needing quick procedures involving minimum instrumentation. Radiographs are also exposed and processed in the quick-check area.

INFORMATION AREA—DENTIST AND HYGIENIST

This area type includes an area for each dentist and a separate and unique area for each hygienist. Information areas are used for consultations and discussions with dental patients. Patients sitting here are face to face with the dentist or hygienist, sitting at approximately the same eye level. They are just far enough apart so their knees don't touch. A table between patient and dentist supports discussion aids. This area is designed to be conducive to effective communication, and is an improvement over the usual practice of dentists and hygienists discussing important things with the patient reclined in a dental chair.

These multifunctional areas are used both as the doctors' and hygienists' private offices and as patient discussion areas. The spaces are highly functional and comfortable. Special design features allow these areas also to be used for patient recovery rooms.

TREATMENT AREA

As with all other areas, the total space required for the treatment area is dictated by the space required for the activities in the area, not by the equipment.

The length of the treatment area, 11 feet minimum, is determined by combining the length of the tallest patient, the area occupied by the dentist, the walkway space for the assistant behind the dentist, and the extension of the arms in washing hands. The width of the treatment area is determined by combining the thickness of the assistant, the width of a patient at the shoulders, and walkway space sufficient for the patient to freely enter and exit.

Of all the areas in the dental office, it is important that this one not be spatially compromised. According to performance logic, the treatment area must be 11 feet long. Many medical arts buildings have rooms only 10 feet long.

LABORATORY AREA

This area contains stations for pouring and trimming models, casting gold, trimming and finishing, and ceramic processing. In addition, each dentist has a station always available for procedures such as trimming dies and making wax patterns. These stations don't take up much space, and they greatly increase the capacity of the office.

HUMAN MAINTENANCE AREA

This area includes space for the staff break room, lockers, and toilets.

SETTING MAINTENANCE

This area includes space for cleaning supplies, inventory, and miscellaneous storage. It is the first of the machine-centered areas located in the back half of the office.

MACHINE-CENTERED, AUTOMATED AREA

This area is for machine-centered stations that do not require the direct attention of an assistant or dentist. Automation in dentistry continues to have a profound impact, and it is just a matter of time before practical applications are developed. In the long-term future of ergonomic office design, it is important to prioritize this type of area over types that require an operator.

MACHINE-CENTERED AREA, OPERATOR REQUIRED

This area is for all stations that are machine centered and require a person to operate the machine. This space accommodates autoclaves, business-related copy machines and computer terminals, and optional stations for panographic x-ray machines and CAD/CAM stations for fabrication of restorations. Equipment should be minimized, and the trend should be to increasingly incorporate equipment into the human-centered areas as the equipment size gets smaller and smaller.

UNACCOUNTABLE SPACE

This is space that is unusable because of structural obstacles such as supporting pillars or corners. Windowsills in offices can also constitute unaccountable space. This type of space tends to collect clutter.

Layout of Areas

The layout of the various areas of the office is determined using the human-centered classification of area types. The order of functional areas places patient care areas closer to the entrance of the office than nonpatient areas. This approach, combined with using as few walkways as possible and having a separate staff entrance, conserves space, increases efficiency, reduces traffic flow congestion, and minimizes patients' confusion about which walkway to use.

Typical dental office layouts are the I-type layout, the L-type layout, and the U-type layout.

SIGHTLINES AND VIEWS

The view that a patient has while walking through the office is important. End-of-walkway views should be views of something that looks natural and calming, such as plants, trees, or artwork. Equipment should not be overemphasized. These sightline considerations help in the comparison of different layout options.

Information and Motor Performance Areas

In dentistry there are two basic types of performance: information performance and motor performance. In an office designed according to performance logic, examples of areas for these two types of performance are 1) the doctor's study and discussion area (doctor's office) (Figure 2) and 2) the treatment area (operatory) (Figure 3).

Doctor's Study and Discussion Area Design

The doctor's study and discussion area is a multifunctional area. It serves both as the doctor's private office and as the doctor-patient discussion area. While in most dental offices discussions with patients take place in the treatment area, a dental office designed according to performance logic has an area designed specifically for good communication between people. Generally accepted ideal conditions for communications between two or more people include having each person's eyes at approximately the same level, and sitting face

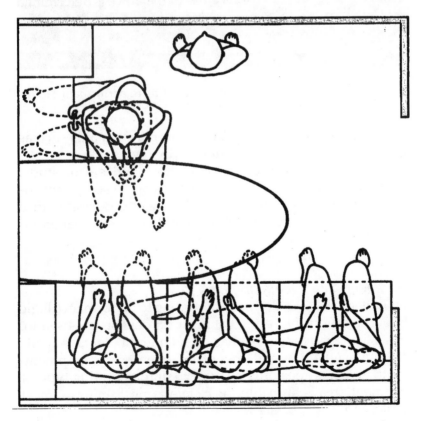

FIGURE 2.—Doctor's study and discussion area.

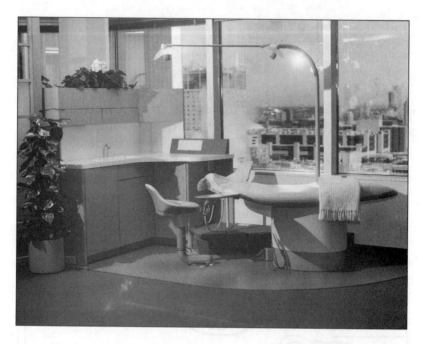

FIGURE 3.—Treatment area designed according to performance logic.

to face across a table that holds communication aids such as models, photographs, brochures, and x-rays.

This area also serves as the doctor's office—for study, phone calls, and the ever-present paperwork. A significant advantage of having this area serve both as the doctor's office and as the patient discussion area is that it gets cleaned up much more regularly!

Treatment Area (Operatory) Design

A treatment area designed according to performance logic differs significantly from what most US dentists are used to. This is largely due to what has been taught in dental schools and the availability and cost of treatment area equipment. Combined with performance logic equipment, this type of treatment area is arguably the cleanest, most uniform, most stable, and least cluttered.

Treatment area designs are commonly differentiated by the number and location of entrances relative to the dental chair, the type of "delivery system,"[1] and the number of sinks in the treatment area.

A treatment area designed according to performance logic has only one entrance. Only one entrance is needed because the space allows for the people using the room (doctor, hygienist, assistant, and patient) to freely enter and leave the room at any time. The assistant is never "locked in" when the patient is in the correct position for treatment. It is not uncommon to find treatment areas designed in such a way that the dental assistant cannot enter and leave without moving instruments or tilting the patient's chair.

The "Dental Bed"

The treatment area designed according to performance logic uses a "dental bed" rather than a dental chair. Although foreign to many dentists, the dental bed is arguably safer than a chair because the gag reflex is actually less in a fully reclined person than in one who is sitting at an angle somewhere between upright and reclined. This approach also positions the patient's mouth in a way that allows the dentist a high level of precision and control with low stress, although it does take some re-learning and adjustment for dentists trained in other approaches.

Positioning of the Dentist

The dentist sits between 11:30 and 12 o'clock for most procedures, rotating freely within the 10:30 to 1:30 range as needed.[2] Again, this seems foreign to dentists trained in traditional approaches and who are more used to the 7 o'clock to 9 o'clock position for working in the patient's lower right quadrant. Without the patient fully reclined it is very difficult, if

---

[1]"Delivery system" is defined here as the location of the handpiece(s), air-water syringe(s), high-volume evacuator(s), and low-volume evacuator(s) relative to the patient. Common delivery systems that are different than the performance logic delivery system are the "over-the-patient," "beside-the-patient," and "behind-the-patient" types.

[2]The right-handed dentist's zone of operation is from 10:30 to 1:30, and the left-handed dentist's zone is from 11:30 to 2:30.

not impossible, to work on the patient's upper quadrants or lower right quadrant.

Concepts and Characteristics

The essence of the philosophy of this office is that the physical setting should allow the two dentists to practice in a way that maximizes the benefits of working together while minimizing the potential pitfalls. This is accomplished in several ways.

Equal Space

The two doctors have equal space. Neither has a larger office, for example. If one office or operatory has a better view, the two dentists simply agree to switch periodically.

Finances

The financial arrangement of who owns what is a separate issue. One doctor can be the owner, with the other an associate employee or independent contractor. Or the two can have a partnership arrangement.

Human-Centered Design

The physical layout of the operatories and other areas is human centered. Each work station in the office is designed for optimal human performance of the task for which the station was designed. Some stations are extremely highly designed and specified, such as the doctor's operatory station. Others, like the staff area, are more loosely designed, although all of the same design principles apply. The order of the stations and areas is such that the human-centered, patient-related ones are closest to the front door.

Human-Centered Performance Areas

Each station and area is determined according to the balanced posture and position of a performer (health care worker or patient) using natural and consistent movements of the hands, fingers, arms, and legs. Equipment and objects within a station or area should not hamper the perception or movements of the performer.

Natural and Necessary Equipment and Equipment Movements

The only functional equipment and objects located within a station or area should be those necessary for activities in that area. The path of motion of a performer, in balanced posture and position, determines the location of the equipment and objects, as well as their direction and distance of motion. The location and distance of motion are determined by frequency of use.

Performance Logic Concept Delivery System

The "delivery system," as defined here, is the location of the handpieces, vacuums, and air-water syringes relative to the patient and providers. The performance logic delivery system is not the typical beside-the-patient, behind-the-patient, or over-the-patient delivery system. In this system, the handpieces, vacuum, air-water syringes, and instrument tray are located and positioned so that they are

1. stabilized in their location so the operator can grasp them comfortably without looking;
2. angulated to minimize regripping; and
3. located out of the way but as close as possible to the patient's mouth (beside and slightly below the headrest, at the shoulder line of the patient.

Proprioceptively Derived Instruments and Human Interface Forms

The instruments, both attached and unattached, have been designed using proprioceptive derivation, a design process in which the specifications of the instrument are derived primarily from the operators' sense of proprioception. This is done using a step-by-step design process that results in optimal human interface conditions. A good, simple example of a proprioceptively derived instrument is a double-ended scaler used to clean teeth. The diameter is relatively small, making rotation and tactile sensation easier. The length is shorter than the typical dental instrument, so the operator does not have to regrip the instrument, after flipping it around, to get the fingers in the right relationship to the working tip. The nickname for proprioceptive-derivation or proprioceptively derived is "pd." In an office designed according to performance logic, the forms (e.g., objects, instruments, handles, switches) most critical to optimal human performance have been "pd'd."

Stabilized Zero-Point in the Operatory

The zero point of the operatory is the patient's mouth (Figure 4). This is possible because the patient support is not a chair. It is more commonly called a dental bed. The dental bed is a stable, nicely padded, ergonomically designed support with a fully adjustable headrest, built-in upper arm supports, and built-in delivery system. It moves up and down.

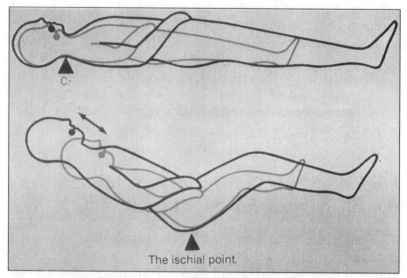

FIGURE 4.—The zero point should be the patient's mouth.

This allows ergonomic refinement in the operatory not possible with a dental chair. With a chair, the zero point is the patient's rear end. With the dental bed, the head is always closer to the desired place, even if the patient has to move up or down a bit. The advantages for the patient and the health care worker are many:

- Less adjustment is needed for the patient to "fit the chair." Children and adults all place their heads in the headrest on their own with little direction.
- The intraoral lighting is better because it is focused on the center of the headrest and doesn't require adjustment—and there are two lights instead of one.
- Impressions are safer and easier because patients gag less (the throat closes in the supine posture, as taught in all CPR courses) and because the person holding the impression is relaxed, with arms and hands balanced.
- The arrangement is cleaner, because the intraoral lights are never touched and the holders for the handpieces, vacuum, and air-water syringes are not on flex-arms.
- The arrangement looks less cluttered and is more soothing to the eye, which commonly leads to less patient anxiety.
- The assistant's stool is attached to a platform next to the patient. The platform is more secure than wheels and allows the assistant to easily rotate from the patients' mouth to the cabinet to prepare materials. This arrangement also keeps the assistant in a predictable location for the dentist (and vice versa).
- The doctor's stool is attached to the floor but can easily be adjusted up and down, as well as forward and backward. It rotates effortlessly around the zero point (the patient's mouth). There are no wheels for floss to get caught in!

Minimal Space

The space occupied by equipment is kept minimal. The equipment's human-interface components, such as switches and handpieces, are located and positioned ideally for the performer, while the supportive parts of the equipment, such as circuit boards and power supplies, are located out of the way in space not occupied by the health care worker.

Easy on the Eyes

Everything in the office has low reflectivity. Even the instruments have a matte finish to prevent stressful glare. Equipment colors are neutral, and equipment labels and logos are minimized or covered up. This way eyes is not strained, and the patient (and health care workers) can enjoy the artwork on the walls, the flowers and plants in the office, or the view out the window.

Process Orientation

The doctors and staff have a high awareness of how they do things, minimizing bending, twisting, and touching things unnecessarily; with benefits ranging from less physical, mental, and ergonomic stress, to improved infection control. With this focus on process, everyone continually looks for ways to better organize and simplify.

Standardized Operatories

Each operatory is basically the same: same equipment, same supplies, etc. This makes scheduling easier and makes the assistant's job easier.

Open Design

There are few doors. This gives a very open and easy feeling to the office. Many patients comment that it doesn't look like a typical dental office, which is partially due to the open design, but also to the colors and finishes used. Patients feel less claustrophobic, and access is improved for wheelchairs and other assistance devices and equipment (Figure 5).

Natural Colors

There is a lot of natural wood in the office, which minimizes the chance that the office will have a dated look years

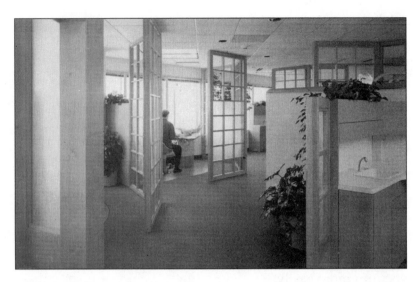

FIGURE 5.—Open-design concept.

in the future. Even the cabinetry looks like wood because of high-quality wood grain plastic laminates.

Designed To Not Show Wear

The surfaces commonly touched or requiring high-level cleaning are covered with high-quality wood grain plastic laminate. Scratches in the wood grain plastic laminate don't show nearly as much as they do in solid-color plastic laminate. The carpet and upholstery can also be chosen to hide lint.

Maintenance Friendly

Table legs and doors are few. This makes cleaning much easier, and there are no wooden chair legs to get marred from the vacuum cleaner. The flooring of the operatories, clinical workstations, and receptionist's station is vinyl, allowing easy cleaning. The flooring of the reception area, office/consultation areas, and all walkways is carpet, making for a quieter, softer, warmer feeling in the office and more comfort for the feet and legs.

Clean

Infection control is improved because finger-hand contacts are minimized.

Angled High-Volume Vacuum

The vacuum instrument used to evacuate water and fluids from the patient's mouth is more angled than the traditional dental vacuum (Figures 6 and 7). The vacuum used in most offices is the type that was originally used in general-medicine operating rooms. The angle is not efficient for dental assistants. Using a vacuum instrument with a greater angle is more ergonomically correct and offers additional advantages such as gentler, more controlled retraction of the patient's lips and cheeks. The patient or dentist also can hold the vacuum more easily.

Interpretive Instrument Tray

Although the dental assistant can participate when the dentist will be using many instruments, he or she cannot determine when the dentist will want every instrument during an appointment. The interpretive instrument tray is fixed at

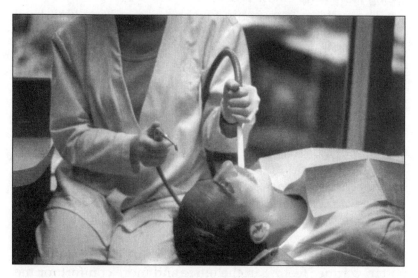

FIGURE 6.—"Traditional" high-volume vacuum.

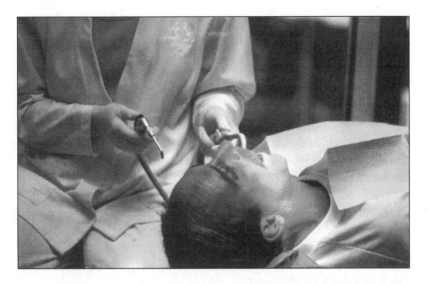

FIGURE 7.—Angled high-volume vacuum.

the shoulder line of the patient on the side opposite from the dental assistant. The mirror, the explorer, and selected other instruments are located on this tray. Because the tray is stabilized in the same location and not on a flex-arm, the dentist can pick up and lay down instruments with minimal looking and a higher feeling of confidence and security.

Third-Finger Finger Rest

Most dentists are taught to use their fourth finger as the stabilizing finger when using a hand instrument such as an explorer or high-speed handpiece. The third finger provides greater control potential. It can be difficult to use a third-finger finger rest with traditional instruments because of instrument design factors such as the presence of ridges or heavy knurl, which force the user to move more than just the fingers to perform a task. The third-finger finger rest also limits the length of motion of the instrument tip.

Reference Posture

In performance logic, the seated dental operator uses awareness-derivation exercises to determine preferred body conditions such as posture and limb position. The body is divided into nine sections to facilitate awareness and sequential self-verification of these preferred conditions (Figure 8).

Seat Height

The ergonomically correct seat height for the dental operator is at or slightly above the height of the lateral point of the head of the fibula. If two operators are to share the same operating stool, such as dentist and assistant, the stool should be set for the taller of the two operators. This is because sitting at a height lower than the lateral point of the head of the fibula will force the person's pelvis to rotate posteriorly, necessitating the use of a back rest. For the working, healthy dental operator, a back rest is not necessary and can actually limit freedom of movement.

Summary

The performance logic approach has been used to determine the design features and characteristics of the dental office described. The organization and specification of the work stations, areas, and instruments was determined using human-

Body Sections	Key Words
1. Feet & lower legs	Cleared
2. Thighs & upper legs	Cleared
3. Pelvic area & lower trunk	Directed (toward your operating point)
4. Upper trunk	Balanced
5. Head	Balanced
6. Shoulders	Loose
7. Upper arms & elbows	Loose
8. Forearms & wrists	Straight wrist
9. Thumbs & fingers	Relaxed 3rd fingers in the "sleeping hand posture"

FIGURE 8.—Nine body sections and keywords to facilitate self-assessment.

centered classifications as a way to have optimal performance conditions and minimal accommodation to equipment. The advantages to the health care workers in the setting are numerous and logically lead to greater comfort, control, and security.

RESOURCES

John C. Wittenstrom, DDS
920 Second Ave. S., Suite 1500
Minneapolis, MN 55402-4014
Tel: 612-339-5363
Fax: 612-339-4435
E-mail: drwitt@drwitt.com

Sachiko Kawaguchi
Human-Space USA Inc.
714 Spoon Court
Arnold, MD 21012
Tel: 410-349-0484
Fax: 410-349-0286

Daryl R. Beach, DMD
LAN Center
Daini Shin Osaka Bldg., 2F
6-3-32 Nishinakajima
Yodogawa-ku,
Osaka 532, Japan

Chapter 14

A Medical-Ergonomic Program for Prevention of Upper Extremity and Back Disorders in the Practice of Dentistry

Margit L. Bleecker, MD, PhD

Abstract

This chapter describes how the dental health care provider can take responsibility for ergonomic interventions, especially at the onset of symptoms. The discomfort experienced in the upper extremities or along the spine at the end of the day is the sentinel sign by which the etiology of the ergonomic stressor can be identified. The medical ergonomic program discussed in the latter part of the chapter empowers the dental health care provider to modify the work environment or technique and thereby alleviate symptoms and prevent future occurrences. The ergonomic problems associated with the practice of dentistry are briefly reviewed in the first part of the chapter.

Introduction

The practice of dentistry involves numerous ergonomic stressors resulting from sustained and awkward postures, repetitive tasks, forceful hand exertions, and vibrating tools. The physical stressors are further modulated by other sources of stress in the profession such as time pressure from a fixed schedule, coping with patient anxieties, and the precision required in the work.[1] An example is the awkward craning neck position that the dentist or dental hygienist often adapts to improve visibility. This position causes cervical discomfort that may be exacerbated by the increased cervical muscle tension with which a dental care worker may respond to a fearful patient.

Prevalence of Symptoms

Symptoms more prevalent among dentists and dental hygienists than among controls include ache, pain, or discomfort in the neck, shoulders, elbows and wrist, or hands.[2] In a survey of almost all licensed Nebraska dentists, 29% experienced neuropathic symptoms of pain (25%) or numbness (15%) and tingling (17%) in the neck and upper extremities.[3] This study, which focused on symptoms in the upper extremity, found the hand to be most frequent site (56%) followed by cervical (46%), thumb (30%), and index finger (26%). However, when symptoms from all body areas are tabulated, low-back disorders outrank symptoms related to the upper back, elbows, wrist, and hands.[4] Dentists as a group complain more of neck-shoulder and low-back problems that are severe enough to interfere with daily activities.[5] Aggregated data from Polish and Norwegian dentists show cervical and lumbosacral pains to be most common.[6,7] Female dentists report more musculoskeletal symptoms than their male counterparts, but the prevalence is no higher than among female office workers.[8]

Surveys in the United States report prevalence of back pain among dentists as one in two, while in the general population the prevalence is one of seven.[9] In Denmark, of 432 dentists, 60% had back and neck pain even when using the sit-down technique.[10] A Canadian study of 465 dentists found 36% currently suffering with back and neck pain while many—62%—had had the problem in the past.[1] These data are consistent with the positive response to questionnaires about back pain in 57% of 487 dentists from the South Carolina Dental Association. Seventy percent of this group noted that colleagues also had back problems.[11]

Risk Factors for Back Pain

Risk factors for back pain in dentists vary among the different studies. Dentists over 44 years of age with low-back pain and the presence of psychosocial problems at the onset of the disability had increased duration of low-back disability.[12] Shugars et al[11] found that age, years in practice, and number of hours in practice per week were not associated with indicators of back pain, but that predisposing factors such as congenital disease, sports injuries, and trauma were strongly correlated with back pain. In a study of Finnish dentists, neck-shoulder or low-back pain and disability was not associated with age, hours worked, working posture, use of an assistant, or bony degenerative changes on x-ray, but was associated with symptoms of occupational stress, work too physically demanding, mental strain, and poor general health ratings.[5] Poor physical condition is associated with weak abdominal muscles that are unable to support a straight spine and that promote a sway-back position, which increases the stress on intervertebral discs and facet joints.[1]

Ergonomic Risk Factors for the Upper Extremities

In the practice of dentistry, ergonomic risk factors for the upper extremities include awkward wrist and finger position, repeated pinch with wrist flexion, vibrating tools, and poor tool design. Both duration and intensity of exposure are important aspects of these ergonomic stressors. Duration of exposure measured in days worked per week and number of years practiced correlated with features of carpal tunnel syndrome among dental hygienists. Intensity of exposure, equated with the number of heavy-calculus patients seen in a day, correlated significantly with all symptoms and the diagnosis of carpal tunnel syndrome. [13] Another high-ergonomic-risk exposure is the use of high-frequency vibrating tools by dentists and dental hygienists that result in a neuropathy.[13] Dentists with pain, numbness, tingling, or loss of muscle control in their neck and upper extremities reported increased symptoms when performing crown and bridge work. These symptoms were relieved or reduced by stretching and resting (halting the dental procedure—59%) or changing posture.[3]

Ergonomic Stressors to the Back

Ergonomic stressors to the back include static postures with forward trunk inclination maintained for two thirds of the treatment hour.[14] Increased intradiscal pressure occurs with this forward trunk inclination in the sitting position.[15] The spine withstands loads best when the lumbar spine is straightened and not in flexion, extension, or rotation. Good chairside posture and overall posture are associated with less back pain.[11] Time spent sitting does not alone correlate with back pain. In fact, upper-back pain is significantly less when 60 to 79% of the time is spent sitting.[11] Posture is frequently compromised when the dentist leans or twists to accommodate poor visibility (see Figure 1). This also applies to dental personnel assisting the dentist, whose line of sight is frequently blocked because of how the fingers are positioned on the mirror handle.[16]

An early intervention program for low-back pain reduced claims of 1-year duration by 56%.[12] Other studies suggest that dentists need physical exercise to handle the physical demands and occupational stress associated with back pain.[5] General exercise and specific exercises for the back most frequently bring relief, suggesting that the underlying etiology for backache in dentists is mechanical.[1]

Accommodations for Ergonomic Stressors

Accommodations for ergonomic stressors should encourage good working posture.[16] Alternating the sitting with standing chair-side posture recruits other muscle groups into use, thereby distributing the strain across many groups.[16] Hours spent sitting is a problem if the trunk is leaning forward, but, if straight posture and lumbar support are used, upper- and low-back symptoms are diminished. Good posture includes shoulders relaxed with elbows close to the body. A conscious effort to incorporate microbreaks into work methodology must be made by dentists since as a group they tend to hold single postures for prolonged periods of time. Long appointments can contribute to sustained postures and therefore should be

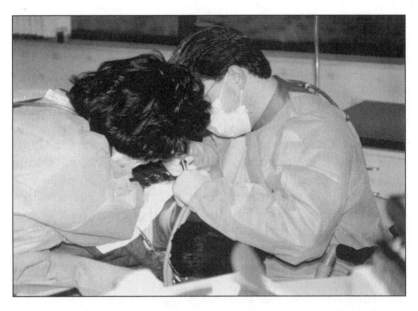

FIGURE 1.—Note the posture adopted by the dentist and the dental assistant to improve poor visibility. Neck and upper back are flexed (dentist) and twisted (dental assistant) and shoulders are abducted.

avoided. Adequate lumbar support from the chair, appropriate positioning of the patient (supine), and correct placement of the dental team are basic to the maintenance of good working posture. The patient's head or neck should be adjusted to improve visibility. Obviously the patient must be kept comfortable which is accomplished by a rolled towel under the neck when forward position of the chin is needed. Placement of equipment or cabinetry within 20 inches of dental personnel diminishes awkward reaching.

Dental scopes that provide a magnified field prevent forward leaning. Poor posture adjustments such as craning, bending and twisting of the neck, bending forward from the waist and elevation of the shoulders result from the attempt to get closer to the work area in the oral cavity. The telescopic loupes are critical in maintaining the necessary distance from the eye to the work area and in increasing size of the viewed object. The angle of the oculars diminishes the need to bend the neck. [16] Magnifiers, used routinely in surgery, should be standard in the practice of dentistry.

A medical-ergonomic program developed at the Center for Occupational and Environmental Neurology addresses the need to incorporate ergonomic interventions as part of medical treatment for ergonomic stressors that occur in the workplace. Classically, the health care provider treats these work-related disorders and places restrictions upon work activities that may exacerbate or interfere with the recovery process. The medical-ergonomic program, instead of limiting the ability to work, identifies and modifies the responsible ergonomic stressors. These alterations may include changes in the work environment or work methodology. The difference in this approach is abatement of the etiology and not just treatment of signs or symptoms. Attainment of long-term health goals requires not temporary restriction of a potential etiologic activity but permanent changes of the causes in the work environment or work methodology.

Prevention in the workplace may be accomplished by primary ergonomic intervention; an ergonomic stressor is identified and abated before a health problem occurs. Even in a well-designed work environment, symptoms may develop because of poor technique or poor work methodology such as the absence of breaks. Therefore, it is critical to link symptoms with the appropriate ergonomic stressors (see Table 1) so that intervention is implemented and the development of a medical disorder is avoided. This point cannot be emphasized enough. If symptoms fluctuate from day to day, the natural inclination is to ignore them. However, they should serve as the red flag that automatically triggers review of the ergonomic stressors associated with the symptom area as outlined in Table 1.

Usually the focus of dental personnel is the completion of the task at hand and not how can this task be completed using sound ergonomic technique. To prevent development of symptoms, a conscious effort must be made to take microbreaks. These include stretching or relaxing the stressed body part for 8 to 10 seconds. For example, leaning back against the lumbar rest with arms hanging at the side dramatically lowers pressure in the lumbar spine, removes traction on the ulnar nerve that occurs with elbow flexion particularly if it is sustained, and removes muscle tension from the shoulder/neck area. Den-

Table 1.—Ergonomic Modifications for Symptomatic Area	
Symptomatic Area	Work Environment or Technique Modification
Back	
low back	Posture—sitting up straight
	Alternate sitting with standing
	Chair—lumbar support, adequate adjustability
	Seated between 10:30 and 11:00
	Patient position—supine, easy adjustability of dental chair
	Dental scopes—prevent leaning forward to improve view of oral cavity
	Avoid long appointments
	Avoid awkward reaching—equipment within 20 inches
	Use foot rest to keep thigh parallel to floor
upper back/ neck	Keep elbows close to the body
	Shoulders should not be raised
	Work close to patient to avoid leaning
	Do not bend to improve visibility
	Fingers holding mirror should be placed away from left corner of patient's mouth (right-handed work)
	Good lighting to improve visibility
	Diminish patient anxiety
	Telescopic loupes
	Adjust patient's head, use neck pillow
	Patient height good for visibility, but dental worker still able to keep elbows close to body
	Keep the neck neutral (straight), place the angles in the work environment
Wrist/Hand	Limit exposure to hand-held tools or work pieces that vibrate
	Use adapters to enlarge tool handles
	Avoid pinch position while flexing the wrist
	Whenever possible try to keep the wrist straight
	Use microbreaks to stretch the fingers

Table 1.—*Continued*	
Wrist/Hand (*continued*)	Avoid long appointments
	Do not schedule sequential patients who require high-force movements of hand and wrist (crown work)
	Use four-handed dentistry
	Fiber-optic light in handpiece to improve visibility
	Telescopic loupes
	Ensure visibility of dental assistant to increase efficiency

tists are predisposed to maintain static upper-body positions that do not allow for recovery of the activated muscle. Therefore, microbreaks need to be programmed into the treatment protocol of a patient. This is particularly important for tasks that require more sustained force in the upper extremities—for example, performing crown or bridge work. The need for microbreaks also applies to dental hygienists whose work schedules are frequently concentrated with no interruptions between patients. Microbreaks, with stretches, should occur throughout the day and should focus on the hand, wrist, shoulder/neck, and low-back regions.

Education covering the underlying general principles of sound ergonomic method is central to the medical-ergonomic program. The dental staff must learn to recognize ergonomic stressors in the office and to relate symptoms to specific problems in the physical layout or techniques used. Repeated pinch activity with the wrist in flexion is to be avoided. As in other professions that require repetitive wrist and hand movements, it is critical to maintain neutral wrist position. Required angles must be incorporated into hand-tool design or adjustment of the work area.

Sustained forceful power grip increases the risk of trigger finger. Extension of the thumb if maintained with sufficient tension, leads to de Quervain's disease, inflammation of the thumb extensor and abductor tendons. Elevation of the shoulders and holding elbows away from the body stresses the upper arm, shoulder, and neck (See Figure 2).

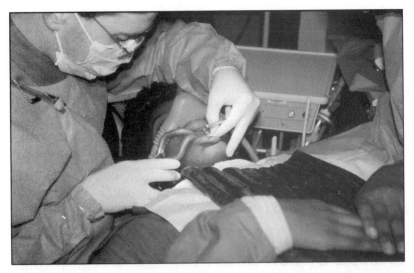

FIGURE 2.—The seating position and the patient height forces the dentist to work with shoulders elevated and elbows abducted to 90 degrees. This posture stresses the upper arm, shoulder, neck and upper back.

Just as the wrist needs to remain in the neutral position, so does the neck. Upper arms and elbows should be close to the body, which is impossible if the patient is positioned too high. The dental health care provider must take the extra time to adjust the work environment to allow for good upper-extremity and back biomechanics. If adequate time is not allowed for each patient, the likelihood of this occurring is greatly diminished.

Example 1—Shoulder/Neck Discomfort

Symptoms in this area respond to nonsteroidal anti-inflammatory drugs (NSAIDs) and thermal modalities (heat or cold). The use of a cervical pillow during sleep maintains appropriate positioning of the neck when gravity is not compressing the vertebral bodies. The obvious ergonomic stressors are those related to bending and twisting the neck to increase visibility. Use of dental scopes and appropriate lighting has to be viewed as part of the treatment, otherwise resolution of symptoms is poor.

To improve visibility, the patient is frequently positioned too high. Working with the patient in this position necessitates elevating the shoulders to bring the arms to the level of the patient. Prolonged contraction of the shoulder and neck muscles in this situation interferes with recovery time for the muscle since the work cycle for this area has now become unduly long. The patient must be lowered so that the dental worker's shoulders and upper arms can relax and the elbows can be aligned close to the body. The act of raising the shoulders and placing the elbows away from the body is done reflexively to accommodate an error in the work environment—namely, the elevated patient.

Example 2—Low-Back Pain

Low-back discomfort is most commonly related to poor posture. An additional factor that contributes to low-back pain is increased body mass; for each additional 10 pounds of weight on the abdomen, 100 pounds of force is generated to the low back. It is important to have good abdominal tone to support the low back. Also, stretching exercises maintain the flexibility of the lumbar spine.

Compromise of the straight spine position results from leaning forward to improve visibility or because the patient is located too far away. Sitting increases intradiscal lumbar pressure, and standing lowers the pressure dramatically. Standing can serve as a microbreak and helps to prevent and alleviate low-back pain. If standing is required for prolonged periods, one foot should be elevated on a low stool to prevent an increase in lumbar lordosis that may increase low back pain. Sitting should occur in a chair with lumbar support, not on a stool. The lumbar support has to be comfortable; it should fit the lumbar curvature, and contact should be maintained with it while the health care provider is sitting.

Example 3—Wrist/Hand Discomfort

Early symptoms in the wrist or hand respond to conservative medical management that includes NSAIDs, icing the affected area for 10 to 20 minutes three times a day, and wearing an elasticized wrist band as a friendly reminder to always keep the wrist in the neutral position. When the wrist is in the neutral position, the pressure in the carpal canal is lowest and the force placed on the flexor and extensor tendons is least.

Stress on the wrist and hand may be directly related to hand-tool design. This is an area of dental practice in which little change has occurred. A pinch position with a flexed wrist cannot be avoided with some hand tools. Working with the hand in this position is a risk factor for the development of carpal tunnel syndrome because it increases carpal canal pressure. Tools need redesign with larger handles and incorporation of angles to allow the wrist position to remain neutral. Vibrating hand tools, which are known to damage the median nerve at the wrist, may be modified to diminish the vibration. Wearing a padded glove to absorb the transmitted vibration would interfere with the dexterity required by the dental health care professional who already is wearing gloves required for universal protection.

Holding the hand tool with more force than necessary is a common error. This increased pinch force is also maintained throughout the work cycle and not just for the required time. The presence of vibration may also lead to an increased pinch grip. To monitor the presence of unnecessary muscle force, a portable biofeedback unit can be used. Surface electrodes placed over the muscles to be monitored are connected to a unit the size of a beeper. Settings may be adjusted so that when muscle force beyond an acceptable range is exceeded, a tone is heard. Use of a portable biofeedback machine helps to identify poor technique and can be used during the period of neuromuscular retraining. It initially feels awkward when changing a learned motor skill, but the use of a portable biofeedback machine may expedite this process.

The dentist should learn not to maintain the "action ready" position when waiting for the dental assistant to complete a task. It is better to perform a hand or wrist stretch during this microbreak. Microbreaks must be incorporated into the work methodology. Dental workers should pace themselves. Patients should not be scheduled back to back for crown work since this work requires sustained high-force movements of hand and wrist.

Example 4—Thumb Discomfort

Discomfort of the thumb is handled in the same way as discomfort of the wrist, with NSAIDs, icing, and special effort to avoid the stress that extension or abduction with force places on the thumb tendons. The thumb is at a higher risk than other digits in the hand because the use of hand tools places stress on the thumb extensor and abductor tendons. For example, when removing heavy plaque, the dental hygienist must maintain sustained force on the thumb. Enlarging the tool handle diminishes the pinch force exerted by the thumb. Rest breaks and attention to patient scheduling are critical for treatment and prevention. Relaxation of pinch force during the work cycle allows recovery. The habit of maintaining the pinch force even when not actively using the hand tool should be broken. Nonoccupational activities that should be temporarily modified include lifting or grabbing bulky items such as large books, which forcefully extends the thumb. A two-handed lift without thumb extension is one possibility.

If a keyboard or mouse is used at work or at home, the tendons in the thumb may continue to be aggravated if the space bar is depressed with the thumb extended rather than in the neutral position. Clutching the mouse may dramatically increased the force exerted on the thumb. The mouse should be used with the hand opened and relaxed. Even grabbing clothes from the washer or dryer may aggravate the thumb. To remove stress to the thumb only a few items should be picked up at one time. Constantly aggravating the symptomatic area will prolong the recovery time.

Nonoccupational Sources of Ergonomic Stress

The focus on ergonomic stressors at work would be incomplete if it did not include nonoccupational sources of ergonomic stress that may increase the risk of symptom development in the workplace. When sporadic hobby activities are performed without adequate recovery time (e.g., weekend athletics, gardening, woodworking, refinishing furniture, quilting, knitting, playing a musical instrument, or sculpting), the threshold for symptom development in the workplace may be altered. Ergonomic stressors previously tolerated now become a problem. Sound ergonomic principles should be applied to these nonoccupational activities. For instance, appropriate warm-up periods and rest breaks are key. Also, everyday activities such as driving a car present stressors to the low back and upper extremities that must be addressed in the overall prevention program to limit ergonomic stressors in the dental office

Prevention also incorporates physical conditioning that can range from daily stretching for flexibility to strengthening programs, particularly of the muscle groups involved in sitting and standing posture. The abdominal and upper-back groups are two areas most in need of strengthening for good posture. Aerobic exercise programs must be tailored to minimize stress to the low back, a region already at risk in dentistry. Exercise relieves back pain by promoting movement. Also, increased muscle tension from occupational stress responds well to exercise. Prevention of low-back pain does include weight control.

Other modalities for preventing and relieving symptoms are the same as those used by athletes: ice, support of the affected area with an elasticized wrap and over-the-counter anti-inflammatory medications, but the most important step is finding the ergonomic stressor and immediately modifying it.

REFERENCES

1. Bassett S. Back problems among dentists. *J Canad Dent Assoc.* 1983;49:251–256.
2. Akesson I, Lundborg G, Horstmann V, Skerfving S. Neuropathy in female dental personnel exposed to high frequency vibrations. *Occup Environ Med.* 1995;52:116–123.
3. Stockstill JW, Harn SD, Strickland D, Hruska R. Prevalence of upper extremity neuropathy in a clinical dentist population. *JADA.* 1993;124:67–72.
4. Shugars D, Miller D, Williams D, Fishburne C, Strickland D. Musculoskeletal pain among general dentists. *Gen Dent.* 1987; July/August:272–276.

5. Lehto TU, Helenius HYM, Alaranta HT. Musculoskeletal symptoms of dentists assessed by a multidisciplinary approach. *Community Dent Oral Epidemiol.* 1991;19:38–44.
6. Sinczuk WH, Izycki J. Back pain syndromes in dentists. Diagnosis and differential diagnosis. *Med Pr.* 1994;45:71–74.
7. Augustson TE, Morken T. Musculoskeletal problems among dental health personnel. A survey of the public dental health services in Hordaland. *Tidsskr Nor Laegeforen.* 1996;116:2776–2780.
8. Moen BE, Bjorvatn K. Musculoskeletal symptoms among dentists in a dental school. *Occup Med Oxf.* 1996;46:65–68.
9. Norris C. Is your back biting back? *Dent Man.* 1977;17:57–60.
10. Kelstrup BU. Tandlaegerne sidder stadig daarligt. *Tandlaegebladet.* 1977; Marts:162–164.
11. Shugars DA, Williams D, Cline SJ, Fishburne C. Musculoskeletal back pain among dentists. *Gen Dent.* 1984;November/December: 481–485.
12. Van Doorn JW. Low back disability among self-employed dentists, veterinarians, physicians and physical therapists in the Netherlands. A retrospective study over a 13-year period (N = 1,119) and an early intervention program with a 1-year follow-up (N = 134). *Acta Orthop Scand Suppl.* 1995;263:1–64.
13. Macdonald G, Robertson MM, Erickson JA. Carpal tunnel syndrome among California dental hygienists. *Dental Hygiene.* 1988;July/August:322–328.
14. Nordin M, Ortengren R, Anderson G. Measurement of trunk movements during work. *Spine.* 1984;9:465–469.
15. Nachemson AL. Disc pressure measurements. *Spine.* 1981;6:93–97.
16. Pollack R. Dental office ergonomics: how to reduce stress factors and increase efficiency. *J Can Dent Assoc.* 1996;62:508–510.

Chapter 15

Low Back Disorders and Dentistry—Stress Factors and Ergonomic Intervention

Eckardt Johanning, MD, MSc, and Ralph Bruder

Abstract

The prevalence of back disorders and musculoskeletal complaints among dental workers is high, although it may be not higher than in many other occupations with stressors such as awkward body posture and prolonged standing. The pathology and biomechanics of low back disorders are reviewed and specific, recognized risk factors for back disorders such as heavy lifting, awkward spinal posture, and vibration are discussed. An overview of the principles of the medical examination and tests is given. Recent results of ergonomic studies, particularly of dental workers and their equipment and seats, are presented. Modern prevention strategies are described.

Background

Musculoskeletal disorders of the back are a leading cause of occupational injury and disability in industrialized countries. According to the Bureau of Labor Statistics, disorders related to repeated trauma (repetitive work procedures) accounted in 1987 for about 40% of all reported occupational illnesses in US private industry. One million workers suffered from back injuries on the job. In 1993 back disorders accounted for 27% of all nonfatal occupational injuries and illnesses involving sick leave time. One hundred million work days are lost each year as a result of back disabilities. Low back pain disables 5.4 million Americans per year and is the most frequently filed workers' compensation claim. The total compensable cost for low back pain in the United States was estimated in 1986 to be \$11.1 billion.[1] The average cost of a worker's compensation claim was \$8300, which is about twice the average cost for all other claims combined. About one third of American workers are in jobs that may increase the risk of developing back disorders, although the causes of lumbar disorders are complex. In 1989 the National Institute for Occupational Safety and Health (NIOSH) identified musculoskeletal disease as the second leading priority of work-related disorders in the United States. NIOSH called particular attention to the need for instituting treatment and preventive research programs related to "traumatogen workplace hazards."[2,3]

Certain health care industry occupations are associated with a high risk for low back disorders. Female nurses and nursing aids (prevalence = 19%) and maids (15%) were about two and one half times more likely than other female workers to suffer low back disorders. Male construction workers (23%), carpenters (22%), and truck and tractor operators (22%) were nearly as likely to suffer low-back disorders as other male workers.[4,5]

The general back-related epidemiology, the cost to business, and an identification of risk jobs or industries have been recently compiled by a state agency in the United States. The highest composite incidence rates for work-related musculoskeletal injuries (including to the low back) were in "wallboard installation" and "temporary help" (24 of 100 full-time workers), followed by roofing (20), moving company (18), garbage collection (15), nursing homes (14), and beer distributors (13).[6] Dentistry was not specifically mentioned in this report.

Nevertheless, several studies from different countries report on musculoskeletal disorders among dentists. According to these studies, neck and low back problems are common among dentists, although the measured prevalence or rates differ considerably.[7-11] The differences may be related to methodological issues or to differences in the working conditions in different countries.

In some studies, the prevalence was not different from that in the general population, and a clear age-related effect was noticeable. In one study, female dentists were more likely to report musculoskeletal problems (including back disorders) than their male counterparts.[9] Also, a high level of general stressors (psychological and economic factors) reported in many dentistry studies may be a contributing or confounding risk factor for musculoskeletal complaints.[12-16] Musculoskeletal disorders and stress-related strain factors are among the most important reasons for early retirement of dentists, mostly of those older than 50 years of age.[17]

In a questionnaire survey study of 329 employees in the public dental services in a Scandinavian country, 81% complained about "some sort of musculoskeletal discomfort" in the year preceding the survey. Neck discomfort was reported by 47% and low back pain by 49%. However, the rates were not different from those among the general Norwegian population.[11] In a 12-year retrospective disability study, low back claims were the main cause of disability (75%) among self-employed dentists in the Netherlands.[8] In an ergonomic intervention study and questionnaire survey of 466 German dentists, problems primarily of the neck, shoulders, and back were reported. The complaints were associated with daily work duration and individual characteristics of the dentists (age and body height), especially awkward body postures during treatment.[18] Awkward body posture as a risk factor for musculoskeletal disorders among dentists will be discussed later in this chapter.

The physical working conditions and the design of dental office equipment is one reason for awkward body postures of dentists and contributes to musculoskeletal complaints and back disorders. Better ergonomic design of chairs for patients and dentists, and of instruments, may help prevent musculoskeletal stress and disease.[19-21] An alternative example for a patient chair that allows the dentist to place the patient in a better position for oral treatment will be presented and discussed later.[22]

Not included in this review are spinal diseases that are caused by infectious processes, inflammatory systemic disease, bone cancer, rheumatological or metabolic disorders, or other nonmechanical disorders. These types of diseases need to be considered in the differential diagnosis and pathogenesis of any lumbar spine disorder. The reader interested in these issues should consult general low-back or rheumatology textbooks on this topic.[23] The focus here is on occupational and ergonomic risk factors and pathogenesis of spinal conditions and injuries.

Pathogenesis and Etiology of Back Problems

The natural history and pathogenesis of low-back pain and degenerative spinal changes are not fully understood. Often the exact cause of low back disorders cannot be clearly defined. In particular, the correlation among symptoms, clinical, and morphological findings is not consistent. Variations in subjective and objective findings among patients have been described. A multitude of symptoms may result from degenerative disease of the spine. Nevertheless, characterization of clinical pain and neurological examination of sensory changes and weakness can help localize a possible morphological/anatomical lesion and assist in the differential diagnosis. Etiologic research has therefore concentrated on identifying and quantitating several personal and work-related factors.[24,25] Various causes and mechanisms have been discussed. Occupational risk factors for back problems are awkward body posture, heavy lifting, bending, twisting, and repeated loading from vibration and shock, as well as smoking, sedentary lifestyle, and certain psychosocial factors.[26,27]

Understanding of the biochemical and biomechanical properties of the vertebra, discs, and ligaments has been broadened with more refined research methods. Researchers from many disciplines, including bioengineers, basic science researchers, clinicians, and epidemiologists are now involved in the analysis of low-back pain.[28–31] Modern epidemiological research principles have been proposed to improve low back pain research methods and clinical tests.[32]

The cause of low-back pain may be related to the muscular, ligamentous, and skeletal structures of the spine. Degenerative bony growth, disc changes, and herniation may lead to spinal cord or nerve root compression, resulting in sciatica or other neurological complications. Pain can arise from an inflammatory or infectious process or from a tumor, a cancer, a trauma, or a fracture. Several rheumatological conditions, collagen vascular diseases, and postural deformities and genetic skeletal defects can affect the structure, function, and symptomatology of the spine. In about half of the cases, the etiology of the pain remains unknown.[33] For many patients, "normal" physiological aging of the spinal elements—the vertebra, discs, and ligaments—is a potential source of back problems. This "natural" degenerative process can, however, be accelerated and influenced by external factors in the work environment.[34–37]

Although understanding of the relationships between disc metabolism and degeneration and exogenous stress factors is limited, hypotheses have been developed about the etiology of "discogenic pain." One recent cross-sectional study of construction workers reported that progressive degenerative spinal changes were associated with an increased risk of sciatic pain.[38,39] Contributing effects of work on degenerative back disease and low back pain syndrome have been described. Spinal degenerative radiological changes can be seen up to 10 years prematurely in subjects with risk factors.[40]

Occupational Risk Factors for Low Back Pain

Risk Factor: Lifting

In many jobs (construction, nursing homes, hospitals, and package and mail handling) heavy or frequent lifting and carrying of heavy loads complicated by awkward body posture are a normal part of the required tasks. If the load is too heavy or the frequency of lifting exceeds the tolerance, acute or chronic injuries (initially mostly micro-traumata) to the lumbar spine can be the consequence. Among dentistry workers, however, lifting has not been identified as a specific risk factor.

Risk Factor: Vibration

Two forms of vibration exposure relevant for acute or chronic occupational health problems are known: whole-body vibration and segmental or hand-transmitted vibration. Long-term whole-body vibration stemming from engines and vehicles has been identified as an important mechanical stressor causing early and accelerated degenerative spine diseases and leading to back pain and prolapsed discs.[41-44] Poor body posture, inadequate seat support and muscle fatigue have been described as cofactors in the pathogenesis of musculoskeletal disorders of the spine in operators/drivers. High prevalence of back pain, early degenerative changes of the spine, and herniated lumbar disc problems have been consistently reported among vibration-exposed occupational groups: tractor drivers, truckers and interstate bus drivers, crane or earth-moving-equipment operators, and helicopter pilots. Also, among operators of rail vehicles (railroad and subway trains) with relatively low vertical but higher lateral vibration the prevalence of back disorders is high.[45,46] Dentists are typically not occupationally exposed to significant levels of whole-body vibration in vehicles and buildings. Long rides to and from work in automobiles with poor seating and under poor street conditions may be a cofactor in the pathogenesis of back problems.[47]

Prolonged and high hand-transmitted vibration, which can lead to serious vascular and neurological impairment, has been described in construction workers, miners, wood-processing workers, and agricultural workers handling power tools and chainsaws.[48,49] The hand-transmitted vibration risk for dentists from high-frequency drills has not been adequately investigated or established,[50] although a simple survey among colleagues showed that a few dentists had complaints similar or identical to those caused by hand-transmitted vibration.[51] A higher vibrotactile threshold than in the control group has been reported in two studies, but a higher incidence of finger blanching (Raynaud's phenomenon) has not been found.[52] The frequency spectrum and acceleration levels of the vibration generated by dental tools are different from those generated by the tools of forestry and construction workers with a high prevalence of hand-transmitted vibration. Overall, vibration exposure appears not to be a primary source or risk factor for dentists.

Risk Factor: Awkward Body Posture

Repetitive or static awkward body posture resulting from excessive bending and twisting increases spinal stress and disproportionate loading of spinal structures. Work in forced, extreme body posture can lead to temporary or chronic spinal misalignment and neurological-compression syndromes. Back stress from lifting tasks can be complicated, and vibration effects can be aggravated. Prolonged sitting in poorly designed chairs with inadequate lumbar support or adjustability can result in muscular fatigue and low back pain. Intradiscal pressures are significantly higher when an individual is seated than when standing or supine.[53] In fact, the highest intralumbar disc pressure was measured in the forward flexed position when compared with various body postures.[54] Ergonomic job analysis with a check-list approach is useful to assess postural stressors. References and resources have been listed elsewhere.[55,56]

Only a few studies have been conducted of awkward body posture and problems with physical dimensions among dentists. In a Japanese study, body postures of dentists were grouped into three categories according to the "inclination of the body." The most common posture was the right-forward position. It was concluded that the body posture of daily dental care practices was the established cause of work-related complaints among dentists.[57]

Psychophysiological strain parameters were felt to be related to the equipment design and use of the working area of dentists in Germany.[19] Repetitive tasks (such as scaling and root planing) and awkward body posture used to access the oral cavity were identified as factors contributing to musculoskeletal disorders.[20]

In a comprehensive study by German ergonomists, factors that influence and determine body posture were studied.[21] Figure 1 gives some parameters that influence the body posture of dentists.

Electromyographic recordings of certain activities performed during routine dental work showed that the cervical and lumbar spinal muscles particularly were under constant strain. The neck muscles were especially highly fatigued. A posture and movement analysis showed that 11 basic body postures are typical for dentists: seven seated postures and four standing postures. Factors that influence the working posture of dentists (Figure 1). Assessment of these types of body postures with three approaches (biomechanical, psycho-physical, and physiological) indicated that some body postures have a

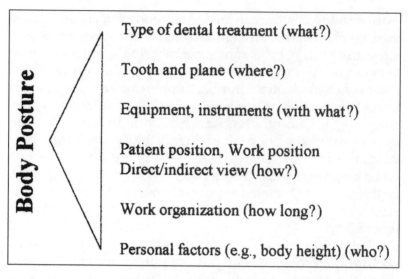

FIGURE 1.—Factors that influence the working posture of dentists.[21]

high stress ranking. An example of a body posture with a high stress ranking is presented in Figure 2.

Diagnosis of Low Back Pain

Medical Screening and Physical Examination

To assess health status and back-related musculoskeletal problems, a detailed clinical examination should be performed to collect subjective and objective data. This should include an investigation of signs and symptoms of spinal abnormalities and movement dysfunction utilizing standardized tests and clinical guidelines.[58,59] The clinical examination should include the following elements:

- an occupational and medical history assessment (demographics, work history/previous employment);
- personal habits (smoking) and behavior (sports);
- medication, medical/surgical and family history; and
- previous musculoskeletal disease or developmental deformity.

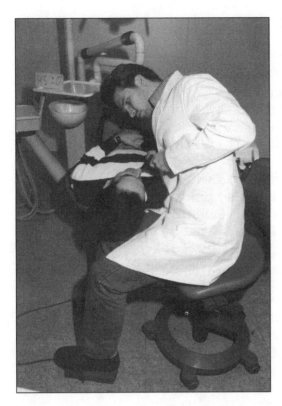

FIGURE 2.—Highly stressing body posture of a dentist during treatment of upper jaw.

Special emphasis should be placed on type, characterization, onset/frequency/duration, aggravating/alleviating factors, and location/radiation of reported back pain. The subjects can be asked to complete a standardized medical/occupational questionnaire. Also useful are pain scales and "pain diagrams," in which the patient indicates areas of pain and other abnormalities on a body chart diagram.

A physical examination should be conducted with special emphasis on the entire spine (neck, upper back, and lower back) with the subjects in standing, seated, and prone positions. A neurological examination should check reflexes and test sensory and motor function, muscle strength, and nerve root inflammation. Functional tests may be useful to detect possible clinical syndromes.

The clinical findings can be summarized by the examining physician into the following diagnostic categories:
- normal,
- minimal, moderate or severe abnormalities involving:

- musculo-ligamentous strain/sprain conditions,
- skeletal problems (specified),
- neurological involvement (sciatica or nerve irritation signs),
- sensory deficits,
- motor weakness,
- reflex changes or), or
- other diagnoses (specified); questionable etiology (specified)

Often a distinction is drawn between acute or chronic low back on the basis of the clinical impression. One of the key questions in a clinical examination is differential diagnosis and whether there is a need for surgical intervention as opposed to so-called conservative (noninvasive) management.

For some laboratory tests such as the measurement of the erythrocyte sedimentation rate, complete blood count and rheumatological markers may be necessary and useful to distinguishing inflammatory, infectious, and malignant back problems from degenerative (spondylosis) back disorders and musculo-ligamentous strain/sprain (mechanical causes).

Imaging and Diagnosis of Disorders of the Lumbar Spine

Computer tomogram scans or magnetic resonance imaging is in most cases not necessary for patients with a simple case of acute low back pain. Plain x-rays films are not sufficiently sensitive and specific enough to detect occupational back disorders, particularly in the early phases of soft-tissue or bony degenerative changes. X-ray films may be helpful to study malalignment of the entire spine. Magnetic resonance imaging and CAT scan are indicated in individuals who require a workup for a differential diagnosis or who need to be assessed for possible surgery, or if initial conservative treatment (about 6 weeks) has failed.

Other Diagnostic Procedures

If patient history or clinical signs suggest nerve-compression problems (radiculopathy) a nerve-conduction study or electromyography (NCS/EMG) or sensory-evoked potentials (SEP) (especially for detection of spinal stenosis) can be useful to study the degree and lumbar level of the involved nerve root. In the early phase, negative results are possible. Discography and myelography are generally not recommended and not necessary in most ambulatory cases.[60]

Treatment of Low Back Pain

In most cases, the clinical care of patients with acute back problems can follow current medical consensus guidelines. Recently, a panel of experts published diagnostic and therapeutic practice standards, which are gaining general acceptance.[60] Pain control medications, short periods of rest, physical therapy, "back school," aerobic exercise (swimming), spinal manipulation, and workplace modification may all be useful to relieve spinal stress and discomfort. In cases of serious, progressive neuro-orthopedic injury and complications, the need for and benefit of surgical intervention should be assessed by the clinician and discussed with the patient. A consensus summary on the diagnosis and treatment of lumbar disc herniation has recently been published.[61] Treatment outcomes depend on many factors: Patient's age, general health, significant comorbidity, and coexposures need to be considered. Certainly smoking should be discouraged. If appropriate, patients may need to be educated about vibration hazards and risky activities (such as prolonged unsupported sitting, heavy lifting, and twisting or bending of the back). They should be encouraged to prevent or minimize any unnecessary further exposure (at work or at home) involving the risk factors described above.

Prevention and Alternative Dental Work Station Design

Primary prevention (before the back pain occurs) should be attempted. A walk-through inspection by an occupational health specialist or ergonomist is often very useful identifying problems with equipment, with set up, and other red-flag conditions. But even in secondary prevention (early diagnosis/screening cases) or tertiary prevention (reintegration of a disabled worker) a better design of the dentist's office can facilitate positive results and improve the treatment outcome (return to work). The results of a workplace analysis can be used to derive design changes. Changing of technical design *and* human behavior are both strategies for minimizing the risk of low back pain. The almost constant sedentary position of dentists is clearly an unfavorable human posture ("static posture"). The missing dynamic in body postures of dentists is one risk factor for spinal discomfort. Thus, frequent changing of the sitting or upright body posture should be attempted by the treating dentist involved in prolonged procedures or between patients. It appears beneficial to do treatments with a high demand for physical strength (e.g., extraction of teeth or crowns) or treatments of a whole mouth (e.g., molding of a part of jaw) in a standing position.

Another aspect of technical design is the determination of adequate environmental conditions (e.g., climatic and lighting conditions). For dental workers, an optimally designed and adjustable work area should include ergonomically designed patient treatment chairs, dental-care worker chairs, hand and foot controls, and instruments.

The working conditions (patient position, physical limitations of chair and equipment) as well as the movement behavior of the dentist should be modified to achieve optimal body posture. A good starting point is to position the patient in such a way that it is possible for dentists to work in a relaxed posture. As a result of laboratory experiments, eight different patient positions have been derived.[21] These positions involve the adjustment of the patient's chair with respect to the angles of head support and back rest, as well as the inclination of the patient's head according to the part of the face (e.g., oral, buccal) and the mouth segment (e.g., upper jaw, left side) of the tooth to be treated.

Figure 3 shows an example of an adequate patient position for treatment of upper jaw and the corresponding acceptable body posture of the dentist.

Positioning of patients is easy with specially designed dental equipment. An example of an ergonomically designed patient treatment chair is shown in Figure 4. A main feature of this patient treatment chair is the integration of a computerized system for positioning the patient. The dentist enters the targeted tooth with a hand- or foot-controlled dialogue technique. Following predefined positions, the angles of the head support and the back rest then automatically adjust in such a way that the dental work can be done with a relaxed (neutral) body posture. The height of the chair is adjusted according to the body height of the dental care worker (which has to be programmed only once into the chair's control system).

As a result of studies in dental offices,[25] it was concluded that eight different treatment positions are not practicable and that some of the positions are uncomfortable for patients. In laboratory experiments, all relevant factors and dental duties were simulated to test different options and survey the treating dentists' satisfaction as well as the patients' comfort. Four

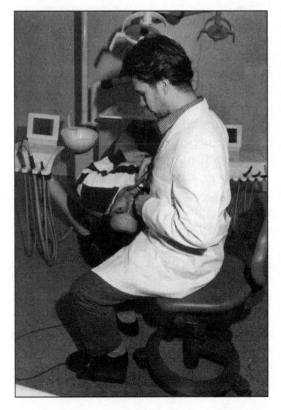

FIGURE 3.—Relaxed body posture of a dentist as consequence of an adequate patient position.

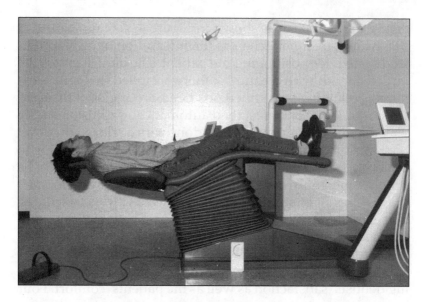

FIGURE 4.—An example of an ergonomic patient treatment chair.

preset patient chair positions were found to be most favorable. These chair positions represent a good compromise between an acceptable body posture for dentists and sufficient comfort for patients.

A special feature of the ergonomic patient treatment chair is the extensive functionality of the foot control. The foot control of different equipment functions appears advantageous in hygiene and infectious control requirements. One conflict that may arise in the design of a foot control is the need to have as many "positions" as possible and still maintain safety. From laboratory experiments it could be derived that it is possible to use four directions for releasing different functions. These four directions are forward- and backward-tilting around the horizontal lateral axis (plantar and dorsal inflection within the upper ankle joint), as well as interior and exterior rotation around the longitudinal axis of the lower leg. It should be noted that the interior rotation around the longitudinal axis of the lower leg is limited to 10°.

Although technical and engineering design of dental work environments is crucial to decreasing the risk of low back disorders, behavioral and motivational factors of dentists should

Table 1.—Adjustment of a Patient Treatment Chair According to the Tooth Being Treated

Tooth to be treated	Angle of back rest (horizontal = 0°)	Angle of head support (horizontal = 0°)
Upper jaw right or left		
Upper jaw middle (oral)	10°	–15 °
Upper jaw/lower jaw		
middle (buccal)	10°	0°
Lower jaw right (oral)		
Lower jaw left (buccal)	10°	5°
Lower jaw right or left		
Lower jaw middle (oral)	15°	5°

not be overlooked. It seems prudent to support ergonomic thinking early during the education of dentists and assistants. Proper postural education and awareness training can promote healthy "movement behavior" and back fitness exercise long before bad habits set in and spinal over-stressing occurs. Dentists are facing many other types of economic and psychological "stressors," which appear to confound musculoskeletal complaints. Stress management programs have been specifically developed for dentists and, according to the literature, are very popular.[62-65]

REFERENCES

1. Webster BS, Snook S. The cost of compensable low back pain. *J Occup Med.* 1990;32:13–16.
2. NIOSH. Proposed National Strategy for the prevention of musculoskeletal Injuries. Pub 89-129. Department of Health and Human Services, NIDSH; 1989.
3. NIOSH. National Occupational Research Agenda. U.S. Dep Health and Human Services, Public Health Service, Centers for Disease Control and Prevention, National Institute for Occupational Safety and Health (NIOSH). 1996 (April, No. 96-115).
4. Guo HR, Tanaka S, Cameron LL, Seligman PJ, Behrens VJ, Ger J, Wild DK, Putz-Anderson V. Back pain among workers in the

United States: national estimates and workers at high risk. *Am J Ind Med.* 1995;28:591–602.

5. Hales TR, Bernard BP. Epidemiology of work related musculoskeletal disorders. *Orthopedic Clinics of North America.* 1996; 27(4):679–709.

6. Work-related musculoskeletal disorders. *Washington State Summary 1992–1994.* State of Washington, Department of Labor and Industries. P417-130-000; October 1996.

7. Sinczuk-Walczak H, I Zycki J. Back pain syndromes in dentists. Diagnosis and differential diagnosis. *Med Pr.* 1994;45(1):71–74.

8. Van Doorn JW. Low back disability among self-employed dentist, veterinarians, physicians and physical therapists in the Netherlands. *Acta Orthop Scand Suppl.* 1995;263:1–64.

9. Moen BE, Bjorvatn K. Musculoskeletal symptoms among dentists in a dental school. *Occup Med.* 1996;46(1):65–68

10. Pollack R. Dental office ergonomics: how to reduce stress factors and increase efficiency. *J Can Dent Assoc.* 1996;62(6):508–510.

11. Augustson TE, Morken T. Musculoskeletal problems among dental health personnel. *Tidsskr Nor Laegeforen.* 1996;116(23): 2776–2780.

12. Bourassa M, Bayland JF. Stress situations in dental practice. *J Can Dent Assoc.* 1994;60(1):65–67, 70–71.

13. Hillman M. Stress and dentistry. *NY State Dent J.* 1995;61(6):50–52.

14. Mazey KA. Stress in the dental office. *J Calif Dent Assoc.* 1994;22(2):13–19.

15. Freeman R, Main JR, Burke FJ. Occupational stress and dentistry: theory and practice. *Br Dent J.* 1995;178(6)part I:214–217;part II:218–222.

16. Reitemeier B. Psychophysiological and epidemiological investigation on the dentist. *Rev Environ Health.* 1996;11(1–2):57–63.

17. Burke FJ, Main JR, Freeman R. The practice of dentistry: An assessment of reasons for premature retirement. *Br Dent J.* 1997; 182(7):250–254.

18. Rohmert W, Mainzer J, Zipp P. *Der Zahnarzt im Blickfeld der Ergonomie* [Dentists in the focus of ergonomics]. *Eine Analyse Zahnärztlicher Arbeitshaltungen* [An analysis of body postures of dentists]. Ed. Forschungsinstitut für die zahnärztliche-Versorgung (FZV). Köln: Deutscher Ärzte Verlag; 1986.

19. Rohmert W, Bruder R. Ergonomic Research and work design for the dentist. In: Singleton WT, Dirkx J, ed. *Ergonomics, Health and Safety. Perspectives for the Nineties.* Leuven University Press 199; 121–142.

20. Bruder R, Rommert W. Ergonomic research of dentists—an example of a cooperation between industrial and university research departments. In: Queinnec Y, Daniellou F, eds. *Design for Everyone. Proceedings of the Eleventh Congress of the International Ergonomic Association.* Paris: Taylor and Francis Publ; 1992:1159–1161. See also Analysis and design of the relationship of patient, dentist, and dental assistant in the work system of dentistry. In: Landau K, ed. *Work Conditions in the Hospital and at Home.* Bayerische Staatsministerium für Arbeit, Familie, und Sozialordnung RB-Nr. 10/91/31, 1991;536–551

21. Pollack R. Dental office ergonomics: how to reduce stress factors and increase efficiency. *J Can Dent Assoc.* 1996;62(6):508–510.

22. Bruder R, Rohmert W. Transfer of ergonomic knowledge in the development of dental equipment. In: *Ergonomics in Computerized Dentistry II. European Society of Dental Ergonomics. Annual Meeting,* July 1995. Den Haag, Netherlands.

23. Borenstein DG, Wiesel SW. *Low Back Pain. Medical Diagnosis and Comprehensive Management.* Philadelphia: WB Saunders; 1989.

24. Frymoyer JW and Gordon SL, eds. *American Academy of Orthopedic Surgeons Symposium. New Perspectives on Low Back Pain.* Chicago; 1989.

25. Riihimaki H. Low-back pain, its origin and risk indicators. *Scand J Work Environ Health.* 1991;17:81–90.

26. Pope MH, Frymoyer JW, Andersson G, eds. *Occupational Low Back Pain.* New York: Praeger; 1984:101–136.

27. Erdil M, Dickerson OB, eds. *Cumulative Trauma Disorders. Prevention, Evaluation and Treatment.* New York: Van Nostrand Reinhold; 1997:441.

28. Nachemson A. The lumbar spine, an orthopedic challenge. *Spine.* 1976;1(1):59–71.

29. Kelsey JL, Hochberg MC. Epidemiology of chronic musculoskeletal disorders. *Ann Rev Public Health.* 1988;9:379–401.

30. Pope MH. Bioengineering—the bond between basic scientists, clinicians, and engineers. The 1989 presidential address. *Spine.* 1990;15(3):214–217.

31. Haldeman S. Failure of the pathology model to predict back pain. Presidential address, North American Spine Society. *Spine.* 1990;15(7).

32. Symposium: research methods in occupational low-back pain. *Spine.* 1990;16(6):665–686.

33. Frymoyer JW. Back pain and sciatica. *NEJM.* 1988;318(5):291–300.

34. Kellgren JH. The anatomical source of low back pain. *Rheum Rehab.* 1977;16(3):3–12.

35. Junghanns H. *Die Wirbelsäule in der Arbeitsmedizin* [The spine in occupational medicine]. Stuttgart:Hippokrates; 1979:I–III.
36. Riihimaki H. Low-back pain, its origin and risk indicators. *Scand J Work Environ Health.* 1991;17:81–90.
37. Boden SD. *The Aging Spine: Essentials of Physiology, Diagnosis, and Treatment.* Philadelphia: Saunders Comp; 1991.
38. Riihimaki H, Wickström G, Hanninen K, Mattsson T, Waris P, Zitting A. Radiographically detectable lumbar degenerative changes as risk indicators of back pain. *Scan J Work Environ Health.* 1989;15:280–285.
39. Riihimaki H, Wickström G, Hanninen K, Luopajärvi T. Predictors of sciatic pain among concrete reinforcement workers and house painters—a five-year follow-up study. *Scand J Work Environ Health.* 1989;15:415–423.
40. Wickström G. Effect of work on degenerative back disease. A review. *Scand J Work Environ Health (Suppl1).* 1979;4:1–12.
41. Dupuis H, Zerlett G. *The Effects of Whole-Body Vibration.* Berlin: Springer Verlag; 1986.
42. Seidel H, Heide R. Long-term effects of whole-body vibration: a critical survey of the literature. *Int Arch Occup Environ Health.* 1986;58:1–26.
43. Hulshof C, van Zanten B. Whole-body vibration and low-back pain. *Int Arch Occup Environ Health.* 1987;59:205–220.
44. Griffin MJ. *Handbook of Human Vibration.* London: Academic Press; 1990.
45. Johanning E, Wilder D, Landrigan P, Pope M. Whole-body vibration exposure in subway cars and review of adverse health effects. *JOM.* 1991;33(5):605–612.
46. Johanning E. Survey results of back disorders and health problems in subway train operators exposed to whole-body vibration. *Scand J Work Environ and Health.* 1991;17(6):414–419.
47. Kelsey JL, Hardy RJ. Driving of motor vehicles as a risk factor for acute herniated lumbar intervertebral disc. *Am J Epidemiology.* 1975;102:63–73.
48. Johanning E, Hulshof C, Christ E. Whole-body and segmental vibration. Chapter 9. In: Erdil M, Dickerson OB, eds. *Cumulative Trauma Disorders.* New York: Van Nostrand Reinhold; 1997:221–250.
49. Palmear PL, Taylor W, Wasserman DE. *Hand-Arm Vibration.* New York: Van Nostrand Reinhold; 1992.
50. Burke FJ, Jaques SA. Vibration white finger. *Br Dent J.* 1993; 174:191.
51. Jaques SA, Burke FJT. Vibration white finger. *Br Dent J.* 1994; 177(8):279.

52. Griffin MJ. Handbook of human vibration. London: Academic Press; 1990:591.
53. Andersson GBJ. On Myoelectric Back Muscle Activity and Lumbar Disc Pressure in Sitting Postures. Goteborg, Sweden: University of Goteborg, 1974. Thesis.
54. Nachemson A. The load on lumbar discs in different positions of the body. *Clin Orthop.* 1966;45:107–122.
55. Perez GM. Applied work analysis for the upper extremity. In: Erdil M, Dickerson OB, eds. *Cumulative Trauma Disorders.* New York: Van Nostrand Reinholt; 1997.
56. Simonton K. *Lessons for Lifting and Moving Materials.* 12/1996 P417-129-000. State of Washington: Department of Labor and Industries; 1996.
57. Kihari T. Dental care works and work-related complaints of dentists. *Kurume Med J.* 1995;42(4):251–257.
58. Roger M. Nelson, project officer. Low Back Atlas of Standardized tests and measures (draft). Morgantown, WV: NIOSH; Dec 1988.
59. Erdil M, Dickerson BO, Glackin E. Diagnosis and medical management of work related low back pain. In: Erdil M, Dickerson BO, eds. *Cumulative Trauma Disorders.* New York: Van Nostrand Reinhold; 1997:441–498.
60. Bigos SJ, et al. Clinical Practice Guideline No 14. Acute Low Back Problems in Adults. Rockville, Md: U.S. Dep Health and Human Services. Public Health Service. Agency for Health Care Policy and Research. AHCPR Publ No 95-0642. Dec 1994.
61. Andersson GBJ, Brown MD, Dvorak J, Herzog RJ, Kambin P, Malter A, McCulloch JA, Saal JA, Spratt KF, Weinstein JN. Consensus summary on the diagnosis and treatment of disc herniation. *Spine.* 21(24S):75S–78S.
62. Mazey KA. Stress in the dental office. *J Calif Dent Assoc.* 1994;22(2):13–19.
63. Freeman R, Main JR, Burke FJ. Occupational stress in dentistry: theory and practice. Part I: Recognition. *Br Dent J.* 1995; 178(6):214–217 and Part II: assessment and control. *Br Dent J.* 1995;178(6):218–222.
64. Reitemeier B. Psychophysiological and epidemiological investigations on the dentist. *Rev Environ Health.* 1996;11(1–2):57–63.
65. Pollack R. Dental office ergonomics: how to reduce stress factors and increase efficiency. *J Can Dent Assoc.* 1996;62(6):508–510.

Chapter 16

Diagnosis and Medical Management of Work-Related Neck and Upper Extremity Musculoskeletal Disorders in Dental Care Workers

R. Herbert, J. Dropkin, S. Levin, P. Marino, F. Gerr, and E. Kolber

Abstract

Dental care practitioners are often exposed in their work to biomechanical hazards such as repetitive motion and nonneutral joint position, and are consequently at risk for the development of work-related upper-extremity musculoskeletal disorders. This chapter provides introduction and background information on the diagnosis and treatment of work-related musculoskeletal disorders in dental care workers. It describes clinical features of specific conditions such as nerve entrapment disorders, occupational disorders of the neck and brachial plexus, shoulder disorders, tendinitis, and hand-arm vibration syndrome. The chapter also provides information on what to include in an occupational and medical history (e.g., demographics, symptom history, review of systems and social history); physical examination (e.g., range of motion, sensory testing and reflex testing); and laboratory evaluation (e.g., basic blood and urine testing, electrodiagnostic studies, and radiologic evaluation). The last section addresses the management of work-related musculoskeletal disorders, including both medical management (e.g., rest, immobilization) and workplace intervention.

Introduction

Work-related upper extremity musculoskeletal disorders, which comprise a heterogeneous group of diagnoses, are being increasingly recognized as a significant cause of morbidity and lost productivity among workers in the United States. These disorders include carpal tunnel syndrome and other nerve entrapment disorders; disorders of the tendons and tendon sheaths, including lateral and medial epicondylitis; de Quervain's disease and tendinitis of the flexor and extensor tendons of the hand; hand-arm vibration syndrome, and disorders of the neck, upper back, and shoulders. Dental care practitioners who are exposed in the course of their work to ergonomic hazards including repetition, awkward and static postures, forceful exertions, mechanical stresses, and vibration are potentially at risk for the development of work-related musculoskeletal disorders.

In this chapter, we describe the spectrum of work-related musculoskeletal disorders that a dental care professional may develop and provide an overview of the appropriate occupational and medical histories, physical examination, and specialized diagnostic testing needed to 1) render a correct diagnosis, 2) ascertain work relatedness, and 3) determine appropriate therapy for dental care workers with work-related musculoskeletal disorders. Clinical features of specific disorders and the medical management of work-related musculoskeletal disorders in dental care workers are then discussed.

Background

Dental work is often performed with the upper extremities in unsupported, awkward postures and the cervical spine in nonneutral positions.[1] Because of these postures, over time the shoulder and neck regions are subject to high stationary loads, which can cause musculoskeletal symptoms following prolonged exposure.[1]

Hagberg reported in a study of dentists conducted in South Wales that the prevalence of musculoskeletal disorders in the neck was 18%.[2] In a survey of self-reported pain in the previous six months, 27% of dentists reported having experienced neck pain. Twenty-four percent of South Wales dentists reported neck disorders occurring since they began working.[2] A Finnish study showed that 50% of dentists had cervical spondylosis compared to 31% in a reference group of farmers.[2]

Swedish dentists had a greater risk of developing right shoulder musculoskeletal disorders compared with clerks.[2] In a study of Finnish dentists, the shoulder was the body part in which pain most frequently occurred; 42% of dentists had pain 6 months before the survey.[2] In another study of Finnish dentists, 13% experienced glenohumeral joint (shoulder joint) osteoarthrosis.[2]

Dental work also requires repetitive movement and nonneutral postures of the hands. South Wales dentists reported 23% of musculoskeletal disorders in the hands occurring since beginning dentistry.[2] [Younger dentists experienced 10% more and older dentists experienced 22% more right hand pain than the clerks.][2]

Additionally, Raynaud's syndrome has been linked to work with high-speed rotating handpieces and ultrasound equipment, such as those employed by dental care workers.[1]

Clinical Background

While there is general consensus that upper-extremity musculoskeletal disorders are responsible for a significant burden of occupational disease, the literature with respect to prevalence and incidence of specific work-related musculoskeletal disorders in dental care workers is limited. Thus, this chapter will focus on the diagnosis and management of the spectrum of work-related musculoskeletal disorders for which dental care workers may be at risk on the basis of their known exposures.

Despite the limited literature focusing on dental care workers, it is usually possible in the clinical setting to render a specific diagnosis and, on the basis of the exposure history, to ascertain work relatedness. This requires a systematic approach to diagnosis and recognition that workers frequently present with multiple work-related musculoskeletal disorders. To avoid omission, the evaluation should begin at the neck and proceed down to the fingers and include evaluation of soft tissue, joints, and neurological systems. Once a precise diagnosis or diagnoses has been made, work relatedness is ascertained, according to general principles of occupational medicine (i.e., relation of symptoms to work, history of work-place exposures to ergonomic factors likely to contribute to the condition, presence of similar condition, and presence of similar conditions among coworkers).

Workplace modifications coupled with rehabilitation are an integral component of treatment. The Occupational Safety and Health Administration (OSHA) has recently produced guidelines for the control of musculoskeletal disorders in the meatpacking industry.[3] Similar guidelines for other industries are expected to follow.

Clinical Features of Specific Conditions

Nerve Entrapment Disorders

CARPAL TUNNEL SYNDROME

Carpal tunnel syndrome occurs following compression of the median nerve as it passes through the carpal canal in the wrist, and is characterized by neuritic symptoms such as pain, paresthesia, and numbness in the cutaneous distribution of the median nerve. Physical signs include diminished cutaneous sensibility to vibration, light touch, and pin prick in the distribution of the median nerve, as well as abnormal two-point discrimination. Thenar muscle weakness and atrophy as well as Phalen's sign (reproduction of hand symptoms following 1 minute of wrist flexion) or Tinel's sign (electric shock sensation radiating into the hand upon tapping the wrist) are classically described physical examination findings in carpal tunnel syndrome. Electrodiagnostic studies are currently the "gold standard" for the evaluation of suspected carpal tunnel syndrome. Prolongation of the distal motor latency of the median nerve, slowing of median sensory conduction velocity across the wrist, and denervation of the abductor pollicis brevis muscle are electrophysiologic findings highly suggestive of carpal tunnel syndrome.[4,5] The combination of symptoms, signs and electrodiagnostic findings is the most valid means of diagnosing carpal tunnel syndrome.[4,6-9] Carpal tunnel syndrome has been suggested to be an occupational hazard among dental care workers.[10] In general, cases of mild carpal tunnel syndrome and some cases of moderate carpal tunnel syndrome can be managed nonsurgically, at least initially. Nonsurgical management should include cessation of inciting occupational and nonoccupational exposures, night splinting with neutral splints, physical therapy and/or occupational therapy, and nonsteriodal anti-inflammatory drugs (NSAIDs) as tolerated, unless medically contraindicated (see Figure 1).

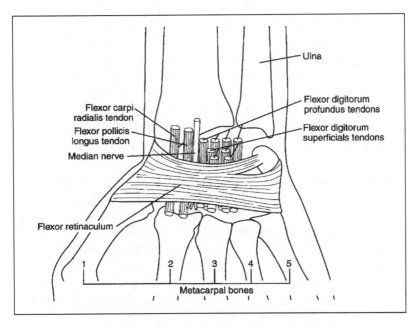

FIGURE 1.—Carpal tunnel syndrome: Carpal tunnel syndrome occurs following compression of the median nerve as it passes through the carpal canal in the wrist.

ULNAR NEUROPATHY

This condition most commonly occurs secondary to compression or injury at the elbow. The nerve may also become entrapped just below the elbow in the antecubital tunnel between the heads of the flexor carpi ulnaris muscle. In addition to compression in the elbow, the ulnar nerve can also be compressed at the base of the palm as it passes through Guyon's canal.

Symptoms of ulnar neuropathy generally include pain, numbness, and/or tingling in the distribution of the ulnar nerve fourth and fifth digits. Motor symptoms are less common, but may include loss of control of the fifth digit or lateral instability of the fingers. Symptoms of ulnar entrapment at the elbow are often exacerbated by flexion and may be relieved by extension of the elbow.[6] Physical examination findings include either a positive elbow flexion or wrist extension test (development of pain, numbness or tingling in the ulnar nerve distribution with elbow flexion or wrist extension in 3 minutes or less). Ulnar sensation should be tested (two-point discrimination and light touch). Motor findings may include weakness of pinch strength between the thumb and adjacent digits, impaired coordination of the thumb and other digits, impaired strength of grip, and asynchrony of finger flexion.[6] As with median nerve entrapment, nerve conduction studies should be performed; however, electrophysiologic abnormalities can occur in clinically "normal" subjects.[6] Workers whose jobs involve sustained flexion at the elbow, with pressure on the ulnar groove are potentially at risk for development of ulnar entrapment of the elbow.[11] Chronic compression of the ulnar nerve at or below the wrist may also result in chronic compressive neuropathy. Occupational groups potentially affected include those whose work involves prolonged periods of gripping dental tools in the palm of the hand.[6] Treatment for ulnar neuropathy includes avoiding leaning on the elbow, physical therapy and/or occupational therapy, and NSAIDs as tolerated. The elbow extension splint is the most commonly used splint for this disorder.[6] Generally, the splinting objective is to position the elbow in extension in order to remove tensile (traction) forces imposed on the ulnar nerve when the elbow is flexed (see Figure 2). This splint is best tolerated at night.

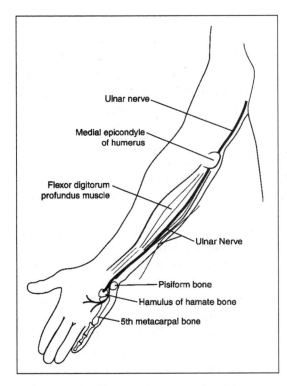

Ulnar nerve

Medial epicondyle of humerus

Flexor digitorum profundus muscle

Ulnar Nerve

Pisiform bone

Hamulus of hamate bone

5th metacarpal bone

FIGURE 2.—Ulnar neuropathy: This condition most commonly occurs secondary to compression or injury at the elbow. In addition to compression in the elbow, the ulnar nerve can be compressed at the base of the palm.

Occupational Disorders of the Neck and Brachial Plexus

Disorders of the neck that can present as upper-extremity pain include tension neck syndrome, cervical radiculopathy, cervical spondylosis, and thoracic outlet syndrome.

TENSION NECK SYNDROME

Tension neck syndrome, also called tension myalgia, is a complex of pain, tenderness, and stiffness of the cervical musculature and trapezius muscles, with the physical findings of muscle spasm. Pain caused by cervical muscle contraction may not always be located in the neck. It can radiate between the shoulder blades, down the arms or up to the occiput. In addition to tenderness on palpation and spasm of posterior neck muscles, physical examination generally reveals limited rotation of the neck. In occupational epidemiologic studies, criteria for the diagnosis of this condition include:

1. neck pain or stiffness, muscle tightness, and palpable hardening and tender spots on the neck coupled with pain on resisted neck lateral flexion and rotation[12];
2. a constant feeling of fatigue or stiffness or both in the neck, plus one or more subjective symptoms such as neck pain or headache, signs of palpable hardening or at least two tender spots or both, and muscle tightness in neck movements; and
3. a variety of symptoms such as pain, tenderness, and stiffness of muscles, as well as signs of hardened bands of nodularities and muscle spasm generally originating from a trigger point for the pain and numbness (referred to the reference zone), without the common boundaries of nerve distribution.[13]

Treatment of tension neck syndrome involves physical therapy and consists of stretching tightened muscles and massaging hyper-irritable regions. Ultrasound and electrical muscle stimulation can also be used to increase blood flow and decrease muscle spasm. Iontophoresis (injection of chemicals through the skin and into the muscle with electrical voltage rather then with a needle) can be used to reduce muscle spasm. Other treatment alternatives include ice massage, moist heat, stretching and strengthening exercises (in chronic cases), aerobic exercise, "spray and stretch," and trigger-point injection.

CERVICAL SPONDYLOLYSIS

Cervical spondylolysis is a degenerative condition involving osteoarthritis of the cervical spine. Common symptoms of cervical spondylosis include stiffness, limitation of movement, crepitus on active or passive movements of the neck, muscle spasm, and localized pain and tenderness. Lateral flexion, rotation, and extension are generally more limited than vertical flexion. Pain is usually in the upper-middle cervical region and may be referred to the occiput, scapula, or shoulders. On radiographic examination, the most obvious findings are reversal of the normal cervical lordosis, narrowing of the intervertebral disc spaces, and osteophytosis.[14] Of note, however, is that in a survey of 50 patients, all of them over 50 years of age, and none of them with neurological complaints, 75% showed radiologic evidence of narrowing of the cervical spinal canal caused by posterior osteophytosis (bone spurs) or narrowing of the intervertebral foramina, indicating that radiologic changes may be inadequate for a diagnosis of cervical spondylosis.[15] Definitions of cervical spondylosis that have been used in occupational studies include the following:

1. pain localized to the neck, tenderness and palpation interspinally, and localized pain in the neck during movements, as well as reduced mobility and spondylosis degeneration confirmed by x-ray[16]; and

2. degenerative changes in the cervical spine, radiographically seen as spurs or reduction in disc height.[17] Hagberg and Wegman found dentists (in two studies) to be at increased risk of cervical spondylosis. Treatment of cervical spondylosis involves restoring the normal lordosis to the cervical spine. This can be accomplished by posture-retraining exercises and segmental strengthening of the posterior neck muscles followed by restoration of the muscular balance of the cervical spine.[18]

CERVICAL DISC DISEASE

Cervical disc disease includes a spectrum of conditions ranging from disc degeneration to disc herniation. Cervical disc herniation may involve both the exiting nerve root and the spinal cord. Cord compression is uncommon, except in patients with spinal stenosis or massive rupture of a disc. The sites of most frequent disc herniation include C-5 to C-6 and C-6 to C-7.

Cervical disc disease usually begins with a stiff neck and splinting of the neck muscles, along with discomfort on the medial side of the scapula. Radicular paresthesia or pain is present when the root is more severely compressed. The symptoms are worsened with particular movements of the head and neck, and are often alleviated by holding the arm elevated and flexed behind the head (unlike patients with shoulder disease, who maintain the arm in a dependent position, avoiding elevation, abduction or excursion at the shoulder joint). In general, with nerve root involvement, there may be tingling in the proximal part of the associated dermatome, distal sensory loss, and, in some cases, wasting or weakness of muscles supplied by the affected nerve root or diminished reflexes along the nerve root distribution. C-5 lesions are characterized by pain in the shoulder along with a dermatomic sensory diminution, with weakness and atrophy of the deltoid. The clinical picture of C-6 lesions includes paresthesias of the thumb and depression of the biceps reflex, with weakness and atrophy of that muscle. The pattern of C-7 lesion includes paresthesias that may involve the index and middle finger and even the thumb, with atrophy and weakness of triceps, wrist extensors, and pectoral muscles. C-8 provides intrinsic muscle sensation and function in the hand and fourth and fifth fingers.[19]

In the Hagberg and Wegman study, cervical syndrome or cervical disease was diagnosed by the presence of pain in the neck radiating to the arm, with a segmental distribution. In general, the management of cervical disc disease should involve the neurologist, neurosurgeon, or physiatrist. Conservative management may include periods of rest, anti-inflammatory agents, use of a cervical collar, and physical therapy, in addition to cessation of inciting workplace exposures.

THORACIC OUTLET SYNDROME

Although most authors agree that this is a fairly rare condition, the standard medical literature is quite contradictory about the frequency and diagnostic criteria for thoracic outlet syndrome. The term thoracic outlet syndrome, which was first suggested by Rob and Standove in 1958,[20] describes a number of symptom complexes that arise from the compression of the neurovascular bundle (brachial plexus, subclavian artery and subclavian vein) as it passes from the neck to the arm. The thoracic outlet consists of the space between the inferior border of the clavicle and the upper border of the first rib, which is compartmentalized by the scalene muscles. For anatomic reasons, the various components of the neurovascular bundle can be compressed at several sites. Additionally, several other factors may contribute to the narrowing of the thoracic outlet. Increased muscle bulk can cause less space for the neurovascular structures, increasing the risk of developing thoracic outlet syndrome. Several congenital factors, such as cervical ribs, may be related to this condition. Additionally, prior fracture of the clavicle with malunion or nonunion and excessive callous formation results in impingement upon the subadjacent neurovascular structures.[14]

The signs and symptoms of thoracic outlet syndrome vary, depending on whether the brachial plexus, the subclavian artery, or the subclavian vein is compressed. There may be both vascular and neurological components, although generally there is very little overlap between symptoms of vascular and neurologic origin.[6]

Compression of the brachial plexus is associated with pain, numbness, and paresthesias. Additionally, there may be associated motor symptoms. Pain is usually localized in the neck and shoulder regions, radiating to the suprascapular region. Paresthesias present as numbness and tingling in the ulnar nerve distribution and in the median cutaneous nerve of the forearm. When present, motor symptoms consist of a sensation of weakness and clumsiness of the fingers. Activities involving abduction of the shoulders can cause worsening of the symptoms. A screening test for this condition is reproduction of neurologic symptoms upon abduction and external rotation of the arm.

Arterial symptoms, which are less common than neurologic symptoms, include pain, weakness, coldness, and fatigue of the arm. The radial pulse may be dampened or absent in different arm maneuvers. Abduction or elevation of the arm may exacerbate the symptoms. Three clinical maneuvers that may be useful in assessing arterial involvement are:

1. In the costoclavicular maneuver, the patient is asked to adduct scapula on the nonaffected side, forcing the clavicle against the first rib. In this test, symptoms should be reproduced with diminished radial pulse to confirm the diagnosis.
2. In the hyperabduction maneuver, the patient abducts his or her arm above the head. When the neurovascular bundle is compressed under the coracoid process and pectoralis minor muscle, symptoms should be reproduced, along with reduction in pulse.
3. In Adson's test, the patient is asked to inhale and turn the head to the affected side. In a positive test, the radial pulse is reduced.

The diagnosis of thoracic outlet syndrome is often a diagnosis of exclusion. Patients in whom this diagnosis is suspected should be sent either to a neurologist or to a vascular surgeon for a second opinion. If this diagnosis is suspected, a chest x-ray should be performed to rule out an apical lesion of the lung, and x-rays of the cervical region should be obtained to look for the presence of bony abnormalities. A subclavian arteriogram may document subclavian artery compression in patients with radial pulse abnormalities. In other patients, electromyography or nerve conduction studies may be useful. However, decisions about the evaluation should be made in concert with a neurologist or other appropriate consultant. The treatment of thoracic outlet syndrome involves physical therapy for stretching anterior upper quadrant muscles, strengthening of the posterior upper trunk and shoulder girdle muscles, and posture retraining exercises to reduce forward head posture and promote a more neutral cervical spine (see Figure 3).

Shoulder Disorders

The shoulder is the most mobile joint in the body.[21] Pain in the shoulder, with loss of mobility of the joint, often leads to disability, lost work time and even early retirement.[22] Shoulder pain should therefore prompt early diagnosis and treat-

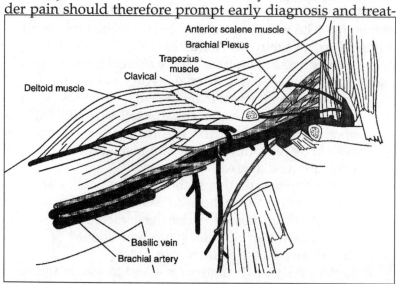

FIGURE 3.—Thoracic Outlet Syndrome: Symptoms arise from the compression of the neurovascular bundle (i.e., brachial plexus, subclavian artery, and subclavian vein) as it passes from the neck to the arm.

ment. It is especially important in the management of shoulder pain and dysfunction that pain arising from the shoulder itself be differentiated from pain referred from another source (e.g., the neck, or abdominal or thoracic viscera).

The principal causes of shoulder pain thought to be associated with work-related stressors include trapezius myalgia; rotator cuff tendinitis (pericapsulitis, subacromial bursitis, supraspinatus tendinitis); rotator cuff tear; bicipital tendinitis; and adhesive capsulitis (glenoid capsulitis).

Trapezius Myalgia

This condition is associated with a history of exposure to static loading in the shoulder-stabilizing muscles over a long period of time (as can occur in highly repetitive work). Patients offer complaints of pain and tenderness localized to the descending part of the trapezius muscle, especially on the side most exposed to the static load.[23] This condition is frequently seen in combination with the "tension neck syndrome" described elsewhere in this paper. Physical examination will sometimes demonstrate local muscle hardening and trigger points along the muscle insertion.[13] Treatment of trapezius myalgia generally includes physical therapy or medical massage therapy, with trigger-point work; a home stretching program; and amelioration of awkward postures and other inciting factors in the workplace. Additionally, biofeedback and the use of home ice/heat regimens may be useful.

Rotator Cuff Tendinitis

Rotator cuff tendinitis is a common cause of pain in the shoulder associated with repetitive motion. The structure most frequently involved in the underlying pathology is the supraspinatus tendon, which is subject to repetitive overload because of forceful muscle contraction when the shoulder is required to sustain or move heavy loads. Supraspinatus tendinitis can proceed through the entire spectrum of reversible inflammation, angiofibroblastic degeneration, fibrosis, calcification, and exostosis formation.[24] Tears of the fibrotic tendon (torn rotator cuff) are common, especially in patients in their fifth and sixth decades of life. The role of possible impingement and consequent ischemia of the cuff when the tendon is compressed between the greater tuberosity of the humerus and acromion during abduction is a subject of debate.[25]

Occupational activities associated with rotator cuff tendinitis include excessive or forcible shoulder exertion, repetitive activities with the shoulder in rotation and the arm elevated, overuse in overhead work, and repetitive pulling or lifting.[12]

The most frequently reported symptom caused by rotator cuff tendinitis is pain, generally localized along the anterior lateral aspect of the acromion, accompanied by functional impairment secondary to the pain. Abduction of the shoulder between 60 and 90 degrees results in increased pain ("the painful arc").

Physical examination should include both active and passive range of motion of the glenohumeral joint, as well as shoulder depression, elevation, and scapular protraction and retraction. Forcible passive flexion of the arm will often produce shoulder pain in cases of cuff tendinitis, as will forward flexion of the humerus to 90 degrees with internal rotation of the arm. Pain with movement of the arm above 90 degrees is common. Palpation of the rotator cuff may reveal tenderness at the insertion of the tendons on the greater tuberosity of the humerus. There is often a significant loss of strength when comparison is made with the unaffected side.

Computer-assisted arthrography with contrast medium, sonography, and magnetic resonance imaging may be of value in the assessment of this syndrome when the history and physical examination suggest the diagnosis. Patients for whom this diagnosis is being considered should be referred for orthopedic consultation.

In rotator cuff tendinitis, the treatment approach includes prevention of further overuse of the shoulder, without complete immobilization of the joint. Failure to maintain mobility of the shoulder can result in the development of adhesive capsulitis (or "frozen shoulder"—see below). Ice application has been used during the period of acute inflammation, along with NSAIDs. Local injection of steroids can be effective in reducing acute inflammation. Within two weeks of an acute "flare-up" and after the patient's pain has begun to subside, rehabilitation exercise with low resistance should be considered (with careful limitation on the resistance load). Some have found high-voltage electrical stimulation of the shoulder to be of benefit.[24] Rehabilitation efforts should be directed toward strengthening the musculature of the entire shoulder.

As is the case with other musculoskeletal disorders, the indications for surgery to remove the degenerated fibrotic tissue include failure to improve with an active rehabilitation program, a loss in the overall quality of life, constant pain without activity, and persistent weakness, atrophy, and dysfunction. Before surgery is contemplated, adequacy of the rehabilitation effort should be reviewed.

Prevention must focus on limiting the amount of work performed with the arms raised overhead or to 90 degrees. Education of the workforce and front-line supervisory personnel is necessary to modify work practices (see Figure 4).

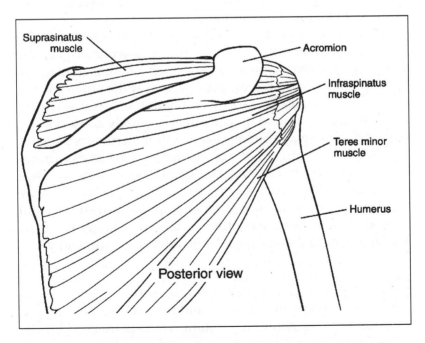

FIGURE 4.—Rotator cuff tendinitis: The structure most frequently involved in rotator cuff tendinitis is the supraspinatus tendon.

ROTATOR CUFF TEARS

Most rotator cuff tears occur from degenerated tendons, with no identifiable episode of major trauma. Again, pain in the shoulder, especially with attempts at abduction, and weakness or absence of abduction are the most common presenting symptoms and signs. MRI is frequently employed to assist in the diagnosis. Management generally involves the same approach as for rotator cuff tendinitis, with a trial of physical therapy and anti-inflammatory agents, and surgery is considered only after a conservative approach has proved ineffective.

BICIPITAL TENDINITIS

Inflammation of the biceps tendon is associated with pain in the anterior of the shoulder, made worse with flexion of the elbow against resistance. Pulling and lifting, especially lifting with arms overhead, and resisted elbow flexion with the shoulder in abduction and rotation are among the risk factors associated with bicipital tendinitis.

Physical examination usually reveals pain elicited in the anterior of the shoulder when the patient attempts to flex the elbow against the examiner's resistance. There is tenderness to deep palpation in the bicipital groove at the anteromedial aspect of the shoulder. X-ray examination may show calcification in the tendon. Management is generally conservative, with physical therapy and the use of anti-inflammatory agents.

Complete rupture of the biceps tendon produces a protuberant ball of contracted muscle over the belly of the biceps, a characteristic deformity. Generally, there is a history of acute overloading of the muscle in an attempt to lift heavy weight immediately before the rupture occurs. In younger workers, reattachment of the tendon is often attempted surgically.

ADHESIVE CAPSULITIS (FROZEN SHOULDER)

Adhesive capsulitis causes, and in part results from, immobility of the glenohumeral joint. There is marked limitation of motion, with severe pain produced by attempts to flex or abduct the shoulder. This is often progressive, since the experience of pain in the shoulder on motion leads to a spontaneous "splinting" of the joint, with conscious as well as reflex restriction of voluntary motion. The condition may follow an acute shoulder injury or may represent the outcome of recurrent episodes of rotator cuff tendinitis.

Treatment involves rehabilitation, with a range of passive motion exercises designed to gradually increase the mobility of the glenohumeral joint. (Such exercises should be used in most cases of acute or chronic shoulder injury to avoid the development of adhesive capsulitis.) Anti-inflammatory agents, electrical stimulation, and heat and/or ice treatments have also been employed. When mobilization of the joint is not accomplished by this kind of conservative regimen, noninvasive manipulation of the shoulder under general anesthesia will often result in considerable improvement of range of motion. That improvement must be maintained by persistent performance of mobilizing exercises.

Tendinitis of the Elbow, Forearm, and Wrist
As described by Gerr et al,

Tendinitis and tenosynovitis refer to inflammation of the tendon and tendon sheath, respectively. Both are associated with the occurrence of pain during physical maneuvers that place the tendons in tension. The diagnosis of tendinitis is based on the presence of pain on palpation of the affected tendon, pain localized over the tendon in motion, and the presence of warmth, swelling and tenderness of the tendons on palpation.[26]

Tenosynovitis can progress to stenosing tenosynovitis, characterized by narrowing of the tendon sheath[27] that results in triggering movements of the digits ("trigger finger"). Although the most commonly affected tendons are the dorsal extensor of the wrist, the extensor carpi ulnaris, and the long abductor and short extensor of the thumb (de Quervain's disease),[28] any muscle-tendon unit of the extremities can be affected[27] (see Figure 5).

DE QUERVAIN'S DISEASE
De Quervain's disease, or stenosing tenosynovitis of the abductor pollices longus and extensor pollices brevis, generally

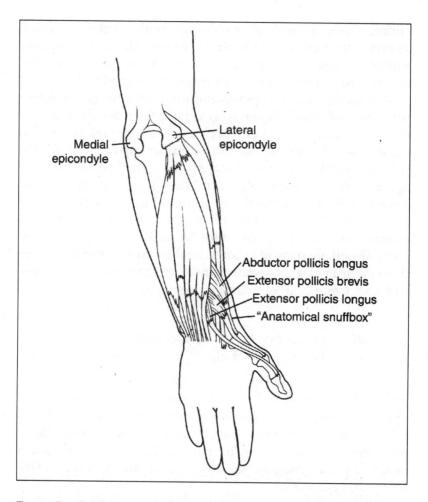

FIGURE 5.—De Quervain's disease: De Quervain's disease, or stenosing tenosynovitis of the abductor pollices longus and extensor pollices brevis, usually manifests swelling over the "anatomical snuffbox."

manifests as pain and swelling over the radial styloid (in the area of the anatomic snuffbox). The pain may radiate up the forearm or down into the thumb. Physical examination reveals pain over the radial styloid when the wrist is passively moved into ulnar deviation with the thumb abducted in the palm. Weakness of resisted extension is often noted. Occupations that require combinations of hand twisting, wringing (in the 19th century, this entity was known as "washerwoman's sprain"), and forceful gripping may increase the risk of developing this disorder.[11]

There is a range in severity of symptoms and time course of the disease and recuperation period. This range is from a more transient to a more persistent and chronic form of tenosynovitis that requires more invasive therapy. Some milder cases may respond to rest, anti-inflammatory agents, splinting with a thumb orthosis, and ergonomic adjustments of the work station and movements. Other, more advanced cases may require local steroid injection and progressive physical therapy/occupational therapy with an exercise program for gradual strengthening. The most commonly used splints are the thumb spica splint (sometimes referred to as a long opponens splint) and radial gutter splint that includes the thumb.[29] Generally splint objectives involve the following: 1) thumb spica splints rest the two inflamed thumb tendons, reducing shearing forces (internal forces tangential to the section on which it acts) between the tendons and bony prominences in the wrist while immobilizing the wrist and hand; and 2) radial gutter splints also rest the two thumb tendons, but allow some motion of the wrist and provide greater hand function. In severe, chronic cases, surgical debridement has been used.[30]

EXTENSOR CARPI RADIALIS LONGUS AND BREVIS TENDINITIS

Tendinitis of the extensor carpi radialis longus and brevis ("oarsman wrist") may result from De Quervain's tenosynovitis. The presentation is one of pain, tenderness, swelling, and crepitus with active tendon motion. This crepitus has been described as a "leatherlike rub or squeak" with wrist flexion and extension that is palpable and sometimes audible in the region of the intersection of the radial wrist extensors and the first dorsal compartment muscle belly. Finkelstein's sign (a test for stenosing tenosynovitis of the intrinsic thumb muscles) may be positive. It has been postulated that these areas are also relatively hypovascular and are perhaps less able to respond to the repetitive stress of work hypertrophy. That is why this entity is seen with repetitive flexion and twisting motions. Treatment is similar to that for De Quervain's disease with rest, anti-inflammatory medications, and ergonomic adjustment as first steps.[30] The most commonly used splint is a wrist immobilization splint in extension (sometimes referred to as a wrist cock-up splint).[31] Generally, the splint objective is to position the wrist extensor tendons in a relaxed position, or "on slack," reducing tensile forces.

FLEXOR CARPI ULNARIS TENDINITIS

The most common type of tendinitis on the flexor side of the wrist is flexor carpi ulnaris tendinitis, in which the patient experiences pain over the tendon in the wrist which is exacerbated by wrist flexion and ulnar deviation against resistance. The treatment is the same as for other tendinitis disorders. The most commonly used splint is the wrist immobilization splint in neutral or 0 to 10 degrees of extension.[32] Generally, splint objectives are to rest the flexor tendons by limiting wrist motion and to limit tensile (traction) forces on the tendons. (see Figure 6)

TENOSYNOVITIS OF THE FLEXOR PORFUNDUS OF THE INDEX FINGER AND FLEXOR POLLICUS LONGUS

The usual presenting complaint with this type of tenosynovitis is one of aching or burning in the distal forearm and hand. This may be confused diagnostically with carpal tunnel syndrome. On physical examination, extension and flexion of the thumb across the palm with fingers extended reproduces the pain. Treatment is the usual regimen for tenosynovitis. However, this form of tenosynovitis may progress to an adhesive tenosynovitis, restricting separate use.

The most commonly used splints are the hand and finger-based splints.[33] The general splint objective is to block finger motion in order to decrease the frictional forces that occur between tendons and between tendons and other digital structures.

EPICONDYLITIS

In the elbow, lateral epicondylitis ("tennis elbow") is more common that medial epicondylitis ("golfers' elbow"). The majority of cases of epicondylitis are not due to sports, de-

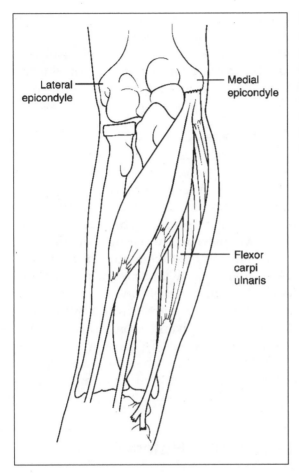

Lateral epicondyle

Medial epicondyle

Flexor carpi ulnaris

FIGURE 6.—Flexor carpi ulnaris tendinitis: The most common type of tendinitis on the flexor side of the wrist is flexor carpi ulnaris tendinitis.

spite their names. Patients with lateral epicondylitis generally report pain in the area of the lateral epicondyle and extensor muscle mass that is exacerbated by a forceful grip, lifting with palm down, wrist extension, and racquet sports.[34] Physical examination reveals the presence of pain to palpation of the lateral epicondyle that is exacerbated by resisted wrist extension with elbow extended. Patients with medial epicondylitis have pain in the area of the medial epicondyle and flexor muscle mass exacerbated by resisted flexion of the wrist and fingers with elbow extended (see Figure 6).

Workers at risk of developing epicondylitis may include those with jobs that involve repetitive, forceful wrist and elbow movement.[35,36] Treatment is similar to other tendinitis disorders, with rest, anti-inflammatory medication, and alteration of workplace ergonomic factors recommended.

A device known as a Lateral Epicondylitis (tennis elbow) strap or a counterforce brace is used to help reduce forces to the extensor tendon origins on the elbow region[37] (see Figure 6).

Hand-Arm Vibration Syndrome

This disorder of blood vessels and peripheral nerves is caused by transmission of vibration to the hands and arms.[38] It has also been called white finger, vibration white finger, occupational Raynaud's disease, and vibration syndrome.[39] The vascular component of the disorder is characterized clinically by cold-induced vasospasm, indistinguishable from Raynaud's disease. The neurological component is characterized clinically by abnormal sensory and motor function and likely involves injury to both nerve fibers and mechanoreceptors. Treatment of hand-arm vibration syndrome includes keeping the body temperature high and avoidance of cold exposure, smoking, and additional hand-arm vibration exposure. Analgesics and NSAIDs, along with neutral wrist splints at night can be used to treat concomitant ulnar and median neuropathy.[40]

Occupational and Medical Histories

Occupational and medical histories are key elements in establishing a correct diagnosis and formulating an appropriate treatment plan for workers with complaints of upper-extremity pain. The occupational history is used both to ascertain work relatedness of the patient's condition and to investigate which workplace interventions will be most suitable for treatment of musculoskeletal conditions of occupational origin. A detailed medical and symptom history is vital to rendering a proper diagnosis of the cause of the patient's upper-extremity symptomatology; additionally, it is used to screen for the presence of systemic conditions that may predispose the patient to developing certain upper-extremity diseases. The history of the worker with a possible upper-extremity disorder of occupational origin should therefore include the information outlined below.

Demographics

As in any medical history, the patient's age and gender should be recorded. Additionally, the dominant hand should be specified.

Occupational History

The occupational history should focus on the presence or absence of exposure to the following workplace factors that may be associated with the development of upper-extremity musculoskeletal disorders: repetitive movements, use of force, work in an abnormal (nonneutral) posture, and inadequate rest periods. The physician should obtain a description and—where possible—a demonstration of all movements performed by the worker in the course of his or her work. The rate at which movements are performed should be estimated, and the frequency and duration of rest breaks should be noted. Additionally, the worker's posture (including the position of both upper extremities) while performing work should be noted. A description of the work station should be obtained. The physician should inquire about adjustability of the chair, work station, and tools. Although it is rarely feasible to obtain a videotape of the patient performing his or her job, workers can usually have a photograph taken of themselves at work. This can be very useful in developing an understanding of the ergonomic stressors faced by the patient. A detailed description of all tools used in the patient's job should be obtained; the history should specify which upper extremity is used and should describe the types of upper-extremity movements required by the tool, how well the tool "fits" the worker's hand, how much force is subjectively required to operate the tool, and whether the use of the tool results in exposure to vibration. Any recent changes in work station design or work pace that may be related to the onset of illness should be noted.

A description of the work pace should be obtained. As treatment of many upper-extremity disorders can require slowing of work pace or initiation of rest breaks, the physician should ask about the presence or absence of factors such as piece-rate work and productivity requirements that may affect treatment plans. As in an occupational history, the number of years at the present (or pertinent) job should be noted; additionally, the number of years performing work at other jobs with similar exposures should be recorded. The history should include the number of days and hours worked as well as the number of hours per day spent performing relevant activities.

In addition to investigating workplace exposures that may be related to the patient's condition, the physician should inquire about nonwork activities that may also involve exposure to cumulative trauma. To avoid inadvertently overlooking such exposures, the history should routinely include questions about housework and care of young children; hobbies (e.g., knitting, playing musical instruments); and exercise/recreation (e.g., weight lifting, rowing).

Symptom History

A detailed systematic symptom history is crucial in establishing a proper diagnosis. The goal of the history is to ascertain the anatomic location of the pain or other symptomatology and to determine whether the condition is due to inflammation of tendons and tendon sheaths, focal nerve entrapment or compression, primary neurologic disease, rheumatologic disorders, infection, neoplasm, or another condition. The physician should elicit a description of the nature of the symptoms, as well as the location, the radiation (if any), the duration, and both exacerbating and helpful factors. Information on prior modes of treatment should be ascertained. The physician should bear in mind that patients may have more than one condition simultaneously. In workers with exposure to repetitive motion of the upper extremity, it is not uncommon to see double crush syndromes (compression at both the cervical spine and within the upper extremity itself—i.e., at the carpal tunnel) or coexistent nerve entrapment and tendonitis. Additionally, the physician should be on the lookout for systemic diseases such as diabetes mellitus and tuberculosis, which can present initially as upper-extremity disorders.

Patients should be asked if they experience pain, aching, stiffness, or burning in any of the following areas: neck, shoulder, upper arm, elbow, forearm, wrist, or fingers and hands. The date of onset of symptoms and any inciting factors should be noted, as should symptom intensity, duration, frequency of episodes, and exacerbating and palliative factors. The physician should inquire about the presence of numbness or tingling in any digits of either hand, and should note which digits are affected. Classically, but not invariably, individuals with carpal tunnel syndrome report symptoms of numbness or paresthesias in the first three digits of the hand; in those with ulnar neuropathy, these symptoms classically occur in the fourth and fifth digits. Individuals who report numbness and tingling should be asked if they are awakened at night by the symptoms. Patients should be asked about muscle strength through questions about difficulty in performing tasks such as turning keys, opening bottles, and grasping door knobs.

Medical History

The medical history should focus on obtaining information about prior musculoskeletal disorders or neurologic conditions that may be related to the present condition and, should cover prior history of upper-extremity or neck trauma or surgery. Additionally, the history should screen individuals for the presence of conditions that may predispose to the development of carpal tunnel syndrome and, in some cases, tendinitis.

The medical history should therefore include the following:
1. a history of musculoskeletal disorders (fracture of either upper extremity, cervical radiculopathy, thoracic outlet syndrome, "tennis elbow," "golfer's elbow," tendonitis, de Quervain's disease, carpal tunnel syndrome, ulnar nerve entrapment, bursitis, osteoarthritis and rheumatoid arthritis, and upper-extremity trauma
2. a history of surgical procedures in the neck or upper extremities
3. a history of the following conditions, which predispose individuals to developing carpal tunnel syndrome: diabetes mellitus, rheumatoid arthritis, osteoarthritis, gout,

hypothyroidism, sarcoidosis, tuberculosis, lupus, scleroderma, and kidney disease
4. reproductive history (for women): current pregnancy, use of oral birth control pills or estrogen replacement therapy, menopause
5. prior hospitalizations; and
6. current medication(s).

Review of Systems

To ensure that possible systemic illness is not overlooked, a standard, comprehensive review of systems should be performed.

Family History

The family history should focus on the presence or absence of neurologic or connective-tissue disease among immediate family members.

Social History

Alcohol consumption should be noted if there is any suspicion of a generalized peripheral neuropathy. A smoking history should be obtained, particularly if the diagnosis of hand-arm vibration syndrome is being considered, symptoms suggestive of Raynaud's phenomenon are present, or neck pain is present (as Pancoast's tumor can occasionally present as neck pain). For all patients in whom a work-related upper-extremity disorder is suspected, the social history should provide the physician with information about factors in the workplace and home environment that may affect elements of treatment, such as emotional stress at work or home or economic factors that may render the worker unable to take time off from work for physical therapy or rest breaks.

Physical Examination

Because of the possibility of systemic illness presenting as an upper-extremity disorder, the physical examination should include examination of the skin (e.g., for butterfly rashes), eyes, oropharynx, thyroid gland, chest, abdomen, lymphatic system, and nervous system. More specifically, neck and upper-extremity physical examination for musculoskeletal disorders should include the following:

1. visual inspection of the neck, shoulders, elbows, wrists, metacarpal phalangeal joints, proximinal interphalangeal joints, and distal interphalangeal joints for joint deformities, swelling, or other signs of inflammation;
2. visual inspection of the hands, with specific attention to the mass of the thenar and hypothenar eminences, bilaterally
3. palpation of the cervical area of the neck and upper back for muscle spasm
4. palpation of the shoulders, elbows, medial and lateral epicondyles, wrists, metacarpal phalangeal joints, proximal interphalangeal joints, and distal interphalangeal joints for tenderness, crepitation, swelling, warmth, or other signs of inflammation, as well as for nodules;
5. palpation of the thenar and hypothenar eminences of both hands to assess muscle mass, palpation of the palmar fascia for nodules, and palpation of the flexor and extensor tendons of the hand.
6. recording, in degrees, of passive and resisted range of motion ; grading of strength during resisted motion with the 1 to 5 point scale; recording of pain, when present, along with location and nature; serial assessment of grip strength (grip-strength dynamometry is useful):
   a. neck—flexion, extension, rotation (head turning to right and left shoulders), and left and right lateral bending (ear to shoulder)
   b. shoulders—abduction (arm lifted outward from side of body up over head), internal and external rotation, flexion (forward elevation), and extension (backward elevation)
   c. elbows—flexion and extension
   d. wrists—flexion, extension, supination, pronation, and ulnar and medial deviation
   e. hand/fingers—flexion into a full fist, extension, abduction, and adduction of the fingers; and
   f. thumb—flexion, extension, abduction, and adduction of the thumbs

7. sensory testing of the upper extremities by testing vibration sensation with a 128 Hz tuning fork in the second and fifth digits of each hand and assessment of sensation in each of the dermatomes of the arm
8. testing of the deep tendon reflexes in the biceps, triceps, and brachioradialis tendons and
9. provocative maneuvers when the history or physical examination raises the possibility of carpal tunnel syndrome, de Quervain's disease, ulnar neuropathy, or thoracic outlet syndrome:
   a. Phalen's maneuver (for carpal tunnel syndrome),
   b. Tinel's maneuver (for carpal tunnel syndrome),
   c. Finkelstein's test (for de Quervain's disease),
   d. elbow flexion test (for ulnar nerve entrapment),
   e. Adson's test (for thoracic outlet syndrome),
   f. hyperabduction maneuver (for thoracic outlet syndrome),
   g. costoclavicular maneuver (for thoracic outlet syndrome), and
   h. abduction/external rotation test (for thoracic outlet syndrome).

Laboratory Evaluation

Laboratory evaluation may be necessary to confirm the presence of specific disease entities or to rule out some of the nonoccupational systemic illnesses. These evaluations can include the following:
1. basic blood and urine testing;
2. specialized blood testing;
3. electrodiagnostic studies; and
4. radiologic evaluation with plain x-rays, computed tomography scan, or magnetic resonance imaging.

Basic Blood and Urine Testing
These tests can reveal many systemic conditions that can cause musculoskeletal pain, joint swelling, or neuropathy:
- Serum chem can screen for undiagnosed diabetes, the "predisposition" to gout (uric acid levels greater than

9 mg/dL yield up to 80% probability of developing gout), and hyperlipidemias (which have associated musculoskeletal disorders).
- Complete blood count can reveal an anemia, which may be associated with collagen vascular diseases, or an elevated white blood count, which can be associated with an infectious process.
- Sedimentation rate is elevated with collagen vascular diseases, inflammatory bowel disease, and infectious processes.

If there is suspicion of a collagen vascular disease, a complete blood cell count, a sequential multiple analyzer (this is not a term in usual use) and an erythrocyte sedimentation rate should be obtained. If carpal tunnel syndrome is diagnosed, an SMA should be performed along with complete blood cell count, an erthyrocyte sedimentation rate test, and thyroid function tests. Also, if clinically indicated, rheumatoid factor, antinuclear antibody, and Lyme titer should be determined.

Electrodiagnostic Studies

Electromyography and nerve conduction velocities are useful in diagnosing the nerve compression syndromes. They are the "gold standard" in the diagnosis of carpal tunnel syndrome.

Electrodiagnostic studies are generally recommended for patients with symptoms of nerve compression (i.e., numbness, parasthesias, muscle weakness, muscle wasting) if there is any question of diagnosis or if conservative therapy does not lead to improvement of symptoms.

Radiologic Evaluation

Plain x-rays, computed tomography scan, and magnetic resonance imaging are useful in diagnosing several conditions:
- Plain x-rays are useful in evaluating the possibility of degenerative joint disease, rheumatoid arthritis, or other joint diseases and should be obtained if the history or physical examination suggests joint involvement. Subclinical fractures may also be diagnosed; therefore, x-rays should also be obtained in individuals who have

sustained traumatic injuries. Evaluation of individuals who are found to have cervical radiculopathy should include x-rays of the cervical spine. X-rays are also warranted to rule out a cervical rib in the case of thoracic outlet syndrome (an extra rib located in the cervical spine may lead to thoracic outlet syndrome). Shoulder films can be useful if there is a possibility of calcific tendinitis.

- Computed tomography scans have been very useful in the diagnosis of degenerative disease of the spine with subsequent nerve impingement. Patients with cervical radiculopathy should be evaluated with either computed tomography or a magnetic resonance imaging of the cervical spine in addition to plain x-rays.

- Magnetic resonance imaging scans have been useful in evaluation of the cervical spine for disease not seen on plain film or computed tomography. It is a good modality for visualization of soft-tissue herniation of the cervical discs. It is also used to evaluate possible rotor cuff tears.

Management

The proper management of upper-extremity musculo-skeletal disorders of occupational origin requires that

1. a correct diagnosis be made
2. appropriate medical treatment be initiated, and
3. modifications be made in the work station and/or work process, so that exposure to ergonomic stressors is reduced.

The goal of treatment is to allow patients to remain employed, or to enable them to return to work as quickly as possible (i.e., to maintain function), while reducing or eliminating symptomatology and preventing disease progression. Treatment of this group of disorders generally involves a team approach to care. The role of the occupational-medicine physician is to establish the diagnosis, often in conjunction with other medical specialists; to coordinate and monitor the efficacy of medical treatment and provide referral to physical therapists or other specialists as needed; and to ensure that appropriate workplace modifications are made, which will often involve contact with ergonomists, union officials, and employers. While a detailed discussion of the management of specific upper extremity disorders is beyond the scope of this chapter, certain general management principles are discussed below.

Medical Management and Rehabilitation

Once a precise diagnosis has been made and the extent of the illness has been characterized, a treatment plan should be developed. With the exception of certain nerve entrapment conditions, such as carpal tunnel syndrome with electromyographic evidence of muscle wasting, the initial approach to treatment should be conservative. Tendinitis, tendon sheath inflammation, carpal tunnel syndrome without evidence of muscle damage, tension neck syndrome, and cervical radiculopathy are all conditions in which inflammation contributes to symptomatology, and in which initial treatment modalities, aimed at the acute phase, differ from subsequent treatment modalities. Successful management thus requires frequent re-evaluation, with follow-up visits every 1 or 2 weeks, during which the time efficacy of the treatment should be evaluated and the management plan modified.

The initial approach to the management of these disorders should include the elements discussed below.

REST

The goal of rest is to limit exposure to both occupational and nonoccupational ergonomic stressors and, hence, to interrupt the inflammatory cycle. The manner in which this goal is achieved will vary, depending on the severity of symptomatology, the type of condition being treated, and the ease with which effective workplace modifications can be implemented. Some individuals will require a period out of work, whereas others may be able to alter their work in such a way that they can continue (e.g., by taking frequent, brief rest breaks and/ or by altering either the work process or the work station).

Social work involvement is often critical in ensuring that patients are able to comply with physicians' advice regarding removal from work or frequent rest breaks, as these interventions can have significant adverse economic and social implications for patients.

IMMOBILIZATION

Splinting programs are routinely prescribed as part of treatment for upper-extremity work-related musculoskeletal disorders. A splint is a temporary device that is used not only to immobilize, "but also mobilize, position, and protect a joint or a specific body part."[32] Splints for overuse musculoskeletal disorders can be effectively employed to reduce shearing, compression, and tensile forces to muscles, tendons, and nerves. In a general sense, the objectives of a splinting program for the treatment of soft-tissue injuries, are based on the redirection of forces and facilitation of healing. This approach is applicable in the treatment of musculoskeletal pain of the dental care worker.

There are commercially available and custom-made splints. Commercially available splints are prefabricated, "off-the-shelf" devices that may be obtained from a pharmacy or surgical supply store or mail order company with the assistance of a physical or occupational therapist. Many new soft splints are available that provide support and allow partial or restricted movement.

Occupational therapists, along with physical therapists who specialize in hand therapy, constitute a large segment of the professionals who fabricate custom-made splints. These splints are made directly on the body from low-temperature thermoplastic materials that become malleable in water when heated to between 135° and 180°. They are generally semiflexible or rigid.

One type of splint has no inherent advantage over another. Advantages of commercially available splints include price and availability of soft, very flexible splinting designs. Advantages of custom-made splints include the ability to ensure better fit and the ability to customize splint components.

The effective implementation of a splinting program involves the consideration of a number of factors. Prior to obtaining and using a splint, a diagnosis should be made indicating the specific soft tissue that is injured. Wearing a splint that covers the region of the discomfort may not in actuality address the specific structure that is causing the problem. Before using a splint, there should be consideration as to the optimal position, degree of immobilization, and ranges of restricted motion desired, in relation to splint conception, design, and function. New materials and products are available that allow this type of control in both prefabricated and custom-made splints; this ability contrasts sharply with the rigid-immobilization splints of the recent past.

Wearing time and use are additional issues to be considered. Motion of a key joint such as the wrist is very important in the performance of various dynamic, functional hand activities. As a result of the physical demands of the dental worker, the wrist is frequently positioned in awkward and extreme postures. It may seem reasonable to employ a splint for the main purpose of restricting movement to nonharmful, neutral postures. However, immobilization of a joint normally used to perform dynamic, hand-intensive activities can have significant effects on other parts of the body. It is not, therefore, recommended that splinting be used for the sole purpose of immobilizing or restricting joint motion and confining the segments of the upper extremity when constant wrist movement for task performance is great. This recommendation applies to all levels of intervention, whether as prevention or as a treatment. Isometric, static muscle contraction that is performed against the confines of a rigid splint may serve as another source of strain to soft-tissue structures. Motion that is blocked at one joint will inevitably be carried out by another joint or by the use of awkward, compensatory postures. Integrating the use of neutral, nonawkward splints, however, is known to be of benefit for rest during breaks and positioning at night while sleeping. For the dental practitioner, this implies that wearing rigid splints while performing dental tasks is not likely to be beneficial and may in fact be harmful. Moderately rigid splints used on the nondominant hand may be better tolerated.

Soft or flexible splints employed during activity may have therapeutic value in that they help to support painful structures while allowing nonpainful, nontraumatizing ranges of motion to occur. Unfortunately, soft splints are often made of materials that cannot tolerate sterilization procedures and therefore are not feasible for use when sterile conditions are necessary. Flexible fabric and soft splints, however, may be used effectively during rest breaks and during active motion activities to provide support for inflamed structures when sterile conditions are not necessary. Thermoplastic splints can undergo effective sterilization.

A good splint fit is critical. Compression or shearing (frictional) forces imposed on delicate anatomical structures can result from splints that are either too big or too small. Unintentional restriction of joint motion is another possible outcome of a poorly fitting splint. Respecting bony prominence and vulnerable soft-tissue structures will improve the comfort of the splint and reduce the risk of secondary injury or irritation from the use of a splint that does not fit well.[41] Individuals with significant nerve injuries may not have normal cutaneous sensation (feeling) which can result in decreased perception of stresses to the skin and superficial structures. Individuals suspected of having sensory loss should, therefore, visually inspect the hand after wearing a splint, to look for areas of redness or abraded skin that signify excessive pressure.

Splints and splint programs should be modified throughout the healing stages of an injury. Greater immobilization is generally recommended in the acute stages of an injury, as well as during acute inflammatory periods that may occur in subacute stages. Less immobilization allowing greater freedom of movement and facilitating the process of tissue remodeling is generally recommended in later stages of healing. In the treatment of overuse musculoskeletal injuries, total immobilization like that required to facilitate bone healing is not generally considered necessary or even desirable. Motion is physiologically important in preserving joint and soft-tissue structures. There is a great deal of evidence in the research literature that structural and biochemical changes occur after only brief periods of immobilization of muscle, tendon, nerve, and joint structures.[42] Excessive or inappropriate use of splints over a period of time can worsen soft-tissue problems by causing musculotendinous shortening, atrophy, and adhesion (scar) formation. The natural kinetic (movement) chain, consisting of the numerous upper-extremity joints and the brain, is also compromised by excessive immobilization. The judicious use of splints, however, to strategically control movement, reduce forces, and support joint and soft-tissue structures, can be beneficial in the treatment of the musculoskeletal injuries of the dental practitioner.

ANTI-INFLAMMATORY AGENTS

During the acute phase of upper-extremity disorders characterized by inflammation, nonsteroidal anti-inflammatory agents should be prescribed unless there is a medical contraindication. Baseline renal function (creatinine and urine dipstick) should be checked prior to initiation of the anti-inflammatory agents in patients who are 40 years of age or older, and should be periodically monitored in such patients. As it takes 2 to 3 weeks for the full effect of the NSAID to be felt, patients should remain on one medication for that period unless side effects develop; after 3 weeks, if no improvement has occurred, a different type of NSAID should be tried.

ELECTROTHERAPY

There are a variety of electrotherapeutic modalities that can be used to help restore muscle to its normal functioning.

- *Ultrasound* is used to produce sound waves which then generates heat that is absorbed by different local tissues.[43] Indications include soft tissue shortening, subacute and chronic inflammation and muscle guarding or trigger areas.[43] Effects include increases in local metabolism, local vasodilatation, increase in muscle relaxation, connective tissue extensibility, and increase in membrane permeability and sedation of sensory nerve endings.[43] *Phonophoresis* is a modality that "injects" molecules of medicine into the skin, muscles and nerves through ultrasound transmission.[43]
- *Electrical muscle stimulation* provides exercise to muscles if the subject has difficulty actively contracting the muscle.[43] Electrical stimulation is used on innervated muscle to strengthen muscle, decrease disuse atrophy, improve

mobility, increase circulation and provide proprioceptive feedback in a muscle.[43] It is used for denervated muscle to maintain nutrition of the muscle, increase blood flow, decrease fibrotic changes in the muscle and diminish muscle atrophy.[43] Indications include injuries to peripheral nerves, inhibition of muscle activity secondary to joint pain and effusion, possible disuse atrophy, and conditions involving limitation of joint range of motion.[43]

- *Transcutaneous electrical nerve stimulation (TENS)* neuromodulates pain through a spinal neurochemical mechanism.[43] Indications include acute and chronic painful conditions.[43]
- *Iontophoresis* uses direct electrical current to slowly introduce "ions of medicine" locally into the skin and surrounding tissues.[43] Indications include post-traumatic edema, trigger points, acute and subacute inflammation, and peripheral circulatory decifit.[43]
- *High volt pulsed galvanic stimulation* effects include pain relief, reduction of muscle guarding, promotion of blood flow, production of relaxation, promotion of fast tissue healing, improvement of fibroblastic activity, reduction of edema and muscle reeducation.[43]
- *Interferential stimulation* effects include relief of pain, production of muscle contraction that may lead to strengthening of muscle, increase in blood flow and muscle relaxation.[43]

PASSIVE AND/OR ACTIVE ASSISTIVE RANGE OF MOTION

Gentle joint-play oscillations/mobilizations and traction can relieve pain and muscle guarding to permit early movement of the extremity and cervical spine in the acute phase. In the chronic phase, more aggressive joint mobilization can be performed to increase the extensibility of the joint. Active assistive range of motion (ROM) can maintain existing range of motion or increase it.

MASSAGE

Transverse friction massage helps form a mobile scar, assists in the resolution of the inflammatory process, and promotes maturation at the healing site through enhanced blood flow to the damaged area.[18] Soft-tissue mobilization decreases muscle spasm, reduces fibrous bands separating muscle fibers, decreases fibrous thickening around vessels, reduces the likelihood of hemorrhages, increases blood flow, and helps restore metabolic balance within soft tissue.[18]

EXERCISE (INCLUDING HOME EXERCISE)

During the acute phase of illness, exercise of affected areas should be avoided. However, in some conditions, gentle stretching exercises may be initiated. After resolution of acute symptoms has occurred, an isometric/isotonic exercise program to strengthen muscles in the affected and surrounding areas may be appropriate. Postural awareness for the upper trunk and upper extremities should be employed so that the dental care provider can tell the difference between good and poor posture. Home exercise should consist of stretching and strengthening exercises, including flexibility and endurance regimes. Generally, the exercise program should be developed for, and taught to the patient by, a physical therapist/occupational therapist.

HEAT, COLD, WHIRLPOOL, AND PARAFFIN

During the acute phase of an inflammatory condition, ice massage should be frequently applied to the affected area. Subsequently, ice and/or heat (either superficial or deep) should be applied. Whirlpool is used to increase circulation, reduce swelling, and control pain. Hot paraffin is used to increase blood flow and for pain control.

JOINT, TENDON, OR BURSA INJECTIONS

Local injections either of steroids or of nonsteroidal antiinflammatory agents may provide temporary relief of symptoms in certain upper-extremity disorders such as epicondylitis; in certain other tendonitis disorders; and in certain cases, in carpal tunnel syndrome. Patients for whom this treatment is being considered should be referred either to a physiatrist or to an orthopedist.

EDUCATION

Instruction in the appropriate use of the neck and/or upper extremity is important for avoidance of activities that may stress the damaged area while the healing process is taking place.

Workplace Intervention

Medical management without modification of the work station, tools, and/or work process is inadequate for the treatment of upper-extremity musculoskeletal disorders of occupational origin. While, ideally, an ergonomist will be involved in job analysis and redesign of the tools, work processes, and work stations, this service is often not readily available. Thus, it is often left to the occupational-medicine physician to establish the probable cause of the patient's condition and to develop a plan for alterations at the patient's work site in order to prevent ongoing exposure to the ergonomic stressors that have resulted in the patient's condition. A detailed discussion of the appropriate approach to redesigning of tools, work stations, and job is provided by Putz-Anderson.[11] In summary, the goal of work place alterations is to "make the job fit the person, not the make the person fit the job."[11] As outlined by Putz-Anderson, appropriate workplace solutions include the following:

1. *Modifications designed to minimize extreme joint position and, hence, reduce stress on joints and tendons.* The general goal is to design work processes so that joints are held at the midpoint of their range of motion (for example, wrists should be kept straight). Examples cited in Putz-Anderson for keeping the wrist in neutral position include alteration of tools or controls (e.g., bending the shaft of a hand tool), moving the part, and moving the worker (e.g., changing a seat height to position the worker differently with respect to a patient).

2. *Modifications to reduce the use of excess force.* This generally involves equipment redesign so that the force required either is reduced or is spread out over a larger area or to stronger muscle groups. While the occupational medicine physician will not be redesigning tools,

he or she may be able to offer simple, practical suggestions such as increasing the handle diameter of tools.

3. *Modifications to effect reduction of highly repetitive movements.* Approaches suggested by Putz-Anderson include task enlargement, so that each worker has more variety in the tasks performed, and mechanization or automation, to reduce human repetition. The occupational-medicine physician will generally recommend more limited measures such as frequent rest breaks.

While it is useful to have access to an ergonomist, this access , unfortunately, is not always available. The occupational-medicine physician will be called upon to issue recommendations to patients regarding workplace modifications suitable for prevention of upper-extremity musculoskeletal disorders. Examples of appropriate recommendations that an occupational medicine physician might make include

1. frequent rest breaks,
2. bending a tool to keep the wrists neutral, and
3. adjusting the height of a chair to minimize strain on the neck and wrists of a worker.

REFERENCES

1. Milerad E, Ekenvall L. Symptoms of the neck and upper extremities in dentists. *Scand J Work Environ Health.* 1990;16:129–134.
2. Hagberg M, Hagberg C. Risks and Prevention of Musculoskeletal Disorders among Dentists. In: *Occupational Hazards in the Health Professions.* Boca Raton, FL: CRC Press; 1989:324–330.
3. Occupational Safety and Health Administration. *Ergonomic Program Guidelines for Meatpacking Plants.* United States Department of Labor; 1990.
4. Kimura J. *Electrodiagnosis in Diseases of Nerve and Muscle: Principals and Practice.* 2nd ed. Philadelphia: F.A. Davis; 1989.
5. Stevens JC. AAEE minimonograph #26: The electrodiagnosis of carpal tunnel syndrome. *Muscle and Nerve.* 1987;10: 99–113.
6. Dawson DM, Hallett M, Millender LH. *Entrapment Neuropathies.* Boston: Little, Brown and Co; 1983.
7. Phalen GS. Carpal tunnel syndrome. *J Bone Joint Surg.* 1966; 48A:211–228.

8. Sandzen SC. Carpal tunnel syndrome. *Am Family Phys.* 1981;24:190–204.

9. Spinner RJ, Bachman JW, Amadio PC. The many faces of carpal tunnel syndrome. *Mayo Clin Proc.* 1989;64:829–836.

10. McFall DB, et al. Carpal tunnel syndrome: treatment and rehabilitation therapy for the dental hygienist. *J Dental Hygiene.* 1993;67:3.

11. Putz-Anderson V. *Cumulative Trauma Disorders: A Manual for Musculoskeletal Diseases of the Upper Limbs.* London: Taylor and Francis; 1988.

12. Silverstein B. The Prevalence of Upper Extremity Cumulative Trauma Disorders in Industry. PhD thesis. Ann Arbor: University of Michigan; 1985.

13. Waris P. Occupational cervicabracial syndromes. *Scand J Work Environ Health.* 1975;5(suppl 3): 3–14.

14. DeLisa J. *Rehabilitation Medicine: Principles and Practice.* Philadelphia: JB Lippencott; 1988.

15. Pallis C, Jones AM, Spillane JD. Cervical spondylosis. *Brain.* 1954;77:274.

16. Dimberg L, et al. The correlation between work environment and the occurrence of cervical brachial symptoms. *JOM.* 1989; 31(5): 447–453.

17. Hagberg M, Wegman DH. Prevalence rates and odds ratios of shoulder-neck diseases in different occupational groups. *Brit J Ind Med.* 1987;44:602–610.

18. Hertling D, Kessler RM. *Management of Common Musculoskeletal Disorders.* 2nd ed. Philadelphia: JB Lippincott Company; 1990.

19. Rowland LP. *Merit's Textbook of Neurology.* Philadelphia: Lea and Febiger; 1989:400–408.

20. Rob CG, Standove NA. Arterial occlusion complicating thoracic outlet syndrome. *Brit Med J.* 1958;2:709–712.

21. Kapandji IA. The shoulder measurement of joint movement. *Clin Rheum Dis.* 1982;8:595–616.

22. Anderson JAD. Industrial rheumatology and the shoulder. *Brit J Rheum.* 1987;26:326–327.

23. Larson S. Chronic trapezius myalgia. *Acta Orthop Scand.* 1990;61:394–398.

24. Nirschi RP. Prevention and treatment of elbow and shoulder injuries in tennis players. *Clinics in Sports Med.* 1988;7:289–308.

25. Ellenbecker TS, Derscheid GL. Rehabilitation of overuse injuries of the shoulder. *Clinics in Sports Med.* 1989;8:583–604.

26. Gerr R, Letz R, Landrigan PJ. Upper extremity musculoskeletal disorders of occupational origin. *Annual Review of Public Health.* 1991.

27. Kurppa K, Waris P, Rokkanen P. Peritenditis and tenosynovitis. *Scand J Work Environ Health.* 1979;5(Suppl 3):19–24.
28. Cailliet R. *Hand Pain and Impairment.* 3rd ed. Philadelphia: FA Davis; 1982:119.
29. Poole BC. Cumulative trauma disorders of the upper extremity from occupational stress. *Journal of Hand Therapy.* 1988;1:172–180.
30. Dee R. *Principles of Orthopedic Practice.* New York: McGraw Hill; 1989.
31. Tenney CG, Lisak JM. *Atlas of Hand Splinting.* Boston: Little, Brown and Company; 1986.
32. Coppard BM, Lohman ML. *Introduction to Splinting.* New York: Mosby; 1996:2.
33. Evans RB, Hunter JM, Burkhalter WE. Conservative management of the trigger finger: a new approach. *Journal of Hand Therapy.* 1988;1:59–68.
34. State of the art review. *Occupational Medicine.* 1990;4(3):427.
35. Punnett L, Robbins JM, Wegman DH, Keyserling WM. Soft tissue disorders in the upper limbs of female garment workers. *Scand J Work Environ Health.* 1985;11:417–425.
36. Viikam-Juntarq E, et al. *Scand J Work Environ Health.* 1991;17:38–45.
37. Powell SG, Burke AL. Surgical and therapeutic management of tennis elbow: an update. *Journal of Hand Therapy.* 1991;4:64–68.
38. National Institute for Occupational Safety and Health. *Criteria for a Recommended Standard: Occupational Exposure to Hand-Arm Vibration.* US Department of Health and Human Services, Centers for Disease Control; 1989.
39. Cherniack MG. Raynauds' phenomenon of occupational origin. *Arch Int Med.* 1990;150:519–522.
40. Herington TN, Morse LH. *Occupational Injuries: Evaluation, Management, and Prevention.* St. Louis: Mosby; 1995:414–418.
41. Fess EE, Philips CA. *Hand Splinting.* 2nd ed. St. Louis: Mosby; 1987.
42. Kannus PJ, Jozsa P, Renstrom P, Jarvinin M, Kvist M, Lehto M, Oja P. The effects of training, immobilization and remobilization on musculoskeletal tissue. *Scand J Med Sci Sports.* 1992;2:100–118.
43. Hayes KW. *Manual For Physical Agents.* 4th ed. Connecticut: Appleton & Lange; 1993.

Chapter 17

The American Dental Association and Dental Ergonomics: Research, Observations, and Activities

Albert H. Guay, DMD

Abstract

There currently is considerable interest in ergonomically related illnesses or injuries in the dental workforce, particularly cumulative trauma disorders, despite the low prevalence of these disorders.

The American Dental Association (ADA) has commissioned independent qualitative and quantitative research to objectively describe and quantify the potential ergonomic risks to dentists and dental hygienists while providing dental treatment. In addition, ADA has surveyed dentists, hygienists, and dental assistants to gather information about ergonomics-related disorders. When potential risk postures, the length of time and the frequency of these postures, and the force exerted are considered, it is apparent that dental workers are at low risk for work-related ergonomic disorders.

Ergonomics-related problems in dental workers are very complex. For a complete understanding of ergonomics in the dental office and the logical development of preventive and abatement remedies, all three components of the ergonomic equation must be considered—the worker, the job, and the work site. Programs to prevent and control ergonomics-related disorders should include education, personal factor control, work site modifications, job modifications, and continuing research.

ADA has been active in several ergonomics arenas to assure that the dental office can continue to be a safe, healthy, and comfortable place to work.

The dental profession and the support industries that manufacture dental equipment and supplies have long been interested in improving the ergonomic environment of the dental office to protect the well-being of dental workers, to improve office efficiency, and to increase patient comfort. The old picture of the dentist and auxiliary personnel at work standing and, with shoulders canted at 45 degrees and neck severely flexed, leaning over a patient who is sitting bolt upright in a dental chair has been radically changed through the application of sound ergonomic principles. Dental equipment has been redesigned to allow the patient to recline while being treated and the treatment team to sit comfortably while working.

Despite these significant advances, there is increased interest in workplace ergonomics and associated illnesses, particularly cumulative trauma disorders. These are disorders of soft tissues caused or precipitated by repetitive, sustained, or forceful efforts or movements of the body or parts of the body over time. These disorders are also referred to as repetitive strain injuries, repetitive stress injuries, repetitive motion injuries, repetitive trauma disorders, upper-limb musculoskeletal disorders, the overuse syndrome, among other terms. In addition, there is continuing interest in neck, shoulder, back, and leg disorders that may be related to work in the dental office.

This increased interest is understandable, since cumulative trauma disorders are an ever-increasing problem across American workplaces. They account for about two thirds of the 500 000 workplace illnesses reported each year. The number of reported cases is growing each year, having increased over 900% in the past 10 years. Workers' Compensation claims for these disorders cost American businesses $20 billion in direct costs and more that $100 billion in indirect costs in 1995. They cause more lost workdays, on average, than most other injuries and comprise about one third of all Workers' Compensation claims.[1]

Because of the obvious implications for workers' safety, health, and comfort and the economic implications for American business and workers' compensation programs, the Occupational Safety and Health Administration (OSHA) of the

US Department of Labor is seeking to ameliorate these problems through adoption and enforcement of standards, along with state occupational safety and health agencies where they have jurisdiction.

The Problem

The literature on illnesses in the dental office related to ergonomic problems is not at all clear and varies considerably. An extensive review of the literature on ergonomics related to dental practice is presented elsewhere. Nevertheless, certain studies bear noting here. Armstrong and Lifshitz summarize the current situation well:

The relationship between many ergonomic problems and their causes simply is not understood well enough to predict with certainty the risk of a problem occurring in a given work situation. Furthermore, it is not always possible to determine if a proposed control measure will indeed remedy a problem.[2]

The literature that does exist generally demonstrates one or more of several flaws: a survey format that relies on self-reporting, lack of longitudinal data, lack of an adequate control sample, extremely small sample size, or use of diagnostic tests of questionable validity. The extreme variability of results from investigations of similar design engender severe doubts about the validity of the conclusions drawn. For example, the prevalence of carpal tunnel syndrome, a cumulative trauma disorder, among practicing hygienists is unknown, according to Huntley and Shannon[3]; their review of the literature records prevalence reports ranging from 1% to 54%. McDonald et al,[4] and Osborne et al,[5] report the prevalence of carpal tunnel syndrome to be between 6% and 7% among hygienists.

Many of the recommendations for the prevention of ergonomic illnesses in workers point to personal attributes of workers such as fitness, personal stress reduction, the presence of predisposing factors, and proper work mechanics rather than workplace modifications.

The list of factors that can predispose a dental worker to cumulative trauma disorders is long. Some of these factors

are relatively rare; many occur very often in the general population. Some factors are common to both sexes, while others
are found only in females. The following have been identified
as predisposing factors:

- traumatic injury to the specific body part;
- age, perhaps—the relationship is not clear;
- arthritis and nonspecific rheumatoid disorders;
- certain metabolic disorders such as diabetes mellitus;
- hypo- and hyperthyroidism;
- certain endocrine disorders;
- neoplasms;
- Paget's disease, acromegaly;
- myxedema, gout;
- being overweight or obese;
- "trigger finger" and "tennis elbow;"
- extensive vehicle driving;
- knitting, crocheting, sewing;
- playing tennis and other racquet sports;
- bowling;
- typing and computer use;
- current or recent pregnancy;
- use of oral contraceptives;
- postmenopause;
- hysterectomy, particularly with removal of the ovaries; and
- estrogen replacement therapy.

One can see in this list of myriad predisposing factors several common activities, conditions, or states of health. One
can also see that combinations of these factors in a single individual would not be unexpected. Many are under the direct
control of the individual. This information confounds any
definitive determination of the etiology of ergonomics-related
disorders in dental workers.

A common strategy employed in industry to prevent or
resolve ergonomic problems is job rotation for workers who
perform functions that have components presenting some
degree of potential risk. Because of the nature of dental care
and the requirement that most dental workers, other than
dental assistants, be licensed, job rotation is usually not an
option. Dental hygienists cannot prepare teeth for crowns with

the dentist assisting, and the dental assistant cannot do deep scaling and root planing.

Musculoskeletal Disorders in Dental Practice

Mandel,[6] citing other sources, claims that dentists average 1.9 days lost from practice because of illness each year, while the average American worker loses 5 days from work per year. This comparison is a strong indicator of the relative health of the profession and, by extrapolation, the relative safety of the average dental office as a worksite.

Dentists report a 60% prevalence of musculoskeletal discomfort of some sort and a 30% to 70% prevalence of back pain.[6] A survey by Basset[7] reported the same experience with back pain for dentists and hygienists. In the general population, 60% to 80% of adults report having had musculoskeletal discomfort, mostly back pain, at one time or another. Diakow says back pain is "an almost universal occurrence in all civilized societies."[8] This comparison of the prevalence of back pain in dentists and hygienists with the general public indicates, for back pain at least, that nonoccupational causes are as likely an etiologic determinant. Shugars and Miller cite five risk factors for back pain, none related to the workplace: obesity, poor general physical fitness, inadequate rest, poor mechanics in body movement, and high personal stress levels.[9]

Lehto et al report a lifetime incidence of neck pain in 45% of male dentists and 67% of female dentists studied and of shoulder pain in 50% of male dentists and 72% of female dentists.[10] Fifteen percent of the female and 12% of the male dentists worked standing up. Stockstill et al state that neck pain afflicts "nearly all" people at some time.[11]

Leg and feet problems in dental workers appear to be insignificant.

Ergonomic problems of the hand and wrist and problems with the elbow will be discussed in some detail below.

Some authors contend that a correlation exists between some dental procedures and certain cumulative trauma disorders, particularly carpal tunnel syndrome. However, there have been few objective studies that attempt to ergonomically analyze and quantify the individual components of tasks performed by dental workers. Failing an understanding of those tasks in such detail, cause-and-effect relationships will remain speculative, and remediation and prevention strategies will continue to be based on trial and error.

To better understand cumulative trauma disorders and objectively evaluate the ergonomic risks to dental workers in relationship to specific tasks, the American Dental Association (ADA) commissioned two independent ergonomic studies of dental workers. In 1995, Humantech, Inc., of Ann Arbor, Michigan, conducted two studies, *Ergonomic Risk Assessment of Dentists and Dental Hygienists* and *Ergonomic Hazard Evaluation of Dental Hygienists*, which were reported on in the *Journal of the American Dental Association.*[12]

Ergonomic Analysis

Dentists

The first step in the evaluation of the ergonomic impact of work performed by dentists must be a qualitative and quantitative evaluation of the individual tasks that make up the dentist's work routine. Certain treatment procedures that represent the majority of work performed by dentists were analyzed to identify ergonomic risk factors. An evaluation system, the Baseline Risk Identification of Ergonomic Factors (BRIEF) survey, was designed to provide a quantitative statement of the number and degree of severity of ergonomic issues for each operation selected (e.g., preparing teeth for crowns and preparing and restoring teeth with filling materials). This assessment of the posture, the force exerted, the duration of the force, and the frequency with which the postures occur for each of the body parts studied provides an in-depth ergonomic study of each job analyzed.

Seven body parts were analyzed for identified postures that posed ergonomic risk for cumulative trauma disorders:

1. the hand, left and right; } (LH, RH)
2. the wrist, left and right,

with the following ergonomic-risk postures for the hands and wrists:

- a pinch grip,
- flexion greater than 45 degrees,
- extension greater than 45 degrees,
- radial deviation,
- ulnar deviation, and
- finger pressing;

3. the elbow, left and right (LE, RE), with the following ergonomic risk postures:
   - forearm rotation and
   - full extension;
4. the shoulder, left and right (LS, RS), with the following ergonomic risk postures for the shoulders:
   - the arm raised greater that 45 degrees and
   - the arm behind the back;
5. the neck, with the following ergonomic risk postures:
   - the neck inclined forward greater than 20 degrees,
   - the neck inclined backward,
   - the neck twisted, and
   - the neck bent sideways;
6. the back, with the following ergonomic risk postures:
   - the back inclined forward greater than 20 degrees,
   - the back twisted, and
   - the back bent sideways (shoulders not parallel with floor);
7. the legs, with the following ergonomic risk postures:
   - squatting,
   - kneeling, and
   - standing on one leg.

The 16 dentists analyzed while performing the study procedures demonstrated ergonomic risk postures for the observed body parts as indicated in Table 1. Eight dentists were studied preparing teeth for crowns and eight were doing restorations.

A summary of the BRIEF study of dentists while they are preparing teeth for crowns and while they are preparing and restoring teeth with filling materials indicates that dentists demonstrate ergonomic-risk postures that could place them at risk for cumulative trauma disorder in the following body parts:

- left and right hands,
- left and right wrists,
- left elbow (marginal),

- left and right shoulders,
- neck, and
- back.

Table 1.—Percentage of Dentists Demonstrating Ergonomic Risk Postures

	LH	RH	LE	RE	LS	RS	Neck	Back	Legs
Crowns	100%	100%	0%	0%	50%	25%	100%	100%	0%
Filling	100%	100%	12%	0%	62%	25%	100%	100%	0%

Posture, however, is only one factor in overall risk. The intensity of the force exerted, the frequency of the exposure, the duration of the exposure, and the susceptibility of the individual are other factors that must be considered in quantifying the overall risk for ergonomics-related disorders.

As a part of the ergonomic analysis, the dentists in the study were asked about any history of pain or discomfort in the body parts studied. Table 2 indicates the prevalence of pain or discomfort reported.

Table 2.—Dentists Reporting Pain or Discomfort

	LH	RH	LE	RE	LS	RS	Neck	Back	Legs
Dentists	12%	31%	6%	12%	12%	20%	43%	62%	0%

Dentists were also asked whether they were currently receiving, or had ever received, medical care for any of the body parts studied. Table 3 describes the prevalence of such medical care.

Table 3.—Dentists Receiving Medical Care

	LH	RH	LE	RE	LS	RS	Neck	Back	Legs
Dentists	0%	0%	0%	0%	6%	0%	18%	18%	0%

It is interesting to note that dentists sought medical care for pain or discomfort only for the back, neck, and left shoulder. For right-handed dentists, these body parts are relatively static and are not directly involved in movements related to the performance of the operations studied. They are postural and probably should not be classified as cumulative trauma disorder illnesses.

The three sections of the analysis, when considered together, give some indication of the total ergonomic-risk postures for dentists as they perform the operations under study. The following body parts at some time assume high-ergonomic-risk postures as dentists perform crown preparations and restore teeth:

- left and right hands,
- left and right wrists,
- left and right shoulders,
- neck, and
- back.

Hygienists

Much attention has been given of late to potentially work-related ergonomic illnesses among dental hygienists, particularly cumulative trauma disorders. According to the American Dental Hygienists Association, 98% of hygienists are female; however, many of the tasks performed by hygienists are also done by dentists, 88.3% of which currently are male.[13] Most authorities report that cumulative trauma disorders affect women more frequently than men. Silverstein et al[14] had difficulty in determining the confounding effect of gender on cumulative trauma disorders in industry for several reasons, some affecting women but really unrelated to gender *per se* (the height of work stations, for example). Generally, they reported a "job-adjusted" ratio of 3:1 in these disorders between women and men. Women appeared to be at greater risk at some tasks, but not all.

Because of this interest, the ADA-commissioned research studied the tasks performed by dental hygienists in considerably greater detail than those done by dentists.

The BRIEF analysis described in the study of dentists was done identically for 15 hygienists. Table 4 reports the results of the BRIEF analysis for hygienists.

Table 4.—Percentage of Hygienists Demonstrating Ergonomic Risk Postures

	LH	RH	LE	RE	LS	RS	Neck	Back	Legs
Hygienist	93%	93%	0%	0%	73%	67%	100%	100%	0%

A summary of the BRIEF study of dental hygienists performing the tasks associated with dental hygiene indicates that hygienists demonstrate ergonomic-risk postures that could place them at risk for cumulative trauma disorders for the following body parts:
- left and right hands,
- left and right shoulders,
- neck, and
- back.

In addition, the surveys of reported pain and discomfort and receipt of medical care were done for the hygienists. Table 5 indicates the prevalence of pain or discomfort reported. Table 6 reports on hygienists who received medical care.

Table 5.—Hygienists Reporting Pain or Discomfort

	LH	RH	LE	RE	LS	RS	Neck	Back	Legs
Hygienist	18%	40%	7%	7%	18%	25%	47%	50%	0%

Table 6.—Hygienists Receiving Medical Care

	LH	RH	LE	RE	LS	RS	Neck	Back	Legs
Hygienist	0%	7%	0%	0%	0%	0%	7%	20%	0%

When considered together, the three sections of the analysis give some indication of the total ergonomic-risk postures for hygienists as they perform their duties. The following body parts at some time assume high ergonomic risk postures as hygienists work:

- left and right hands,
- left and right wrists,
- left and right shoulders,
- neck, and
- back.

This list of body parts at risk is identical for dentists and dental hygienists.

An in-office ergonomic-hazard evaluation was done of seven dental hygienists while they performed routine dental hygiene tasks. This analysis used objective measures to determine ergonomic risk exposure to several body parts during four subtasks of hygiene practice:

- probing,
- scaling,
- polishing, and
- flossing.

This hazard analysis used detailed posture analysis, biomechanical measurement techniques, and time-weighted averages for all of the subtasks to compile a composite ergonomic-risk profile for dental hygiene.

Several ergonomic analysis procedures were used:

- direct real-time electromyographic measures of dynamic muscle activity for key muscles,
- real-time goniometric measurement of hand/wrist postures,
- video analysis,
- ergonomic risk analysis,
- task analysis on working times for each subtask, and
- time-weighted averaging of ergonomic risk factors.

The ergonomic hazard evaluation used both objective methods (posture risk assessment) and biomechanical measurements (electromyography and goniometry) to determine the ergonomic risk for cumulative trauma disorders for the body parts studied. The posture risk assessment was done by ergonomists from video tapes using a modified Rapid Upper Limb Assessment (RULA) survey. Its correlation with cumulative trauma disorder symptoms has been established.[15]

A goniometer like the one illustrated in Figure 1 was attached across the wrist joint and electrically measured the following:
- wrist flexion and extension,
- wrist ulnar and radial deviations,
- the frequency of hand/wrist movements, and
- the amount of time spent in specific postures.

The maximum grip force was measured by an electromyography monitor. Surface electrodes were placed on the wrist flexors and extensors and their activity monitored, recorded as a percentage of the maximum grip force (% MVC), during the performance of the several work tasks by the hygienists who were studied.

The RULA system and the EMG-goniometer measures both predict the ergonomic risk for the body parts studied, and the information they generate can be used interchangeably.

It is generally thought by ergonomists that, for tasks that are repetitive or are performed over long periods of time, muscle forces that are more than 20% of the force exerted in maximum voluntary contractions (MVC) for the hands/wrist increase the risk of fatigue to muscle and tendon units. Such fatigue can cause pain and discomfort and increase the risk of

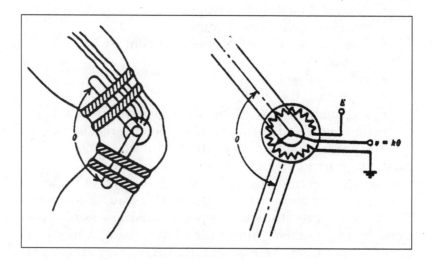

FIGURE 1.—Sample goniometer and schematic.

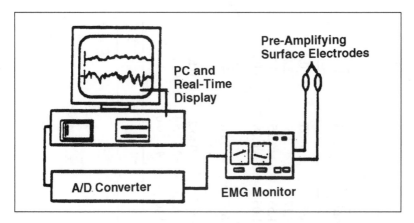

FIGURE 2.—Electromyographic measuring system schematic.

cumulative trauma disorders. Forces below 10% MVC are considered to be more desirable.[16]

Of the four muscles measured (left and right flexors, left and right extensors) for the four tasks studied (probing, scaling, polishing, flossing), 2 of the 16 subtasks (4 x 4) showed force measurements at or above 20% MVC. They were the right flexor during flossing (20% MVC) and the right extensor during polishing (22.5% MVC). Eleven others measured between 10% and 20% MVC, and three measured below 10% MVC. This signifies that few procedures hygienists perform require using muscle forces that can be considered to pose significant ergonomic risk.

The final factor in establishing the ergonomic hazard of the various body parts while performing a set of procedures is to consider the relative amount of time spent in doing each of the procedures. This will establish a time-weighted risk score for each body part studied for each procedure studied. The results of this ergonomic hazard analysis are presented in Table 7.

Both hands and the back are classified as being at moderate risk for cumulative trauma disorders, and the elbows, shoulders, and neck are classified as being at high risk.

The time factors used in the ergonomic risk analysis were derived only from the observed percentage of time hygienists spent doing the four tasks enumerated and did not take into account the amount of time spent at these tasks in relation to

Table 7.—Time-Weighted Ergonomic Hazard Analysis

Subtask	Left Hand	Right Hand	Left Elbow	Right Elbow	Left Shoulder	Right Shoulder	Neck	Back
1.1	0.74	0.64	0.28	0.3	0.55	0.5	0.55	0.4
1.2	4.05	3.85	1.92	1.58	3.08	3.17	2.5	2.25
1.3	2.03	1.9	0.96	0.79	1.54	1.58	1.25	1.13
1.4	1.28	1.25	0.45	0.45	1.03	1.05	0.78	0.7
Sum	8.04	7.64	3.61	3.13	6.2	6.3	5.08	4.48
Low Risk	0 to 4	0 to 4	0 to 2	0 to 2	0 to 3	0 to 3	0 to 2	0 to 3
Moderate Risk	4.1 to 8	4.1 to 8	2.1 to 3	2.1 to 3	3.1 to 5	3.1 to 5	2.1 to 4	3.1 to 5
High Risk	8.1 to 12	8.1 to 12	3.15 to 5	3.1 to 5	5.1 to 7	5.1 to 7	4.1 to 6	5.1 to 7

Subtask key: 1.1 = probing, 1.2 = scaling, 1.3 = polishing, 1.4 = flossing the total amount of appointment time. Without this consideration, a distorted view of total risk exposure results, since hygienists also spend time doing tasks during the average hygiene appointment (listed in Table 9) other than the four studied ergonomically.

ADA surveyed 135 hygienists at its 1994 Annual Session about the nature of dental hygiene practice. The time of an average hygiene appointment for adult and child patients is presented in Table 8.

The percentage of hygiene appointment time spent on the several tasks performed by hygienists for both adult and child patients is given in Table 9.

Table 8.—Average Hygiene Appointment Time

Appointment Time—Child		Appointment Time—Adult	
29 min. or less	6.8%	44 min. or less	15.6%
30 min.	70.9%	45 min.	32 %
31–40 min.	8.5%	46–59 min.	16 %
41 min. or more	13.7%	60 min.	33.6%
		61 min. or more	2.5%
average : 32 minutes		average : 50 minutes	

Table 9.—Hygiene Appointment Tasks

Task	Adult Patient % (±)	Child Patient % (±)
Patient Administrative	8.4% (5.1)	7.5% (4.1)
Operatory Preparation	9.2% (5.6)	8.5% (5.0)
Radiographs	6.2% (3.5)	7.7% (9.8)
Ultrasonic Scaling	18.5% (13.3)	4.6% (10.4)
Hand Scaling and Root Planing	31.3% (17.3)	16.2% (17.4)
Polishing	10.5% (7.2)	20.6% (19.1)
Fluoride Treatment	3.4% (3.3)	7.6% (5.1)
Sealants	3.6% (6.7)	20.8% (20.0)
Oral Hygiene Instruction	9.5% (10.8)	10.5% (12.9)
Other	9.4% (7.4)	11.9% (10.0)

The procedures done by hygienists that pose the highest potential ergonomic risk for cumulative trauma disorders are hand scaling and tooth polishing. The average time per procedure data indicate that hygienists spend 21 minutes in a 50-minute adult hygiene appointment doing those procedures and 12 minutes in a 32-minute child hygiene appointment. The substitution of ultrasonic scaling for hand scaling also may reduce the overall risk exposure.

The variation of tasks associated with the average hygiene appointment may be considered to be the equivalent of "job rotation" in the dental office for the purposes of preventing cumulative trauma disorders. The hygienist performs several different "jobs" during a typical hygiene appointment, some of which pose no ergonomic risk (e.g., taking and developing radiographs, making patient appointments, etc.).

At the same Annual Session, hygienists were surveyed about their experience with physical symptoms related to their work. Recall the question of the reliability of self-reporting surveys when judging the significance of this survey. The findings from 131 hygienists surveyed are reported in Table 10.

Hygienists were asked, "During or at the end of your work day, do you regularly have pain, tingling, or numbness in [body part]?" and "Have symptoms prevented you from working?"

In this group of hygienists, 4% (6 of 131) were diagnosed by a physician as having a cumulative trauma disorder. On average, 19.4% of hygienists reported discomfort in each of

Table 10.—Ergonomically-Related Symptoms in Hygienists		
Body Part	Symptoms	Prevent Working
Fingers	46.9%	2.6% 3/113
Hand	49.6%	2.6% 3/113
Wrist	43.4%	0.9% 1/113
Forearm	22.1%	0.9% 1/113
Shoulder	51.8%	2.6% 3/113
Neck	59.1%	5.3% 6/113
Back	59.3%	8.8% 10/113

five non-work-related activities (e.g., sports, gardening, etc.). Seventy-seven percent of the hygienists surveyed reported hormonal or weight-related predisposing factors.

Several conclusions can be drawn from this information:

1. During the performance of some tasks related to the practice of dental hygiene, certain body parts may assume postures for a limited time that could place them at risk for ergonomic problems.
2. The tasks that present the greatest level of ergonomic risk are hand scaling and tooth polishing.
3. The highest level of risk and reported discomfort are for the back and the neck, body parts that are not directly involved in the performance of therapeutic tasks, but are postural.
4. Hands and wrists are described as being at moderate postural risk.
5. Hygienists spend a minority of appointment time performing tasks that place body parts at risk; 42% (21 minutes out of 50 minutes) for adult visits and 37% (12 minutes out of 32 minutes) for child visits.
6. The intensity of muscular effort exerted does not pose significant risk.
7. The prevalence of cumulative trauma disorders in hygienists is low (physician-diagnosed, causing loss of work time, or self-reported), although some "symptoms" are reported by about one-half of the hygienists surveyed.
8. Non-work-related predisposing factors for acquiring cumulative trauma disorders are very common among hygienists, and individual hygienists probably present several simultaneously.

Dental Assistants

Dental chairside assistants were also surveyed at the 1994 ADA Annual Session. As with dental hygienists, dental assistants were asked, "During the day or at the end of your work day, do you regularly have pain, tingling or numbness in [body part]?" and "Have symptoms prevented you from working?" The findings from 107 assistants surveyed are reported in Table 11.

Table 11.—Ergonomics-Related Symptoms in Dental Assistants		
Body Part	Symptoms	Prevent Working
Fingers	28.7%	0.0% (0/107)
Wrist	22.6%	0.1% (1/107)
Hands	35.3%	0.1% (1/107)
Forearm	16.4%	0.0% (0/107)
Shoulders	42.5%	0.1% (1/107)
Neck	47.1%	0.2% (3/107)
Back	50.0%	0.2% (3/107)

In this group of dental assistants, one individual was diagnosed by a physician as having a cumulative trauma disorder. On average, 19.6% of dental assistants reported discomfort in each of five non-work-related activities (e.g., sports, gardening, etc.). Sixty-five percent of the dental assistants reported the presence of hormonal or weight related predisposing factors.

Comprehensive studies of ergonomic risk were not done for dental assistants because of the rarity of ergonomics-related problems uncovered in the screening survey.

Implications for Dental Practice

It is apparent that the greatest number of ergonomics-related problems for dentists, hygienists, and dental chairside assistants occur in the back and the neck. To a significant extent, the shoulders also present similar problems. These difficulties are postural and are not directly related to the accomplishment of the tasks that these providers routinely do. The disorders probably should not be classified as cumulative trauma disorders since they do not involve the performance of rapid repetitive movements over an extended period of time. If anything, they should be classified as sustained, nonforceful, postural problems.

Considerable efforts have been expended by the dental profession, dental equipment manufacturers, ergonomists and time-motion analysts to modify the design of dental equipment and instruments, change the positions of patients and practitioners with respect to each other, modify dental office design and the placement of equipment, and introduce stress-reducing "four-handed dentistry." Instruction in this concept is part of the standard curriculum in dental and dental auxiliary education, although instruction in ergonomics per se may not always be a part of the curriculum. Unpublished dentist survey data from ADA indicate that, although about one quarter of dentists have at some time attended ergonomics seminars or training programs, 38% believe that the training they received in dental school regarding ergonomics was adequate. This assessment varies significantly with the years since graduation. Dentists who graduated between the mid-1970s and the mid-1980s are most likely to feel their dental school ergonomic training was adequate (43%). Among those who graduated between the mid-1950s and the mid-1960s, the percentage who felt their ergonomic training was adequate was lowest (28%). Educational efforts must continue and expand to further reduce posture-related problems in the dental office.

The prevalence of cumulative trauma disorders among dental workers is low. Although efforts must continue to further reduce the occurrence of these disorders in dental workers, the temptation must be resisted to quickly categorize all back, neck, shoulder, and upper-extremity disorders found in dental workers as work related. Personal worker attributes have been identified as being important in the prevention or development of ergonomics-related disorders, and the list of factors that predispose a worker to these disorders is long and comprises many factors that are commonly found in the general population. Work tasks or the workplace environment may play a minor role in the occurrence of ergonomics-related disorders in some individuals.

Changes in the tasks performed, the workplace environment, or work routine may be ineffective in preventing ergonomics-related disorders in some individuals in the face of the overwhelming influence of other factors. Limiting the time spent using a handpiece in preparing teeth for crowns may have little effect in reducing hand/wrist cumulative trauma disorders for a dentist who is a racquet sports enthusiast. Modifying the design of the handle of dental scalers may be irrelevant in preventing cumulative trauma disorders for a hygienist who exhibits several predisposing factors. Can the "blame" for ergonomics-related disorders be placed only on the tasks dentists and dental hygienists perform, without regard for predisposing factors? Should changes in the predisposing factors, most of which are elective on the part of the worker, be discounted in favor of workplace changes, which may be a minor factor in the etiology of the disorder and difficult to implement?

Success in the reduction of cumulative trauma disorder by modifying any of the several factors that may play a role in the etiology or exacerbation of these disorders will be directly related to the relative role each factor plays in any individual. All three components of the ergonomic equation must be considered—the employee, the job, and the workplace (including the tools used for the job)—for a complete understanding and a logical development of preventive and abatement remedies.

When ergonomics-related disorders in a dental office are being considered, several determinations should be made, much like those for any worksite:

- The incidence of ergonomically related disorders reported by employees should be considered.
- A qualitative and quantitative job analysis should be done, or applicable existing analyses should be used, to determine the ergonomic risk levels for dental workers for the tasks they routinely perform.
- Tasks that present significant ergonomic risk should be identified.
- Information from the above studies should be correlated to estimate the role of the workplace in any observed ergonomics-related disorders.

Current knowledge about ergonomics-related illnesses and injuries is insufficient, and the variety of factors involved is too great to justify the adoption of any rules that apply to all workplaces, particularly dental offices. Certain steps can be taken, however, to prevent and control these disorders in dental workers when they occur. They fall into five categories: education, personal-factors control, work site modifications, job modifications, and research.

Education

The importance of employing sound ergonomic practices in the daily practice of dentistry should be taught to all dental workers during their initial training programs (see Chapter 11, "Human-Centered Ergonomics"). These sound practices should be taught and their observance noted as an element of student appraisals. In addition, education in this field should continue throughout the working life of the individual. According to the data available, worker posture is a critical factor. Good posture habits should be taught initially and reinforced periodically. On-the-job trainees should also receive information on this subject.

Personal Factor Control

Employees should be informed of the factors characteristic of an individual worker that have been identified as having a bearing on the development of ergonomics-related disorders. With this knowledge they then will have the opportunity to reduce or eliminate those factors under their control.

Work Site Modifications

Dentist employers should always be seeking ways to modify the layout of the dental operatory and equipment placement and design to reduce ergonomic stress on dental workers (see Chapter 13, "Ergonomically Correct Design Concepts of a Functioning Dental Office"). Although laudable progress has been made over time, improvements are always possible. It would appear, however, that additional improvements will be marginal because of the already low incidence of work-related disorders among dental workers. Instrument design appears to be the most fruitful area for improvement.

Job Modifications

With an understanding of the risk factors inherent in the tasks dental workers do, modifications in job routines may be helpful. For example, hygienists may alternate scaling and polishing tasks rather than scaling the entire mouth and then polishing all of the teeth; less stressful sequencing patterns for hand scaling might be developed to reduce the duration of stress on specific muscle groups; etc.

Research

Additional research is needed to understand ergonomics-related disorders and their relation, if any, to specific work and work sites. Transfer of information learned from such research to the dental operatory should be as rapid as possible.

ADA Activities

The American Dental Association has been involved in activities related to dental workers' health, safety, and comfort. The association has engaged in early discussions with OSHA over an ergonomics standard and will continue to advocate policies that are based on sound science and a reasonable understanding of the dental workplace. It is hoped that the research the association has sponsored will contribute to this outcome.

To help to better understand the dental workplace and any potential ergonomic risks facing dental workers in the performance of dental care, the association has undertaken and also has sponsored clinical research in this area. The surveys of dental workers cited above are being done on an annual basis so that trends, if developing or changing, can be detected as soon as possible. The task analysis already completed under the sponsorship of the association will be a valuable tool for dentists to use in evaluating the tasks they and their auxiliary personnel perform for potential ergonomic risks.

ADA has been an active participant in the American National Standards Institute (ANSI) Z365 Committee on Ergonomics. This committee has worked for about 6 years to develop a *voluntary* ergonomics standard. The committee is made up of members representing government, labor, business, industry, science, and the health professions. The association also participates in the Ergonomics Coalition organized by business and industry. The coalition is supporting research in the area of ergonomics and hopes to provide both ANSI and OSHA with information and advice in the development of any voluntary or mandated ergonomics standard.

ADA continually sponsors educational programs for all members of the dental work team in the form of publications, including the *Journal of the American Dental Association*, lectures and seminars. At the Annual Session of the Association, the latest designs of equipment and instruments are exhibited. Programs are also developed and presented for the entire dental team on providing efficient treatment for dental patients that is ergonomically safe for dental workers.

The other parties in the dental care system also have an important role to play to ensure that the dental operatory is a healthy, safe, and comfortable place to work. The dental schools and the training programs for dental auxiliaries should educate students about the importance of ergonomic considerations for all dental workers in providing dental care. Good work habits should be taught from the outset; it is easier to start off with good habits than to break bad ones. Research into ergonomic issues for dental workers should be a part of each school's research agenda.

Manufacturers and suppliers of dental equipment and instruments should have an understanding of the ergonomic implications of the design of dental equipment and instruments. Through their research and development activities, more ergonomically safe and efficient equipment can be made available to the profession. They should also educate the users of their products and monitor the ergonomic effects of their products on dental workers.

Conclusion

The prevalence of ergonomics-related disorders, particularly cumulative trauma disorders, is low among dental workers. This is a result of the efforts of all segments of the dental profession to make the dental operatory a safe, healthy, and comfortable place to work.

An in-depth and dissecting objective analysis of the work tasks performed by dental workers indicates that, despite the fact that the hands and wrists of dental workers must sometimes assume potentially high-risk postures in the accomplishment of the fine manipulations required to provide dental care, the frequency, duration, and intensity of those activities place dental workers at low overall risk for the development of cumulative trauma disorders. The greatest ergonomic risk areas—the back, neck, and shoulders—are postural rather than dynamic problems.

The July 1997 National Institute for Occupational Safety and Health (NIOSH) publication, *Musculoskeletal Disorders and Workplace Factors*,[17] concludes from their literature analysis that

- there is a positive association between highly repetitive work and cumulative stress disorders,
- there is a positive association between high forces and cumulative stress disorders,
- there is a positive association between wrist and hand posture and cumulative stress disorders, and
- there is a positive association between a combination of risk factors and cumulative stress disorders.

This analysis indicates the nature of the repetitiveness, the forces exerted, and the postures assumed in the delivery of dental care make it understandable that dental workers are at low risk for ergonomics-related disorders at work.

Ergonomics-related problems among dental workers are very complex. It appears the characteristics of the individual worker often may have a significant bearing on the development of cumulative trauma disorders. This has far-reaching implications, both for the determination of causation and for potential prevention or abatement activities.

Reduction of existing work-related ergonomic disorders in dental workers will only be effectively accomplished through a cooperative effort of educators, practitioners, and manufacturers, with the help of ergonomists and researchers. The dental profession has voluntarily created and maintained a safe, healthy, and comfortable dental workplace. Governmental regulators should allow, and encourage, these voluntary efforts to continue. Monitoring of the ergonomic health status of dental workers should be ongoing, so that any unfavorable changes can be spotted early and appropriate corrective action taken.

REFERENCES

1. Dear JA. Ass't Secretary of Labor for Occupational Safety and Health. Remarks at International Conference on Occupational Disorders of the Upper Extremity. Ann Arbor, MI, October 24, 1996.
2. Armstrong TJ, Lifshitz Y. Evaluation and design of jobs for control of cumulative trauma disorders. In: *Industrial Hygiene Science Series: Ergonomic Interventions to Prevent Musculoskeletal Injuries in Industry.* Chelsea: MI: Lewis Publishers; 1987:111–115.
3. Huntley DE, Shannon SA. Carpal tunnel syndrome. A review of the literature. *Dental Hygiene.* 1988;62(July/August):316–320.
4. Macdonald G, Robertson MM, Erikson JA. Carpal tunnel syndrome among California dental hygienists. *Dental Hygiene.* 1988;62(July/August):322–328.
5. Osborn JB, Newell KJ, Rudney JD, Stoltenberg J. Carpal tunnel syndrome among Minnesota dental hygienists. *J Dent Hygiene.* 1990;64:79–85.
6. Mandel ID. Occupational risks in dentistry: comforts and concerns. *J Am Dent Assn.* 1993;124:41–49.
7. Basset S. Back problems among dentists. *J Canad Dent Assn.* 1993;4:251–256.
8. Diakow PRP, Cassidy JD. Back pain in dentists. *J Manip Physio Thera.* 1984;7:85–88.
9. Miller DJ, Shugars DA. Back pain in dentists: current research and prevention. In: *The Health of the Dental Professional.* Chicago: American Dental Association; 1987:57–63.
10. Lehto TU, Helenius HYM, Alaranta HT. Musculoskeletal symptoms of dentists assessed by a multidisciplinary approach. *Community Dent Oral Epidemiol.* 1991;19:38–44.
11. Stockstill JW, Harn SD, Strickland D, Hruska R. Prevalence of upper extremity neuropathy in a clinical dental population. *J Am Dent Assn.* 1993;124:67–72.
12. Bramson J, Smith S, Romagnoli G. Evaluating dental office ergonomic risk factors and hazards. *J Am Dent Assn.* 1998;129:174–183.
13. *1995 Distribution of Dentists in the United States by Region and State.* Chicago: American Dental Association; 1997.

14. Silverstein BA, Fine LJ, Armstrong TL. Carpal tunnel syndrome: causes and a preventive strategy. *Seminars in Occupational Medicine.* 1986;1:213–223.
15. McAtamney L, Cortlett N. RULA: a survey method for the investigation of work-related upper limb disorders. *Applied Ergonomics.* 1993;24:91–99.
16. Herberts P, Kadefors R, Bronman H. Arm positioning in manual tasks. An electromyographic study of localized muscle fatigue. *Ergonomics.* 1980;23:655–665.
17. Bernard BP, ed. *Musculoskeletal Disorders and Workplace Factors.* Cincinnati, OH: US Department of Health and Human Services, National Institute for Occupational Safety and Health; 1997:5a-1-67.

Chapter 18

OSHA and Ergonomics

Gary Orr, PE, CPE

Abstract

The injuries and illnesses caused by musculoskeletal disorders are covered by OSHA, and employers are subject to penalties if they do not record the injuries on the OSHA 200 log or do not protect workers from recognized hazards. The best way for an employer to protect workers from injury is to integrate ergonomics into the workplace. Effective programs start with planning, so that the basic elements of the program can be tailored to the needs of the company, office, or institution. Management commitment and employee involvement are critical to the success of a program and must be considered in the development of a written plan. Procedures, policies, and materials must be developed for the basic elements of a program, which include work site analysis, hazard control, medical management, and training. While many companies choose to have a separate program to address ergonomics, other approaches that integrate ergonomics into a quality program or a safety and health program have also been successful at reducing musculoskeletal disorders.

Introduction

The Occupational Safety and Health Act (OSHAct) was signed by President Richard Nixon in 1970 and became effective in 1971. Since passage of the act, significant progress has been made in reducing workplace fatalities, injuries, and diseases. The rate of workplace fatalities has been cut by 72% and the rate of workplace injuries by 23%. There is still, however, considerable room for improvement. Workplace injuries and illnesses impose tremendous costs on workers, families, employers, and society. Job injuries alone resulted in costs of more than $120 billion and 125 million days of lost work in 1994.

In the OSHAct, the Occupational Safety and Health Administration (OSHA) was given the authority to establish regulations and enforce compliance by employers.[1] It is important to remember that OSHA's authority is focused on the employer. There is very little in the OSHAct regarding the conduct of workers, and there is nothing pertaining to manufacturers of equipment.

Congress had foreseen situations where existing standards would not address emerging health and safety problems, so a provision in section 5(a)(1) allows OSHA to issue citations for situations for which a standard does not exist but for which the hazards are serious and controls are known. Section 5(a)(1) is often referred to as the "General Duty Clause":

Each employer shall furnish to each of his employees employment and a place of employment which are free from recognized hazards that are causing or likely to cause death or serious physical harm to his employees.

Over the past 25 years the American workforce and workplace have changed, and with those changes have come new safety and health problems. OSHA has not been able to issue regulations to keep pace with new hazards; consequently, over the past 15 years, many citations have been issued under section 5(a)(1). Some of these new hazards include the following:

- Workplace violence is a serious problem. Homicide is the second leading cause of workplace fatalities, and the leading cause of work-related deaths among women workers. Most of these fatalities are a result of robberies and other criminal acts, not assaults by coworkers.
- Serious injuries and illnesses from poor job design (ergonomics) are a significant health concern. Incidents associated with repeated trauma accounted for 615 000 cases serious enough to result in lost workdays.[2]

OSHA divides work-related incidents into injury cases and illness cases. The difference, simply stated, is that injury cases are acute or sudden in nature, whereas illness cases are chronic or cumulative in nature. With regard to employee health, OSHAct states the following:

The Agency shall set a standard which most adequately assures, to the extent feasible, on the basis of the best available evidence, that no employee will suffer material impairment of health or functional capacity even if such employee has regular exposure to the hazard dealt with by such standard for the period of his working life.

In 1992, OSHA announced its intention to prepare a standard to prevent musculoskeletal disorders caused by jobs. These jobs can be characterized by an imbalance between the demands of the job and the capabilities of the workers. Since that time, OSHA has been working with stakeholders to determine how to define a poorly designed job, and to determine the actions employers need to take to fix the job. Clearly, jobs that result in musculoskeletal disorders for all or most workers should be redesigned, but since people design jobs for people and ingenious workers find ways to significantly improve a poorly designed job, it's rare to find a job in which all or most workers are hurt. It is not rare, however, to find industries in which incident rates for repeated trauma are two or more times the national rate. Many people equate poorly designed jobs with a sewing sweatshop or a poultry assembly line with pieces whizzing by at a blurring rate, but other industries also have high rates of musculoskeletal disorders (see Table 1).

Risk Factors

Tasks often linked to muscloskeletal disorders usually expose workers to at least two risk factors (see Table 2).

These risk factors are named in study after study as contributors to upper-extremity and back muscloskeletal disorders. When two risk factors are present simultaneously, then a muscloskeletal disorder is likely for all but a few workers. When an injury occurs, there is usually prolonged exposure to a risk factor. Exposure for several hours per day, day after day means the soft tissues do not have sufficient time to recover, and the result is an injury. That is why many of these injuries are referred to a cumulative trauma disorders. Not all the musculoskeletal disorders come from repeated exposure; for example, high exertion forces have resulted in muscle tears, tendon ruptures, and herniated discs. In many cases the prescription for recovery is to rest the affected joint or muscles.

Table 1.—Industries with High Cumulative Trauma Incidence Rates

Industries with high reported incidence rates of upper-extremity cumulative trauma— Bureau of Labor Statistics Standard Industrial Classification	Industries with high reported incidence rates of back cumulative trauma— Bureau of Labor Statistics Standard Industrial Classification
01 Meat products 209 Misc food and kindred products 225 Knit wear 342 Cutlery, handtools and hardware 363 Household appliances 371 Motor vehicles and equipment 375 Motorcycles, bicycles and parts	242 Sawmills 244 Wood containers 336 Nonferrous foundries 363 Household appliance manufacturer 411 Local/suburban transport 421 Trucking and courier services 422 Warehousing 451 Air transportation 518 Beer, wine, distilled beverages 704 Membership hotels 805 Nursing/personal care 806 Hospitals

Table 2.—Signal Risk Factors

Performance of the same motion or motion pattern every few seconds for 2 hours continuously, or for more than a total of 4 hours, excluding mandatory breaks.
Unsupported fixed or awkward work posture for more than 2 hours continuously, or for a total of 4 hours, excluding mandatory breaks.
Use of vibrating or impact tools or equipment for more than 2 hours of continuous use, or for more than a total of 4 hours.
Using forceful hand exertions for more than a total of 4 hours.
Unassisted frequent or forceful manual handling

Patient: Doctor my elbow hurts when I play tennis.
Doctor: Stop playing tennis for a while

For some people rest is not enough; because of the severity of the injury; genetics (e.g., poor circulation, diabetes); or personal preference (e.g., hobbies, work methods, sleep habits, smoking, etc.) the pain does not go away with rest. For those cases immobilization, anti-inflammatory drugs, therapy, or surgery may be needed.

Controlling Risk Factors

To provide a workplace that is consistent with the intent of the OSHAct, an employer must do more that react when injuries and illness occur in the workplace. Employers must identify employees that are at risk of serious injury. Although debate continues about many issues surrounding ergonomics, most employers can readily identify risk factors. The critical question for most employers is not the existence of risk factors, but the value of the controls, where value is defined as the benefits relative to the cost. When the benefits outweigh the costs, most employers are eager to implement controls; when the benefits are roughly equal to the cost, some employers will cautiously implement controls; however, when the benefits are less than the cost, an employer will allocate only the minimum resources necessary. Before starting an ergonomics program, many employers were skeptical of the authenticity and effectiveness of ergonomics interventions. However, after engineering or administrative controls are implemented, skepticism turns into optimism, which in turn creates more opportunities to improve jobs.

In a traditional classification of control measures, there are engineering controls and administrative controls. The opportunities for engineering and administrative controls differ depending on the stage of the job development (new or existing jobs). Engineering controls are easier to implement in new jobs. With existing jobs, trying to retrofit controls is often costly and requires the workers to change the way they have been doing the job. Engineering and administrative controls are defined as follows:

- *Engineering controls* are the preferred methods of reducing or eliminating exposure to musculoskeletal-disorder risk factors. Engineering controls involve physical changes to the work stations, equipment, production facility, or any other relevant aspect of the work environment to reduce or eliminate the presence of risk factors. Engineering controls are typically permanent controls.
- *Administrative controls* are procedures that significantly limit daily exposure by working with employees on work organization issues such as work schedule or manner in which work is performed. Examples of administrative controls include job enlargement, frequent breaks, and methods training. The limitation of administrative controls is that the hazard has not been reduced, only the exposure, so the controls must be audited periodically to ensure they are in place and effective.

Engineering controls often are understood only as automation or mechanization, but a range of engineering controls should be considered as alternatives:

- *Automation* removes the worker from the hazard. When the worker does not add any value to the procedure other than mechanical energy (no judgment, no qualitative decisions, etc.) then automation may be useful. Automation is usually expensive and is not flexible in meeting changing work requirements
- *Mechanization* provides mechanical power that is directed by the worker. Jobs that require heavy lifting, hard squeezing, or pinching for several hours (see Photo 1), day after day are candidates for mechanical assistance. These systems tend to cost less than automation, but usually between $1,000 and $20,000, so the cost is significant and management should be concerned about value. In addition, mechanized systems that are not well designed can slow down the worker, which leads to worker and employer frustration.
- *Changes to the facility* may help. Glare, hard floors, and temperatures that are too cold can result in awkward postures, reduced circulation or forceful exertions, all

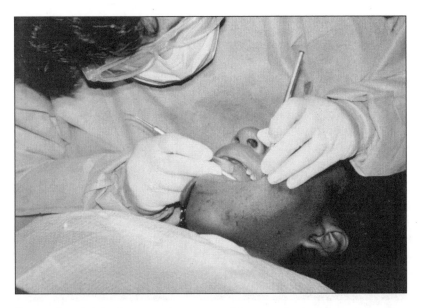

PHOTO 1.—A job that requires several hours of pinching, day after day.

of which contribute to muscloskeletal disorders. Discussions with workers will often highlight problems with the facility.

- *Equipment and tool changes* may help. Equipment that does not adjust and tools that vibrate or create awkward postures are often the source of muscloskeletal disorders. Hand-arm vibration syndrome results in tingling and numbness in the hands. Routine exposure to vibrating hand tools or vibrating equipment can often be corrected with periodic maintenance. Vibration-absorbing material needs to be carefully matched to the frequency of the vibrating source. For example, a vibration-dampening glove may seemed to have stopped the vibration, but may have little effect in preventing hand-arm vibration syndrome if the vibration energy is still entering the hand.
- *Posture* is important. Awkward postures are often caused by equipment that cannot be adjusted or by tools that force the worker into an awkward hand or foot posture (see Photo 2). Awkward postures are not defined by how bad they feel (i.e., contorted postures). They are defined

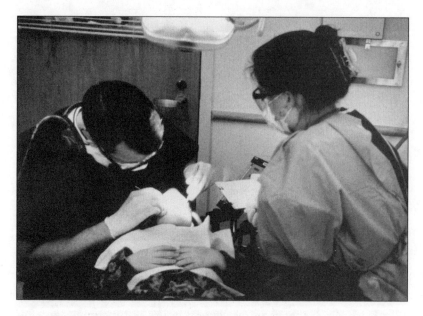

Photo 2.—Awkward hand posture.

relative to neutral postures. A neutral posture is the position of a joint at which the least amount of muscle activity is required to maintain the position. For example, neutral postures are the weight of the head supported primarily by the spine (neutral neck), the elbows close to the waist (neutral shoulder), hands in a handshake position (neutral wrist), and the nose not beyond the toes (neutral back both forward and lateral). When a joint is in both an awkward posture and unsupported, muscle fatigue happens more quickly. Recurring muscle fatigue or tendon exertions without adequate recovery are thought to be primary contributors to muscloskeletal disorders. Hard squeezing or pinching adds to the muscle fatigue and tendon strain. When forceful exertions and unsupported awkward postures are combined in a job, then fatigue limits the time a worker can perform the job.

- Where adjustable equipment and special tools are available to workers, *training* is also needed to ensure that workers understand both how and why the controls are used. Even with adjustable equipment, muscloskeletal disorders can occur when workers are told to get into one posture and to stay there. The best posture is the next posture. When job routines are established, it is important to incorporate frequent changes in posture rather than to set up a "good ergonomic posture" that has to be maintained for several hours.

- A *quick fix* is sometimes helpful. After workers and managers become aware of risk factors, there are generally opportunities to make some improvements to a task. For example, a sterilizer unit that is set back on a counter can be moved closer to the worker (less than a 20-inch reach). Boxes of copy paper and x-ray film can be opened and handled in smaller bundles. Padding can be applied to sharp corners and hard tool handles. Many of the quick fixes already exist in the workplace, as workers have invented ways to make a task tolerable.

Ergonomic Programs

Finding and fixing risk factors is at the heart of ergonomics, but to sustain the effort and achieve the best return on the dollars invested, the employer should consider ways of integrating ergonomics into the culture of the organization. Many employers have chosen to develop an ergonomics program as a way of institutionalizing the process to ensure that jobs continue to be designed for people. In 1990, OSHA published a booklet on ergonomic programs titled *Ergonomics Program Management Guidelines for Meatpacking Plants.*[3] The booklet was developed in response to the enormous number of muscloskeletal disorders in meat-processing plants. The information is written in general terms, however, so that other organizations can read and apply the principles. Recently, OSHA has been working with stakeholders to identify the elements of successful safety and health programs. The elements of an effective safety and health program can be applied to an ergonomics program. On the basis of the information both in the guidelines booklet and from the work of the Safety and Health Programs team, OSHA has begun to formulate the elements needed for a successful program (whether it is a safety and health program or an ergonomics program). The following describes the minimum requirements for an acceptable ergonomics program.

- *Management leadership* means that management understands the principles of ergonomics and the importance to their business, and gives visible support to the ergonomics program. Implementation tools provided by management might include:
  —information,
  —adequate time and training,
  —assigned responsibility and accountability,
  —program review procedures,
  —designation of a person responsible for ergonomics who has some expertise in hazard recognition and applicable OSHA guidelines, and who has authority to order or purchase equipment.
- *Employee participation* means that workers and their representatives are involved in the ergonomics program, inspections of work areas, and the selection/implementation of controls, and that they are permitted to review job analyses. Workers' and representatives' right of access to information is understood by workers and recognized by management. The employer has a documented procedure by which employees can raise complaints of hazards and receive timely employer responses.
- *Contractor safety* means that management provides ergonomic tools, equipment, and facilities to contractors. Management monitors contractor practices in ergonomics and will stop contractor practices that expose host or contractor employees to excessive risk. Management informs the contractor and employees of risk factors present at the facility.
- *Survey and hazard analysis* means that risk factors have been identified for all high-hazard jobs and procedures; analyses are communicated to and understood by affected employees. Hazard analyses are conducted for jobs, tasks, and workstations, where back injuries or repeated trauma illnesses have been reported. There is an implementation plan to control all high-hazard jobs.

- *Inspection* means that competent personnel conduct inspections with appropriate involvement of employees. Items in need of correction are documented. Time periods for corrections are set.
- *Hazard reporting* means that a formal system for hazard reporting exists. Employee reports of hazards are documented, corrective action is scheduled, and records maintained.
- *Accident investigation* means that OSHA-101 is completed for all recordable incidents. Reports are generally prepared with cause identification and corrective measures prescribed.
- *Data analysis* means that injury/illness logs and exposure records are kept correctly, are audited by facility personnel, and are essentially accurate and complete. Rates are calculated to identify high-risk areas and jobs. The employer keeps a history of incidence and severity rates. Workers' compensation claim records and medical visits are analyzed. The results are used to set priorities and evaluate the success of the ergonomics program. Incidence and severity rates clearly show a downward trend or leveling off at rates among the best in the industry.
- *Hazard control* means that appropriate controls (engineering, administrative controls, and personal protective equipment) are in place for significant hazards. Some serious hazards may exist. The employer is generally in compliance with voluntary standards and good practices in the industry. Documented reviews of ergonomic needs for the upper extremity, back, and lower extremity have been conducted. The employer has a method of identifying problem jobs before a work-related musculoskeletal disorder occurs. Engineering controls are commonly used. Administrative controls (e.g., job rotation) are rarely used as long-term solutions for hazardous jobs.
- *Maintenance* means that a preventive maintenance schedule is implemented for areas where it is most needed; it is followed under most circumstances.

Manufacturers' and industry recommendations for maintenance frequency are complied with. Employees are aware that tools need to be maintained to avoid musculoskeletal disorders. Employees know the procedure for replacing tools that are not functioning properly. The employer recognizes the need to have the right tool for the job. The employer or employee will stop an activity if the proper tools are not available.

- *Medical program* means that medical surveillance, removal protection, monitoring, and reporting comply with applicable standards, guidelines, or recommended practices. Employees report early signs/symptoms, without fear of reprisal, for job-related injury or illness. First reports are followed up with a comprehensive screening exam (noninvasive) and appropriate treatment. Alternate-duty jobs have been identified by someone trained in ergonomic job analysis.
- *Ergonomic training* means that training includes OSHA rights and access to information about jobs and ergonomics. The employer attends training in all materials provided to employees under their direction. Employees can generally demonstrate the skills and knowledge necessary to perform their jobs safely. Records of training are kept, and training is evaluated to ensure that it is effective.
- *Program evaluation* means that the ergonomics program is routinely evaluated. The evaluation includes discussions with employees, supervisors, technical and medical staff. Project documentation is reviewed and follow up on implementation and recommendations are reviewed.

Ergonomic Programs—Priorities

Many employees and employers start into ergonomics to solve an immediate problem, such as a carpal tunnel case related to a computer workstation, or as a result of an muscloskeletal disorder that causes a dental hygienist to lose workdays. Information is gathered, a control strategy is formulated, something is purchased, and everyone hopes the problem goes away. Find and fix is part of an ergonomics process; it is not a program.

An ergonomics program starts with planning. In the planning process, decisions are made that will direct the course of the program. The bookends of the planning process are the policy statement and written plan. Planning addresses the who, what, when, where, and how, as well as the question of evaluation. The direction and priorities of a program must be consistent with the philosophy of the business. For example, if management is concerned about rising workers' compensation costs, then a measure of the success of an ergonomics program should be its impact on workers' compensation. Where absenteeism and turnover are critical to management, then the ergonomic program evaluation should measure job satisfaction. Whatever the hot button is for managers, some measure of that element should be integrated into the evaluation metrics (see Table 3).

An ergonomics program does not need to stand alone. Many organizations have started with an ergonomics program that is organizationally separate from other programs. The intent was to stress the importance of muscloskeletal disorders. Other organizations have integrated ergonomics into other existing programs such as safety and health programs and quality programs. With training in ergonomics, those programs, if they are effectively used in the company, can be modified or expanded to include ergonomic issues.

Finally, the use of evaluations is critical to the effectiveness of an ergonomics program. The evaluations must provide the following:

Table 3.—Examples of Measures for an Ergonomics Program	
Activity Measures	Results or Impact Measures
Policy Statement	Incidence rates
Job specific awareness training	Severity rates
Priority jobs identified	Workers' compensation
Controls implemented	Turnover
Technical resource established	Absenteeism
Written plan	Productivity
	Quality of service
	Quality of work life

- Value—employers want to know if the money spent on ergonomics has been beneficial to the company. The benefits are measured in terms that are meaningful to management. For example, if lost workdays do not get the attention of management, but losing a customer because no one was there to answer the phone is important, then those measures should be in the evaluation.
- Direction—the evaluation should provide feedback on the progress of the program in meeting established milestones. When the program is not achieving the desired results, it can be revised to align the activities with the expectations. If the needs of the organization change, then the program and measures can be changed to reflect the new requirements.

In summary, ergonomics balances the job requirements with the capabilities of the worker. Consequently, ergonomics should be considered with *all* jobs. When a worker will suffer material impairment of health or functional capacity with regular exposure to a hazard, then the employer has a legal obligation to eliminate the hazard or reduce the exposure to levels that will not cause impairment. Beyond the legal requirements and possible penalties, it makes good business sense to design jobs with the worker in mind, since injuries and illnesses are reduced and workers are more productive. For most companies, a program is the best way to integrate the necessary changes into the culture of the organization. After extensive planning, implementation, and regular evaluation, companies have found that ergonomics has not only reduced injuries and illnesses, but also has improved morale, with the tangible benefits alone more than paying for the cost of the program.

The contents of this chapter are the thoughts and opinions of the author and do not necessarily reflect the views of the Occupational Safety and Health Administration.

REFERENCES

1. The Occupational Safety and Health Act. Public Law Number 91-596. 91st Congress. S2193; Dec 29, 1970.
2. Occupational Injuries and Illnesses: Counts, Rates, and Characteristics. US Department of Labor, Bureau of Labor Statistics; 1993.

3. *Ergonomics Program Management Guidelines for Meatpacking Plants.* OSHA Publication 3123. US Department of Labor, Occupational Safety and Health Administration; 1993.

FURTHER READING

Akesson I, Lundborg G, Horstmann V, Skerfving S. Neuropathy in female dental personnel exposed to high frequency vibrations. *Occupational Environmental Medicine.* 1995;52:116–123.

Barry RM, Woodall WR, Mahan JM. Postural changes in dental hygienists: four-year longitudinal study. *Journal of Dental Hygiene.* 1992;147–150.

Elements of Ergonomic Programs. Publication number 97-117. US Department of Health and Human Services, Centers for Disease Control and Prevention; March 1997.

Finsen L, Christensen H. Postural loads in the neck and shoulder region during dental work. In: *Proceedings of the 12th Triennial Congress of the International Ergonomics Association. Vol. 2: Occupational Health and Safety.* Toronto: Human Factors Association of Canada; 1994;2:102–104.

Gerwatowski LJ, McFall DB, Stac DJ. Carpal tunnel syndrome: risk factors and preventive strategies for the dental hygienist. *Journal of Dental Hygiene.* 1992;Feb:89–94.

Hjortsberg U, Rosén I, Orbaek P, Lundborg G, Balogh I. Finger receptor dysfunction in dental technicians exposed to high-frequency vibration. *Scandinavian Journal of Work, Environment and Health.* 1989;15:339–344.

Huntley DE, Shannon SA. Carpal tunnel syndrome: A review of the literature. *Dental Hygiene.* 1988;316–320.

Liss GM. Upper extremity symptoms and carpal tunnel syndrome among dental hygienists. In: *Proceedings of APHA Annual Meeting.* American Public Health Association; 1993: 319.

Macdonald G, Robertson MM, Erickson JA. Carpal tunnel syndrome among California dental hygienists. *Dental Hygiene.* 1988;322–328.

Milerad E, Ericson MO, Nisell R, Kilbom A. An electromyographic study of dental work. *Ergonomics.* 1991;34(7):953–962.

Osborn JB, Newell KJ, Rudney JD, Stoltenberg JL. Musculoskeletal pain among Minnesota dental hygienists. *Journal of Dental Hygiene.* 1990;132–138.

Pitchford J. Carpal tunnel syndrome: occupational hazard. *Dental Assisting.* 1985;April:15–16.

Chapter 19

Developing a Comprehensive Ergonomics Program in the Dental Practice

Robin Mary Gillespie, MPH

Abstract

To identify and eliminate ergonomic hazards, each organization must develop a program suited to its size and needs. This chapter follows the recommendations provided by the federal Occupational Safety and Health Administration (OSHA) to employers making a commitment to improving ergonomic conditions and reducing health and safety hazards.

The basic model parallels any good safety program. Employers are responsible for identifying hazardous activities evaluating and correcting risk factors; providing appropriate training; and integrating the issue into other organizational activities, such as purchasing, record keeping, and employee health. Workers are expected to contribute to this process and to follow recommended procedures. Developing a good program is a reiterative process, consisting of program development, task analysis, redesign, implementation, and review phases.

This chapter describes how to start up an ergonomics program in a dental office or small clinic. It lists and explains the steps needed for planning and implementation and provides evaluation, documentation, and training tools.

Introduction

To identify and eliminate ergonomic hazards, each organization—clinic, office, educational institution—must develop a program suited to its size and needs. A consistent approach to potential ergonomics hazards will make the process simpler and more reliable. This chapter follows the recommendations provided by the federal Occupational Safety and Health Administration (OSHA) to employers making a commitment to improving ergonomic conditions and reducing health and safety hazards.*

The basic model parallels any good safety program. Perhaps most familiar to dental offices is the similar approach to bloodborne pathogens.[1] Employers are responsible for identifying hazardous activities; evaluating and correcting risk factors; providing appropriate training; and integrating the issue into other organizational activities such as purchasing, record keeping, and employee health. Workers are expected to contribute to this process and to follow recommended procedures. As illustrated in Figure 1, developing a good program is a reiterative process, consisting of program development, task analysis, redesign, implementation, and review phases. Conscientious attention to each step will produce changes suited to the particular work requirements and conditions, and will keep responding to changing needs.

Table 1 lists 11 steps management should take to establish an effective ergonomics program.

Steps

Step 1: Recognize That Ergonomics Hazards May Exist

The significant risk factors and elevated rates of cumulative trauma disorders in dentistry are documented elsewhere in this book. Responsible employers are willing to address the hazards faced by their workforce. This chapter assumes that you have already taken this step.

---

*A comprehensive description of OSHA's definition of a good health and safety program can be found in the Program Evaluation Profile (PEP), OSHA Notice CPL 2, available from the Directorate of Compliance Programs. Most dental offices would not be expected to address every program element because not all hazards are encountered in such work places; however, the significant categories and levels of achievement are instructive.

PROGRAM DEVELOPMENT	Establish committee –or– Name monitor	Set: Schedule Goals Budget Responsibilities	Train ergonomics monitors
HAZARD ANALYSIS	Review	List tasks	Analyze tasks Analyze work areas
REDESIGN	Redesign: Tasks Work areas	Plan for changes: Purchasing SOPs Remodeling	Develop policies Maintenance Medical management Scheduling Job rotation	Review and revise
IMPLEMENTATION	Training: All staff High-risk Special	Work station changes	Behavioral changes: Procedures Breaks, rest Rotation Scheduling	Maintenance changes Medical management
REVIEW	Evaluate changes Execution quality New hazards	Update records review Update symptoms review Reinspect work stations	Train new staff Refresher training	Revise policy as needed

FIGURE 1.—Ergonomic Program Flow Chart.

Table 1.—The 11 Steps of an Ergonomics Program
1. Recognize that problems may exist and plans to make changes.   2. Establish an ergonomics committee that includes workers.   3. Analyze the work site using inspections, surveys, and records review.   4. Analyze tasks associated with injuries.   5. Redesign jobs that cause chronic injuries; changes may affect staffing, work practices, production rates, and tools.   6. Investigate and buy engineering controls.   7. Schedule and fund maintenance and repairs.   8. Provide training for workers and management on potential hazards, chronic injuries, and prevention. Provide job-specific training for each high-risk job.   9. Provide good medical management, including symptoms analysis and referrals, early noninvasive treatment, appropriate modified-duty and return-to-work programs, evaluation of modified duty for ergonomic stressors.   10. Set and observe time lines for all activities.   11. Carry out regular inspections and ongoing hazard correction.

Step 2: Establish an Ergonomics Committee Including Workers

Start by designating those responsible for carrying out the program. In larger organizations, the most effective committee will represent the range of workers affected and those with responsibility or ability to make changes. In a smaller office, it may be possible to enlist everyone. At a minimum, dentists and support staff should be involved, as well as record-keeping and purchasing personnel. Ergonomics committee members should be selected based on aptitude, interest, and job responsibilities. Participants may be best selected by their peers. In a unionized workplace, procedures may exist for selecting worker representatives.

The ergonomics committee should hold regular meetings. Meeting on paid time will improve participation; it may be required under state wages and hours regulations. A budget for training, reference materials, and possibly consultation is likely to make the program more effective, as well as to show the extent of the organization's commitment.

Make sure to keep your employees tied into the ergonomics process. If you try to solve problems through technical expertise or management prerogative alone instead of enlisting participation from all staff, you may fail to garner support or cooperation. Reporting to staff on problems and proposed changes before final decisions are made will improve acceptance. It will also help head off additional problems that only those workers directly affected by changes might be able to foresee.

Step 3: Analyze the Work Site Using Inspections, Surveys, and Records Review

The first job of the ergonomics team is to determine whether hazards or injuries currently exist. If your budget allows, you may want to hire a professional ergonomist to get started. Ideally, the ergonomist will help you understand the problems you face, not simply provide a technical report.

Analyzing a workplace involves three initial steps: A) records review B) symptoms survey, and C) workplace inspections.

A: REVIEW INJURY RECORDS

Is there a history of health problems caused by excessive physical demands? Identify all cases of muscle strain, carpal tunnel syndrome, tendinitis, and other soft-tissue problems. Look at OSHA injury records, workers' compensation claims, and incident reports. Review other health records such as sick leave and disability to see if problems have occurred that were not properly identified as work-related. If any cumulative trauma disorders are identified, proceed to analyze the work-related risk factors in tasks performed by affected workers, as described under step 4.

In large organizations, it may be useful to calculate the rate of repetitive strain injury by dividing the annual occurrence of problems by the number of workers. This will give you an idea of the severity of the exposures and help estimate the future cost of uncorrected cumulative trauma disorders. In most dental offices, statistics are neither necessary nor especially useful because so few people are employed. You will be able to evaluate the risks and costs simply by examining your current cases.

B: Survey for Symptoms

Many cumulative trauma problems develop slowly. People may work for a long time before reporting symptoms. A survey of the workforce can reveal pain, numbness, and other symptoms that indicate the presence of strain and risk factors before permanent damage has been done. Surveys should be as brief as possible while still providing useful information. If the responses are anonymous, workers may be more likely to tell the truth. Avoiding leading questions—such as whether a symptom is work-related—will garner the most information without putting workers on the spot about problems and their causes.

To avoid skewing your results, make sure everyone in the workforce completes the survey, not just employees with symptoms. Figure 2 shows a frequently used format for surveying for symptoms and active repetitive strain injuries.

C: Inspect the Workplace

Look for risk factors such as awkward postures, sustained positions, contact stress, and vibration. You can use the workplace inspection form (Figure 3) as a general guide, and the workstation evaluation form (Figure 4) to record measurements. In particular, look for workstations that require bending for long periods, that contain hard edges that press on soft tissue, that through visual demands or equipment placement constrict workers into awkward postures, or that are too high or too low for the people using them. Make sure to ask workers what problems they are experiencing with the tools or equipment setup, because they know the job (and its hazards) best. Some signs that ergonomic analysis is needed are listed in Table 2.

Step 4: Analyze Activities Associated with Injuries

When you have identified a task, tool, or work area that is associated with cumulative trauma injuries, you must next figure out what risk factors are associated with the problems. You may have already started this step with your initial inspections. Now you will want to evaluate those

```
                    Symptoms Survey Checklist
                                                 Date____/____/____

Name:_____


_____     _____     _____
Facility                  Department          Job Name

_____     _____     Time on this Job
  Shift                   Hours Worked/Week                years____months_____


    Other jobs you have done in the last year
    (for more than 2 weeks)


_____  _____  _____     _____ months _____ weeks
  Dept          Job#       Job Name                 Time on THIS job

_____  _____  _____     _____ months _____ weeks
  Dept          Job#       Job Name                 Time on THIS job

      (If more than 2 jobs, included those that you worked on most)



          Have you had any pain or discomfort during the last year?
               1) Yes _____   2) No _____   (If NO, stop here)
  If YES, carefully shade in the area of the drawing which bothers you the MOST.













                           Complete The Other Side
```

FIGURE 2.—Symptoms Survey Checklist (front).

areas or jobs in greater detail. This usually requires breaking the suspected tasks down into component activities consisting of single movements or actions. This process is called "task analysis." Use ergonomic task evaluation check lists (Figures 5 and 6) to record each action required to complete a task, then determine whether stressful postures or activities are involved. In addition to the equipment and workstation problems that are visibly obvious, ask whether the task requires repeated movements—commonly, shoulder, arm, or hand movements—that cause repetitive strain.

Symptom Survey Checklist Continued   Page ____ of ___

(Complete a **Separate Page** for each area that bothers you)

Area described on this page: Neck___ Shoulder___ Elbow____ Wrist/Hand____

Upper Back___ Low Back___ Thigh/Knee___ Low Leg___ Ankle/foot____

1. Please put a check by the word(s) that best describe your problem
   __1) Aching   __5) Numbness (asleep) __ 9) Tingling
   __2) Burning   __6) Pain   __10) Weakness
   __3) Cramping   __7) Swelling   __11) Other
   __4) Loss of Color   __8) Stiffness

2. When did you first notice the problem? _____ (month) _____ (year)

3. How long does each episode last? (Mark an X along the line)
        1 hour   1 day   1 week   1 month   6 months
     _____/_____/_____/_____/_____

4. How many separate episodes have you had in the last year? _____

5. What do you think caused the problem? _____
   _____

6. Have you had this problem in the last 7 days? 1) Yes _____ 2) No____

7. How would you rate this problem (mark an X on the line)

   NOW   _____
            None   Unbearable
   IN THE PAST _____
            None   Unbearable

8. Have you had medical treatment for this problem? 1) Yes____ 2) No____

   8a. If NO, why not_____

   8b. If YES, where did you receive treatment?
        1. _____Company Medical   Times in the past year____.
        2. _____Personal doctor   Times in the past year_____
        3. _____Other   Times in the past year_____

   8c. If YES, what treatment? _____

   8d. If YES, did the treatment help?   1) Yes _____ 2) No _____

9. How much time have you lost in the past year
   because of this problem?   _____ Days

10. How many days in the last year were you on
    restricted or light duty because of this problem?   _____Days

11. Please comment on what you think would improve your symptoms

    _____

    _____

FIGURE 2. *Continued*—Symptoms Survey Checklist (back).

Remember that repetition is especially a problem when combined with awkward postures.

Note: If cumulative trauma disorders have already occurred, investing in the services of a professional ergonomist to evaluate hazards and recommend changes may be your wisest step. Preventing additional problems can require significant technical expertise.

WORKPLACE INSPECTION FORM

Work area:_____

Date and time:_____

- Walk through the work area during typical work hours.
- Observe normal work activities. Talk to people if possible.
- Find out if the jobs are done differently at different times of the year, month, day or shift.
- Do a task analysis of each job listed here.

What jobs require:

☐ Heavy lifting, pushing or pulling

_____

_____

_____

☐ Working above the shoulders

_____

_____

_____

_____

☐ Leaning, stooping, bending or twisting

_____

_____

_____

_____

☐ Bent wrists or hands in awkward positions

_____

_____

_____

_____

FIGURE 3.—Workplace Inspection Form (front).

5: Redesign Jobs That Cause Chronic Injuries

Once you know what the problems are, you can reduce or eliminate risk factors using the techniques and concepts covered elsewhere in this book. Table 3 lists areas in which changes may be needed.

☐ Gripping, pinching or grabbing with hands

_____

_____

_____

_____

☐ Contact with hard surfaces or sharp edges

_____

_____

_____

_____

☐ Extreme temperatures

_____

_____

_____

☐ Slippery or uneven work surface

_____

_____

_____

☐ Vibration

_____

_____

_____

☐ Noise

_____

_____

FIGURE 3. *Continued*—Workplace Inspection Form (back).

Try to correct or reduce each risk factor identified. Sometimes the most efficient approach is to start from the beginning, asking yourself what is the best way to do the job rather than attempting to change existing details. Sometimes, however, a few modifications to existing practices will reduce risks to a satisfactory level.

```
┌─────────────────────────────────────────────────────────────────────┐
│                     WORKSTATION EVALUATION                            │
│                   (ATTACH DRAWING OR PHOTOS)                           │
│                                                                       │
│ DEPARTMENT: _____    WORK AREA: _____  │
│ JOB(S): _____  │
│ OBSERVER(S): _____      DATE: _____    │
│                                                                       │
│ MEASURE:                                                              │
│                                                                       │
│ TASK HEIGHT _____   SEATING HEIGHT _____  WORKSTATION HEIGHT _____  │
│                                                                       │
│ REACH HEIGHT _____  REACH DISTANCE: - FORWARD _____ - TO SIDE _____ │
│                                                                       │
│ LIFT HEIGHT _____  LIFT DISTANCE _____   MAXIMUM LIFT WEIGHT _____  │
│                                                                       │
│ STEP OR STAIR HEIGHT _____         VISUAL ANGLE _____              │
│                                                                       │
│ EVALUATE PHYSICAL ENVIRONMENT (GOOD/FAIR/POOR)                        │
│                                                                       │
│ LIGHTING _____  EXITS _____   WALKING SURFACES _____             │
│                                                                       │
│ NOISE _____   TEMPERATURE _____                                    │
│                                                                       │
│ COMMENTS:                                                             │
│                                                                       │
│ 1. _____  │
│ 2. _____  │
│ 3. _____  │
│ 4. _____  │
│ 5. _____  │
│ 6. _____  │
│                                                                       │
│                                                                       │
│ WORKSTATION CLASSIFICATION:      _____ ACCEPTABLE _____ NEEDS CHANGES │
│                                                                       │
│                                  _____ NEEDS MAJOR CHANGES _____ URGENT │
│                                                                       │
│ SUGGESTED IMPROVEMENTS:                                               │
│                                                                       │
│ 1. _____  │
│ 2. _____  │
│ 3. _____  │
│ 4. _____  │
│ 5. _____  │
│ 6. _____  │
└─────────────────────────────────────────────────────────────────────┘
```

FIGURE 4.—Work Station Evaluation Form.

Some corrections will be possible to make immediately. However, the most effective job redesign does not necessarily happen all at once. Frequently, immediate modifications will reduce risk factors, but only more complex changes, involving purchasing decisions and alterations in other practices, will eliminate the hazard. Significant architectural or equipment redesign may need to wait until other major remodeling is scheduled. No matter how difficult the ultimate resolution is, you can almost always

Table 2.—Signs That Ergonomic Analysis is Needed

Crowding
Repeated minor accidents such as bumps or dropping things
Broken equipment
Repetitive or routine work practices

ERGONOMIC TASK EVALUATION

TASK OR PROCEDURE:_____
JOB TITLES: _____   WORK AREA: _____
OBSERVER(S): _____   DATE: _____

JOB TASKS		REPETITIONS/SUSTAINED ACTION			
#	DESCRIPTION	#/MINUTE	#/HOUR	#/SHIFT	DURATION
1					
2					
3					
4					
5					
6					
7					

Attach additional sheets if necessary

Task by Task Evaluation

STRESSFUL MOVEMENT OR ACTION	TASK	1	2	3	4	5	6
Head/Neck Bent							
Wrist Bent Up							
Wrist Bent Down							
Wrist Bent to Thumb (Radial)							
Wrist Bent Towards Elbow (Ulnar)							
Fingers Active							
Fingers Grip							
Forward Body Tilt							
Back Body Tilt/Arch							
Leaning to the side							
Twisting							
Shoulders Raised/Lowered							
Reach above Shoulder							
Reach Behind							
Contact Stress							
Other:							

Is this a repetitive motion job?   YES/NO

What is the risk of repetitive strain injury?   HIGH/MEDIUM/LOW

WHY?   (CIRCLE ALL THAT APPLY) POSITION/REPETITION/FORCE

FIGURE 5.—Ergonomic Task Evaluation.

ERGONOMIC JOB EVALUATION

JOB OR TASK NAME: _____

LOCATION AND DATE OBSERVED:_____

PRESENT?	STRESSFUL MOVEMENT, ACTION OR CONDITION
	Heavy Lifting
	Wrist Bent Up
	Wrist Bent Down
	Wrist Bent to Thumb (Radial)
	Wrist Bent Towards Elbow (Ulnar)
	Fingers Active
	Fingers Grip Forcefully
	Leaning Forward
	Leaning Back, Arching Back
	Leaning to the Side
	Twisting to Lift, Push or Pull
	Shoulders Raised to Reach Work Surface
	Reach or Lift Above Shoulder
	Reach Behind Body
	Contact Stress (tools, surfaces, equipment)
	Head/Neck Bent
	Environmental Conditions (cold, heat, noise, housekeeping)
	Working Conditions (monitoring, overtime, stress)

What is the risk of ergonomic strain or injury?   HIGH   MEDIUM   LOW

WHY?   (CIRCLE ALL THAT APPLY) POSITION   REPETITION   FORCE   CONDITIONS

What health or safety problems or injuries or illnesses have been experienced in this job?

_____

_____

_____

FIGURE 6.—Ergonomic Job Evaluation (front).

institute temporary improvements until ideal solutions can be implemented.

Make sure that your changes do not introduce additional physical demands. Changes should be evaluated for ergonomic safety before *and* after implementation. For best results, changes should not increase workload or time required to

What improvements would you recommend to reduce:

AWKWARD POSITIONS

_____

_____

_____

_____

EXCESSIVE FORCE

_____

_____

_____

_____

REPETITION

_____

_____

_____

_____

CONDITIONS

_____

_____

_____

_____

What problems will you face in improving this task?

_____

_____

_____

_____

FIGURE 6. *Continued*—Ergonomic Job Evaluation (back).

complete tasks, or otherwise burden workers. Changes that make work harder may be resisted.

Remember that this step is not complete until the changes have been both implemented and evaluated.

Step 6: Investigate and Buy Engineering Controls

Better designed tools and equipment represent the most important engineering controls in a dental office. You will want

Table 3.—Ergonomic Risk Factors
Work practices: Changes may be needed in: postures, repetition, force
Equipment: chairs (patient and worker), hand tools
Work surfaces: height, reach distance, match with chairs, storage
Administrative factors: scheduling, production or pacing, task rotation, maintenance
Organizational contributors to stress: overtime, patient demands, staff conflict

to consider whether the new product is comfortable, durable, and appropriate for all users. Ideally, vendors will provide you the chance to use equipment before you buy it. It is sometimes difficult to fit everyone with one chair, for example, so try to work with vendors who will combine products at reasonable prices. If you can, test several choices before committing to significant changes. When final decisions about purchases are made, all users should be involved.

Table 4.—Ergonomic Improvements, Grouped by Time Required for Implementation
Changes that can be made immediately:
Adjusting equipment height, tension, and placement to suit affected workers
Repairing equipment
Changing how equipment is used, including postures, duration, and force
Instituting breaks to reduce length of exposure or repetition
Reminding workers to change postures routinely
Changes that will take longer to develop and implement:
Purchasing better hand tools
Purchasing chairs for staff
Rearranging workspace
Long-term improvements that require planning and capital investment:
Changing counter height and location
Installing new patient chairs
Making extensive architectural changes

Companies that are developing ergonomic tools may be interested in your input if you find limitations or significant advantages to their products. It is sometimes possible to adapt what is currently available by changing handle types, adding padding, or combining characteristics of different products, so don't hesitate to call manufacturers and tell them what you need.

Be warned: The claim "ergonomic" is routinely made for *any* equipment that is round, is soft, or looks funny. (Thanks to Chris Grant of the University of Michigan's Center for Ergonomics for this formulation.) This kind of ergonomics is no improvement unless it meets your needs.

Step 7: Schedule and Fund Maintenance and Repairs

This apparently minor component of a good ergonomics program is, in fact, critical. Worn tools usually require greater force to use, and broken adjustments encourage people to maintain awkward postures. Keeping tools sharp and adjustable equipment running smoothly reduces risks and saves money without major changes. Unfortunately, people rarely fix things on their own or even report problems. Instead they continue working in difficult conditions.

The ergonomics committee should work with those involved in maintenance and repair to identify products and parts that need regular servicing, such as casters or pneumatic controls, or regular replacement, such as blades and drill bits. Routine schedules should be established and records maintained. As for equipment that breaks or wears out, priority should be given to repair needs that affect workplace safety and comfort. Staff should be encouraged to identify equipment that is not working properly and refrain from using it. This approach may require that additional supplies and back-up equipment be available.

Step 8: Provide Training for Workers and Management on Potential Hazards, Chronic Injuries, and Prevention; Provide Task-Specific Training for Each High-Risk Job

Training should be provided to everyone in the organization, whether or not cases of cumulative trauma have been diagnosed or risk factors identified. It should cover basic risk factors, signs of cumulative trauma, and ways to prevent problems. Universal training helps ensure full cooperation in the ergonomics program; this is important in preventing problems that people do not yet take seriously. As an added advantage, training can provide workers with skills to reduce risks outside of work.

Job-specific training for each high-risk job and training for the ergonomics committee members should cover the specific problems identified at the work site, as well as general concepts. This training will integrate the recommendations concerning posture, tool use, breaks, and other changes that develop out of the task analysis. Typical general and high-risk job training outlines are provided in Figure 7. Staff members responsible for purchasing, scheduling, and general safety will profit from training that addresses their role in improving ergonomic conditions, even if they do not provide dental care. An additional training component on computer ergonomics should be provided to office staff.

Step 9: Provide Good Medical Management

Note: This component of your program can also help you to observe requirements of the Americans with Disabilities Act and to make the work site friendly to all staff and patients with physical restrictions.

Cumulative trauma disorders—chronic or developing—may be identified through records review, symptoms surveys, or reports from workers. Staff should be encouraged to report symptoms related to work as soon as they develop, regardless of whether medical treatment is required.

Early and noninvasive treatment is recommended. Even for carpal tunnel syndrome, surgery and other invasive treatments are usually not appropriate in the early stages of disease. While at work, symptomatic workers should be able to apply ice, do exercises, and rest as instructed by their health care providers.

Workers with symptoms—pain, numbness, etc.—should be protected from continued exposure. Sometimes simply resting the affected area and avoiding additional strain is enough

---

General Training Outline
I.   Cumulative trauma rates and problems identified in dental work
II. Risk factors for cumulative trauma injuries—general
III. Causes specific to dental work
IV. Preventive measures
     A. Individual changes
     B. Procedure/task changes
     C. Work station changes
     D. Medical management
V.   Solutions planned for this organization

High-Risk Job Training Outline
I.   Cumulative trauma rates and problems identified in dental work
II. Risk factors for cumulative trauma injuries—general
III. Causes specific to dental work
IV. Preventive measures
     A. Individual changes
     B. Procedure/task changes
     C. Work station changes
     D. Medical management
V.   Hazards identified in this job
VI. Proposed solutions—include discussion/input

FIGURE 7.—Training Outlines.

to prevent a chronic problem, but returning to a biomechanically stressful activity is likely to reignite symptoms. Workers with persistent pain or other symptoms should be evaluated by medical practitioners who are trained in occupational health and ergonomics.

Workers with diagnosed cumulative trauma problems should not return to the working conditions that caused their problems. Before an injured worker resumes work, the tasks and equipment should be analyzed as described above. Workers with ongoing problems should be offered appropriate modified duty. Modified duty activities should also be evaluated for ergonomic stress.

Employers are sometimes concerned that talking about ergonomics can produce symptoms in workers without existing problems. While it is true that injury rates seem to increase when an ergonomics program is instituted, this results from identifying problems before they are debilitating, *not* from placing seeds of psychosomatic illness in workers' minds. Early diagnosis works in the employer's favor by revealing risk factors and ergonomically hazardous activities. You can head off more serious problems if you survey your workforce and refer symptomatic workers to competent health providers who understand how work can cause cumulative trauma disorders.

Step 10: Set and Observe Time Lines for All Activities

Ergonomics is unlikely to be the sole responsibility of anyone in the organization. It can very easily take a back seat to more pressing work demands. Establish and meet deadlines to keep your program on track. End each meeting with a clear statement of who is responsible for what and when results or actions are expected. Committee members may need to be relieved of some other duties while the project is being set up.

Step 11: Carry Out Regular Inspections and Ongoing Hazard Correction

The ergonomics program is not finished when you have corrected your current problems. It is necessary to review records and work stations regularly—perhaps every 3 to 6 months, or when symptoms appear. Target areas where the work practices or workloads have changed. Observe good ergonomic principles whenever you are making new purchases, renovating, or moving.

Conclusion

The specific design of an organization's ergonomics program is less important than its success in identifying and eliminating hazards. If you have already implemented other safety programs—such as OSHA-required hazard communication or bloodborne disease programs—you may know how you want to carry out your ergonomics program. If such activities are too demanding or time consuming for your organization, you may want to begin by enlisting the services of a professional ergonomist. Consult Chapter 20, "Resource Centers," for help in finding local and national resources.

REFERENCE

"Bloodborne Pathogens," 29 CFR 1910:1030.

Chapter 20

Resource Centers

Denise C. Murphy

Abstract

The information in this chapter is designed to assist the reader in learning about various types of ergonomics-oriented centers and courses. Each center is characterized by its goals and objectives, areas of expertise and qualifications of personnel working at the center, and types of services offered.

Some of the centers are university based and offer formal academic degrees in ergonomics-related areas. Other centers offer different learning formats: education may be provided to the dental care worker as a consumer/patient (e.g., the Mount Sinai Center) or as a student enrolled in a training program about the musculoskeletal hazards associated with the practice of dentistry (e.g., the OSHA workshops). Some centers emphasize research, while several centers focus on clinical aspects of biomechanical conditions, including early diagnosis, treatment, and rehabilitation. The thread common to all the centers, however, is the overall goal that unites them—*prevention* of work-related ergonomic disorders.

This chapter may not include every national center where work-related biomechanical disorders are addressed; many hospital-based and university-based facilities also list activities such as "occupational medicine" among their services. Diagnosis and treatment of biomechanical or repetitive disorders would be one of the conditions addressed in that type of clinical setting.

Rather, the chapter presents a sampling of the types of centers that currently exist, primarily within the United States, and that are known to the author. This collection may serve as a "jumping off" point for the reader in exploring the other institutions.

The Mount Sinai/I.J. Selikoff Center for Occupational and Environmental Medicine

One Gustave L. Levy Place, Box 1058
New York, NY 10029
212-241-2582 or 212-241-0176

The Mount Sinai Program to Prevent and Treat Work-Related Musculoskeletal Disorders was established to improve health and create safe work environments. The goals of the program are to reduce lost work time and prevent disability through early intervention and treatment of work-related musculoskeletal disorders. Physicians at the center are experts in the diagnosis, treatment, and prevention of those disorders. They have been successfully treating workers in New York City since 1988. The program is unique because it integrates occupational medicine with rehabilitation, ergonomics, social work, education, and research.

Services

CLINICAL SERVICES

Patients who come to the center receive a thorough clinical evaluation, which includes detailed medical history, detailed occupational history, and complete physical examination. The early treatment of work-related musculoskeletal disorders can minimize injuries, decrease lost work time, prevent disability, and avert surgery. Physicians use a team approach to the management of work-related musculoskeletal disorders. The occupational medical physician may refer patients to

- physical and occupational therapy,
- the occupational ergonomics clinic,
- social work,
- medical massage therapy,
- support groups,
- educational services, or
- vocational rehabilitation.

OCCUPATIONAL ERGONOMICS CLINIC

Proper work station design can prevent work-related musculoskeletal disorders and improve safety and comfort. The ergonomist assesses individual work stations and provides patient education. Keyboard operators simulate their work using a work station at the center. Topics discussed include

- body mechanics;
- work station layout;
- tools, equipment, furniture, system, and job design; and
- work practices.

ERGONOMIC CONSULTATIONS

The staff ergonomist works with facility managers, nurses, industrial hygienists, engineers, and union health and safety representatives to develop ergonomic programs. Services include

- work site analysis to identify preventable ergonomic risks,
- job design/redesign to eliminate or reduce ergonomic hazards,
- training in the recognition and control of ergonomic problems,
- medical management programs and protocols focused on disability prevention, and
- in-house ergonomic programs.

SOCIAL WORK SERVICES

A certified social worker has extensive experience with these disorders and is pioneering creative and innovative services for people with work-related musculoskeletal disorders. Services include

- individual counseling,
- patient support groups, and
- vocational rehabilitation.

PATIENT EDUCATION PROGRAM

The center provides up-to-date information and training about medical problems, occupational ergonomics, voice recognition technology, and social and financial issues.

RESEARCH

The center uses the expertise of the epidemiologists, biostatisticians, and basic scientists in the Department of Community Medicine at the Mount Sinai Medical Center to conduct research on work-related musculoskeletal disorders. The focus is on prevention and treatment of work-related musculoskeletal disorders.

Occupational and Industrial Orthopaedic Center

63 Downing Street
New York, NY 10014-4331
212-255-6690

Located in Greenwich Village in Manhattan, the mission of the Occupational and Industrial Orthopaedic Center (OIOC) is to serve industry and the workforce with clinical, educational, research, and consulting services in the prevention and treatment of musculoskeletal injuries and disorders. OIOC consists of a multidisciplinary team of health care professionals, engineers, ergonomists, and basic scientists. Its four major activities are clinical activity, educational activity, research, and consultation.

Services

The OIOC out-patient clinic offers medical evaluation, functional evaluation, physical therapy treatment and stress management. Clinical programs include
- low back treatment,
- neck treatment,
- stress management and counseling,
- the upper- and lower-extremity program, and
- the return-to-work program.

The goal of the treatment programs is to prevent chronicity and to return the individual to active life and productive work. The clinic offers patients a completely equipped exercise and fitness facility; a variety of rehabilitation modalities including heat, ice, ultrasound, and neuromuscular stimulation; and dynamic and isometric computerized strength-testing equipment. In 1995, the OIOC clinic had a total of 4113 patient visits (an increase of 30% from 1994), and 15 patients participated in the extensive return-to-work program.

Along with clinical services, OIOC provides educational, research, and consulting services. OIOC has been conducting basic and applied research in various areas of musculoskeletal biomechanics. The OIOC research team has a track record in measuring and evaluating parameters of physical performance, muscle recruitment patterns, whole-body vibration exposure, workplace evaluation, ergonomic job analysis, and ergonomic task analysis. The research work conducted at OIOC is supported by federal grants and industry-based projects.

Research

The research facilities and equipment available at OIOC and its Muscle Recruitment Laboratory include a 64-channel general-purpose data acquisition system, analog-digital storage oscilloscope, B200 triaxial dynamometer, BackTracker portable triaxial trunk electrogoniometer, Polhemus 3Spacer tracker, 16-channel electromyography (EMG) system, Bruel and Kjaer human vibration measurement set, Kistler force plate, Natick pull test, biofeedback systems, Polar portable heart rate monitor, Oxylog portable oxygen consumption measuring device, video cameras, and a portable data collection and analysis system.

Personnel

The center's personnel form a multidisciplinary group that investigates new ways of reducing musculoskeletal injuries and occupational stress. Board-certified orthopedic surgeons perform clinical evaluations and treat employees who have these musculoskeletal injuries and disorders. Bioengineers analyze injuries using the principles of engineering, science, and technology. Ergonomists develop methods for work analysis and injury prevention. Physical and occupational therapists develop more effective rehabilitation programs. Epidemiologists quantify the incidence of occupational injuries and the efficacy of preventive programs. Psychologists study effective treatment for pain and ways of evaluating and reducing stress in the workplace.

Formal Academic Study

The Program of Ergonomics and Biomechanics of New York University offers both Master of Arts (School of Education) and Doctor of Philosophy (Graduate School of Arts and Sciences) degrees to those qualified students who seek an advanced understanding of the theory and application of ergonomics and biomechanics disciplines. This unique program is conducted by OIOC at the Hospital for Joint Diseases, which is a member organization of the New York University Medical Center. OIOC is an internationally recognized clinical, research, and educational center that specializes in the prevention and treatment of musculoskeletal and occupational injuries.

Students with backgrounds in medicine, physical and occupational therapy, osteopathy, occupational nursing and medicine, orthopaedic surgery, epidemiology, anthropology, psychology, physics, engineering, and the basic medical sciences are attracted to the program. Students in the program are trained to apply immediate practical solutions to health-related problems and to develop methods for preventing musculoskeletal and work-related injuries.

The primary objective of the program is to prepare the student for an academic and research career. The curriculum is designed to be a well-balanced blend of theoretical, practical, and research skills coursework. The multidisciplinary faculty, with backgrounds in medicine, engineering, epidemiology, physical sciences, human factors, and ergonomics have been carefully selected to support this curriculum.

Bellevue Occupational and Medical Clinic

Bellevue Hospital, Room CD349
27th Street & First Avenue
New York, NY 10016
212-562-4572

The Bellevue Occupational and Environmental Medicine (OEM) Clinic is a university-based OEM clinic and the only OEM clinic in the New York City public hospital system. Bellevue provides clinical OEM services that are accessible to patients and workers who use the public hospitals for medical care. In addition to the clinical component, Bellevue is in the process of developing OEM research and educational programs.

Two categories of diagnosis are commonly seen at the clinic. The "occupational diagnoses" include upper-extremity cumulative trauma disorders, work-related lung diseases such as asthma, work-related upper respiratory disorders, neurotoxic disorders, and work-related skin disorders. The other category, "environmental diagnoses," includes indoor air-related complaints.

General Services

These include

- diagnosis, treatment, and prevention of occupational-related disease;
- diagnosis, treatment, and prevention of environmental-related disease;
- medical monitoring of persons working with toxic substances;
- medical screening for work-related diseases;
- industrial hygiene evaluation of work sites;
- occupational health education;
- medical clearance for respirator use;
- consultations to labor and industry;
- vocational rehabilitation services; and
- access to all clinical specialty services at Bellevue Hospital Center.

Specialized Services

These include

- occupational pulmonary disease evaluations,
- evaluation for small airways disease,
- ergonomics evaluations,
- work site hazards evaluations,
- occupational dermatology, and
- qualitative respirator fit testing.

Nonroutine testing includes methacholine challenge test, high-resolution chest computed tomography, bronchoalveolar lavage, and nerve conduction velocity/electromyogram.

Personnel

The staff includes physicians (including a rehabilitation physician), and industrial hygienist, a health educator, an epidemiologist, a toxicologist (consulting), and a social worker. Training is available to physicians (medical, toxicology fellows, emergency physicians, and primary care physicians); students (medical, epidemiology, graduate students); ergonomics/biomechanics graduate students; groups of workers; and union health and safety staff.

Affiliations

Bellevue is affiliated with the New York University Medical School Departments of Pulmonary and Critical Care Medicine and Environmental Medicine; the New York City Poison Control Center; the New York State Department of Health Occupational Health Clinic Network; and the National Toxicology Program. Bellevue also is an academic awardee of the National Institute of Environmental Health Services.

Research

Research areas include occupational respiratory disease, upper-extremity cumulative trauma disorders, and occupational-disease screening by physicians.

The Lorin E. Kerr Ergonomics Institute

The Department of Work Environment
University of Massachusetts—Lowell
1 University Avenue
Lowell, MA 01854
508-934-3250

The Kerr Ergonomics Institute (KEI) was founded in 1991. The goal of KEI is to develop programs and strategies that promote worker health and improve company productivity. The faculty and associates of KEI promote injury prevention; foster the development of effective work processes; and develop sound industrial and public policy by providing consultation and training to local, national, and international companies and public agencies.

On-going ergonomics research encompasses the fields of engineering, psychology, health sciences, economics, management, labor relations, and policy development. The research investigates ways of achieving sustainable economic development through injury prevention and participatory work redesign.

Technical Assistance

The faculty and associates of KEI can respond to requests for technical assistance in a variety of areas, including

- walk-throughs for hazard identification/stress audits;
- in-depth ergonomic, psychosocial, and biomechanical analysis;
- statistical analysis of worker compensation claims, OSHA 200 log data, and other company records;
- surveillance of work-related musculoskeletal disorders and other stress-related diseases;
- recommendations for job redesign;
- training for workers and supervisors;
- "fitting" trials for work stations and production equipment; and
- policy and technology reviews.

Faculty Research

Topics include

- ergonomic stressors and surveillance in automotive manufacturing,
- job content questionnaire—a psychosocial stress analysis instrument,
- reduction of work-related musculoskeletal disorders among construction workers,
- evaluation of workers' compensation as an economic incentive for injury prevention,
- electromyographic assessment of hand function and muscle control, and
- policy development and multicompany, ergonomic analysis of hazard and intervention.

Formal Educational Opportunities

The Work Environment Program (WEP), an academic and research graduate program, was founded in 1987. The program comprises the Department of Work Environment, the Massachusetts Toxics Use Reduction Institute, the Lorin E. Kerr Ergonomics Institute for Occupational Injury Prevention, the New England Consortium, and the Technology and Work Program.

WEP was created to direct attention to the prevention of work-related illnesses, injuries, and deaths and to promote the health and safety both of workers and of the general environment through research, teaching, and technical assistance. Its concern with the work environment also encompasses the psychosocial stressors of the workplace, which affect workers' health and job performance and employers' productivity.

Because of the complexity of work environment problems and the need for prevention, WEP seeks solutions that integrate the scientific with political, economic, and social approaches. Since its initiation, over $14 million of research funding has been awarded to the program by government, private, and professional sources.

The primary objective of the academic department is to educate scientists to study and evaluate workplace factors that affect the health status of workers and to develop new methods of controlling or eliminating risk. The department awards both master's and doctoral degrees. Its curriculum focuses on identification, quantitative assessment, and prevention of chemical, ergonomic, and other hazards to human health. Current areas of concentration are occupational epidemiology, industrial hygiene, occupational ergonomics, and work environment policy. The doctoral program requires a master's degree or equivalent and a substantial original research dissertation.

The University of Michigan Center for Ergonomics

College of Engineering
1205 Beal Avenue (10E Building)
Ann Arbor, MI 48109-2117
313-763-2243

In the late 1950s, when a formal ergonomics activity was established at the University of Michigan, the science of ergonomics was virtually unknown to the general public. Today the importance of good ergonomics is widely understood, and the University of Michigan Center for Ergonomics stands as one of the leading research centers in the world. The research has been developed in response to the real-world needs of industry, government, and professional groups.

The director of the center defines ergonomics as "the study of what people are required to do on their jobs and how job conditions can be engineered for people." Ideally, ergonomic considerations are an integral part of the design process from inception to completion—from the design of work stations for employees who manufacture the product to the design of the product itself.

Originally established in 1959 as the Engineering Human Performance Laboratory, the center was renamed the University of Michigan Center for Ergonomics in 1980. The center is consistently at the forefront of fundamental and applied ergonomics research, working collaboratively with industry to improve the lives of workers as well as the products they make. For more than 20 years, research has been conducted on human performance, occupational low back pain, occupational upper-extremity cumulative trauma disorders, implementation of workplace ergonomic programs, epidemiology of musculoskeletal disorders, work measurement, and biomechanical modeling. The center has a staff of approximately 30 and operates within the Department of Industrial and Operations Engineering. Annual grants, contracts, and gifts of up to $450,000 each support this research.

Graduate students, research scientists, and research sponsors are drawn to the center both because of its distinguished record of research and because of its extensive resources—state-of-the-art laboratories, test equipment, and computer systems. The center's facilities include individual laboratories for biomechanics, work physiology, cumulative trauma disorders, work measurement, posture and job analysis, vibration, tool studies, and human factors research.

Formal Educational Opportunities

While the Center for Ergonomics may be best known as a research organization, it is closely affiliated with several outstanding academic programs at the University of Michigan. Master's and PhD students in the departments of Industrial and Operations Engineering, Environmental and Industrial Health, and the Bioengineering Program perform their research at the center. An average of 35 graduate students work side by side with professors, scientists, and professionals from sponsoring corporations that are carrying out ergonomics research. The center also offers continuing education courses. These courses give professional ergonomists, engineers, and designers in private industry a way to keep up with the latest ergonomic thinking and research. Sponsors also stay up to date by taking advantage of the products of research performed at the center. An extensive library of publications written by professors and graduate students is available to them, along with recently developed ergonomics software.

Research

Current research projects include
- driver-vehicle interfaces in intelligent vehicle highway systems;
- ergonomics in hotel/resort operations;
- studies of working posture;
- work seat design and evaluation;
- ergonomic design optimization for percussive rivet tools;
- hand vibration, muscle stress, and muscle fatigue; and
- repetitive work and hand work.

In addition, the center is a National Institute for Occupational Safety and Health (NIOSH)–funded educational resource center (ERC) and offers four special graduate education programs:

1. Occupational Safety and Ergonomics,
2. Industrial Hygiene,
3. Occupational Medicine, and
4. Occupational Health Nursing.

Center for Ergonomics and Safety Research

University of Nebraska—Lincoln
175 Nebraska Hall
P.O. Box 880518
Lincoln, NE 68588-0518
402-472-3495

The Center for Ergonomics and Safety Research at the University of Nebraska was established in 1991 to study and improve people's job performance and well-being in relation to their job tasks, equipment, and environment.

At the work site or in the center's research lab, ergonomics professionals will improve workers' job performance and safety. The center performs ergonomic evaluations; provides ergonomic training and information; offers specialized ergonomic learning experiences; and conducts basic and applied ergonomic research.

There are four categories of interest and specialization:

1. Job and work site ergonomic improvement includes
- workplace safety and workers' health;
- ergonomic team building and team processes;
- organizational functions and the effects of organizational change on workers;
- work/rest cycles, shift work, and their impact on workers' productivity and fatigue;
- prevention of cumulative trauma disorder; and
- ergonomic training for employees.

2. Occupational ergonomics include
- manufacturing ergonomics,
- construction ergonomics,
- dental ergonomics,
- retail ergonomics, and
- transportation ergonomics.

3. Hand ergonomics include
- ergonomic assessment of hand tools;
- occupational hand, wrist, and arm injuries;
- effects of vibrating hand-held tools on hands, wrists, and arms; and
- effects of gloves on workers.

4. Ergonomic testing and research include
- nerve conduction screening,
- product prototype evaluation and design, and
- ergonomics of sleep and the sleep environment.

Personnel at the Center for Ergonomics and Safety Research are affiliated with the University of Nebraska—Lincoln Department of Industrial and Management Systems Engineering. Their areas of expertise include ergonomics, quality control, information processing, design of experiments, statistics, ergonomics, safety, and biomechanics.

University of California, San Francisco

The Ergonomics Program
Center for Occupational and Environmental Health
1301 South 46th Street, Building 112
Richmond, CA 94804
510-231-5720

The University of California offers ergonomics consulting services to companies, labor organizations, and government agencies via the Ergonomics Program. In a climate in which cumulative trauma disorders and the associated workers' compensation costs continue to increase, these services are directed toward identifying the risk factors for such disorders and assisting clients in reducing the hazards created by these risk factors.

Examples of the impact of such services are
- the redesign of a manufacturing plant where tasks required repetitive and intense hand maneuvers; the redesign resulted in reduced muscular loading of the shoulder muscles, reduced repetitive pinching, and a reduction in cases of carpal tunnel syndrome and tendinitis;
- the redesign both of work stations and of tasks of court stenographers, which reduced hand and wrist fatigue and increased productivity; and
- a job analysis at a hazardous waste facility, which led to improved materials handling procedures, thereby lowering the risk of back injuries.

Personnel and Services

Consulting services are provided by trained and experienced industrial engineers and health professionals. Services include

- evaluation and modification of video display terminals and other aspects of work stations;
- job evaluations combined with recommendations for modifications;
- tool design to reduce hand and forearm fatigue;
- training of employees and supervisors in ergonomic concepts, proper work break patterns, and exercises;
- review of medical management protocol for employees with cumulative trauma disorders;
- design of an effective ergonomics program to meet in-house needs and satisfy pending OSHA ergonomic regulations; and
- assistance with the evaluation and selection of furniture and hand tools.

Research

The Ergonomics Laboratory in the center is a research laboratory established to increase our understanding of how nerves and tendons are injured; to characterize risk factors for chronic musculoskeletal disorders of the arm, hand, and shoulder; and identify engineering and administrative methods of controlling these disorders. The laboratory also provides consulting to regional companies, unions, and government agencies on ergonomic issues.

Formal Educational Offerings

The Ergonomics Program is located at U.C. Berkeley's Richmong Field Station at the site of various research laboratories, predominantly associated with the College of Engineering. The Ergonomics Program conducts research and consulting to identify risk factors for cumulative trauma disorders and to evaluate interventions for preventing these disorders.

Faculty

The director of the program is a physician with training in biomedical engineering. In addition, two industrial engineers serve as ergonomics consultants and trainers for the program—both are board certified in professional ergonomics. The program occupies 5000 square feet of research space and 1000 square feet of meeting/office space. The laboratory has video and electronic systems for measuring joint position, motion, and force.

The ergonomics track is initially a master's program— a Masters in Science program in Environmental Health Sciences at the School of Public Health. Students interested in the PhD program apply through the Bioengineering Program at U.C. Berkeley and indicate an interest in occupational biomechanics.

The primary objective of the ergonomics program at U.C. Berkeley is to provide practitioners and researchers with advanced training in the principles and concepts of ergonomics. A secondary objective is a breadth of knowledge about related disciplines such as epidemiology, industrial hygiene, safety, and occupational health. A multidisciplinary approach to problem solving and is promoted.

School of Industrial Engineering

Purdue University
1287 Grissom Hall
West Lafayette, IN 47907-1287
317-494-5400

The strength of the program at Purdue University comes from the integration of the knowledge found in many engineering disciplines, because the consideration of human, material, organizational, and technological variables is increasingly critical for the success of modern organizations/institutions.

Industrial engineers traditionally have been concerned with the quality of life of the worker. Purdue continues this tradition by giving students hands-on research and coursework in ergonomics. One senior faculty member is conducting research to develop predictive models for the occurrence of carpal tunnel syndrome, one of the most common disabling injuries experienced by many high-risk workforces (including dental care workers).

As of 1995, the formal educational program included 342 students in the undergraduate program, 106 in the master's degree program, and 72 PhD candidates under the tutelage of 30 faculty members. The emphasis at Purdue is on research, and to support this effort, the institution is currently remodeling 2300 square feet of laboratory space intended for four instructional laboratories—the Human Technology Interface Laboratory, the Ergonomics Laboratory, the Product Usability Laboratory, and the Undergraduate PC Laboratory.

Research

Most relevant to dental care practitioners is a series of research studies conducted by faculty at Purdue's School of Industrial Engineering during the 1970s. The results of these studies were published between 1973 and 1977 and include the following:

- "Pilot study on criteria in cavity preparation—facts or artifacts?"
- "Training dental students in dental amalgam condensation";
- "Use of personality, anthropometry, and vision scores to select students for psychomotor dental performance";
- "Use of 20X microscopes for the psychomotor dental operations";
- "Training in force exertions during condensation of dental amalgam";
- "Perceptual and motor training for the acquisition and retention of psychomotor in dental amalgam restorations: class I in the mandibular first molar";
- "Electromechanical simulator for acquisition of psychomotor skills in cavity preparation";
- "Objective evaluation of quality in cavity preparations";
- "Skills analysis of cavity preparations: class I in mandibular right first molar";
- "A second generation training simulator for acquisition of psychomotor skills in cavity preparation."

Further information about these dental studies may be obtained by contacting Dr. Gavriel Salvendy at Purdue, School of Industrial Engineering.

The Center for Occupational and Environmental Neurology

Childrens' Hospital Professional Building
3901 Greenspring Avenue
Baltimore, MD 21211-1398
410-669-1101
The Center for Occupational and Environmental Neurology (COEN) addresses all aspects of prevention, evaluation, and treatment of health problems in occupational and environmental neurology.

Areas of Expertise
Areas of expertise include
- occupational neurology, neuropsychiatry, and neurotoxicology;
- medical/ergonomic program;
- ergonomic assessment;
- behavioral toxicology;
- occupational neuroepidemiology;
- industrial hygiene;
- biological monitoring; and
- medical surveillance.

Services
The following services are provided:
- neurological and neuropsychiatric evaluation;
- neuropsychological evaluation—for diagnosis, treatment planning, and vocational rehabilitation;
- psychotherapy;
- nerve conduction studies and electromyography;
- auditory, visual and somatosensory evoked potentials;
- quantitative electroencephalography analysis;

- development of medical management and medical surveillance;
- programs for health outcomes related to ergonomic stressors and exposure to neurotoxic compounds;
- risk assessment;
- prevention programs;
- teaching tapes for employees; and
- on-site visits and presentations.

Of most interest to readers concerned with dentistry would be the Medical Ergonomics Program. The four blocks of this program are occupational therapy, management and employee education, abatement of ergonomic stressors, and the Center for Occupational and Environmental Neurology. Some of the activities undertaken as part of this program include training of supervisors, work site visits, provision of educational in-services that focus on prevention, early detection and interventions, medical ergonomic consultations, training of the worker in safe movements and task techniques using biofeedback, use of therapeutic modalities, and diagnostic studies and evaluations.

Educational Resource Centers

The National Institute for Occupational Safety and Health (NIOSH) has developed a program that establishes centers of learning for occupational safety and health throughout the United States. These educational resource centers (ERCs) are located at 27 universities and serve all 10 Department of Health and Human Services (DHHS) regions. Most centers offer formal degree programs in subjects that are pertinent to the field, such as bachelor's or master's degrees in industrial hygiene, occupational health nursing, and ergonomics. In addition, continuing education offerings, which are developed to meet the needs of professionals within their geographical regions, are a critical component of all ERCs. The format, length, and content of the continuing education courses may vary from center to center. The schedule of courses being offered from 1996 through 1997 includes, for example, Reproductive Hazards in the Workplace, Occupational and Environmental Medicine, Clinical

Management of Low Back Pain, Pesticides, and Ergonomics. The formats used range from lecture to hands-on to training small workshops, and the duration of the offering may be anywhere from half a day to 1 week, depending on the topic and outcome anticipated for the participant.

Subject areas include, but are not limited to (1) trend analysis, (2) job analysis, (3) control implementation, (4) control evaluation, (5) medical management, (6) training, and (7) team approach.

In Table 1, the reader will find a list of the ERCs currently in existence, as well as their geographical locations, the names of contact people, and telephone numbers.

The OSHA Training Institute

1555 Times Drive
Des Plains, IL 60018-1548
847-297-9990

The Occupational Safety and Health Administration (OSHA) Training Institute provides basic and advanced training and education courses in safety and health. Course subject matter includes hazard recognition, OSHA policies and standards, and hazard abatement techniques. Courses are designed to build a more effective workforce and to aid in professional development.

Unless otherwise specified, all courses conducted at the institute begin at 8:15 a.m. and end at 4:00 p.m. on the starting date and conclude at 10:15 a.m. on the final date. Most courses last for more than 1 day, and a reasonable tuition is charged to all attendees, who may include federal employees, private sector employees, and other nonfederal governmental employees. Continuing education units (CEUs) are available to participants in courses conducted by the Training Institute in accordance with the administrative and program criteria guidelines that have been established by the International Association for Continuing Education and Training.

Table 1.—Educational Resource Centers (ERCs) as of November, 1996.

Name of Center	Location	Contact Person	Telephone
Deep South Center for Occ H&S*	Birmingham, AL	Cherie Hunt	205-934-7178
Northern California Center for Occ/Envir Health**	Richmond, CA	Barbara Plog	510-231-5645
Southern California ERC	Los Angeles, CA	Ramona Cayuela	213-740-3998
Great Lakes Center for Occ/Envir H&S	Chicago, IL	Leslie Nickels	312-413-0459
Johns Hopkins ERC	Baltimore, MD	Morton Corn	410-955-3602
Harvard ERC	Boston, MA	Kathryn Lord	617-432-3518
Michigan Center for Occ H&S Engineering	Ann Arbor, MI	Patricia Cottrell	313-763-0567
Midwest Center for Occ H&S	St. Paul, MN	Jeanne Ayers	612-221-3992
New York/New Jersey ERC	New York, NY/NJ	Lee Lausten	908-235-5062
North Carolina ERC	Raleigh, NC	Larry Hyde	919-286-3232
University of Cincinnati	Cincinnati, OH	Amit Bwattacharva	513-558-1731
Southwest Center for Occ/Envir Health	Houston, TX	Pam Parker	713-742-4648
Rocky Mountain Center for Occ/Envir Health	Salt Lake City, UT	Donald Bloswick	801-581-4163
Northwest Center for Occ H&S	Seattle, WA	Jan Schwert	206-543-0314

* Occupational health and safety
** Occupational and environmental health

OSHA Training Institute Education Centers Program

In recent years, the demand for OSHA Training Institute courses from the private sector and from other federal agencies has increased beyond the resources of the institute. To address the increased demand, the OSHA Training Institute has established OSHA-supervised educational centers at the 12 nonprofit organizations listed in Table 2.

Each of the 12 centers is authorized and approved to offer nine courses, including the course titled "Principles of Ergonomics." This course introduces the student to the applica-

---

Table 2.—OSHA-Supervised Educational Centers

Location	Center
Ypsilanti, Michigan	Eastern Michigan University/ United Auto Workers
Atlanta, Georgia	Georgia Tech Research Institute
St. Paul, Minnesota	Great Lakes Regional OSHA Training Consortium— University of Minnesota, Minnesota Safety Council, and University of Cincinnati
Manchester, New Hampshire	Keene State College
Kansas City, Missouri	Maple Woods Community College
Washington, D.C.	National Resource Center for OSHA Training—Building and Construction Trades Department, AFL-CIO/West Virginia University
Lockport, New York	Niagra County Community College
Lakewood, Colorado	Red Rocks Community College/Trinidad State Junior College
Arlington, Texas	Texas Engineering Extension Service
San Diego/La Jolla, California	University of California
Seattle, Washington	University of Washington

tion of ergonomic principles for prevention of musculoskeletal disorders. Topics include work physiology, anthropometry, musculoskeletal disorders, video display terminals, and risk factors such as vibration, temperature, manual handling, repetition, and continuous keyboard use. The course features industrial case studies covering analysis and design of work stations and equipment, laboratory sessions in manual lifting, and coverage of OSHA's proposed ergonomic protection standard. The course runs for a total of 4 days, and tuition for the private sector ranges from $415 (in Des Plaines) to $695, depending on which center one attends.

North Carolina Ergonomics Resource Center

703 Tucker Street
Raleigh, NC 27603
919-515-2052

The mission of the North Carolina Ergonomics Resource Center (NC ERC) is to improve the productivity, safety, and well-being of the people of North Carolina, in all sectors of business and industry, including government. By emphasizing applied research and timely delivery of programs, NC ERC identifies, analyzes, and corrects ergonomic deficiencies in the workplace. Its primary goal is to act as a bridge for technology transfer and information exchange between the university, state agencies, and industry.

Three levels of membership are available at NC ERC. Developing members participate in the Ergonomics Voluntary Compliance Program. Depending on size and projected needs, developing members implement the center's Ergonomic Prescription; these members also have access to all of the center's services and programs. Practicing members are those members currently maintaining ergonomics programs; practicing members participate and benefit from the center's general programs, including research and consultation, and have the option of contracting with the center for special services or projects. Associate members include consultants, vendors, and associations that provide ergonomics programs and services in North Carolina.

Programs and Services

COMPLIANCE AND OSHA
The center
- develops, implements, and monitors ergonomics programs, including the Ergonomic Prescription, and
- provides on-site review and consultation.

EDUCATION AND TRAINING:
NC ERC provides education and training in
- office ergonomics,
- basic ergonomics,
- advanced ergonomics,
- ergonomics risk assessment,
- management of musculoskeletal disorders, and
- team ergonomics.

OFFERINGS
NC ERC offers
- monthly workshops/seminars at the center, and
- on-site programs for member companies.

RAPID RESPONSE
The Center maintains a phone-in/mail-in consultation service for members and nonmembers as well as for the public at large. This service answers questions related to ergonomics, suggests sources for ergonomic products, and provides names of practitioners who might be able to respond to a specific need or question.

CENTER LABORATORY
NC ERC uses several state-of-the-art systems for basic and field research in ergonomics. The center's laboratory is equipped with computer-based systems configured to allow for optimum use of resources during data collection and analy-

sis. Specialized equipment and instrumentation are available for conducting one-of-a-kind projects. The laboratory is available to members and affiliates undertaking specific center studies and projects.

THE CENTER STAFF
NC ERC is staffed by experienced ergonomists and health care specialists. These professionals are supported by a team of media, publication, and laboratory specialists.

CENTER CONFERENCES
A fall conference for industry and business provides state-of-the-art updates on ergonomics and related issues. A spring conference for center affiliates and associates reviews ergonomic research, new technology, and applications.

CENTER RESEARCH
Research topics include
- ergonomic risk assessment,
- job design/restructuring,
- workplace design/redesign,
- product design/redesign,
- development of fit-for-work programs, and
- appliance programs.

CENTER PUBLICATIONS
NC ERC publishes the following:
- *ErgoTalk* (center newsletter),
- *ErgoNote* (research bulletin), and
- *ErgoVision* (multimedia training courses).

ERGONOMIC AUDITS
NC ERC provides a full array of audit surveys tailored to meet specific needs and goals:

- Ergonomic audits range from simple walk-through surveys for problem recognition to objective measurement and evaluation of workplaces/jobs to determine the ergonomic soundness of the organization.
- Proposals are developed for ergonomic improvements that address recognized deficiencies.

University of Wisconsin—Milwaukee

College of Engineering and Applied Science
P.O. Box 784/EMS Building
Milwaukee, WI 53201
414-229-4967

The College of Engineering at the University of Wisconsin offers the following services: formal education culminating in undergraduate and graduate degrees or certificates, informal multiday courses, research, laboratory-related activities, and consultation to industry.

Research

For approximately 20 years, the university has been performing research on ergonomics-related issues. The emphasis has been on (1) developing models to analyze jobs in industry and to identify jobs that involve the risk of musculoskeletal disorders, and (2) prevention of injuries in occupational settings. Some of the research projects completed or currently under way include

- revised NIOSH equation for manual lifting (includes software development);
- the Strain Index;
- metabolic Rate Prediction Model;
- 3-D Static Biomechanical Model;
- prevention of injuries to health care professionals (nurses, nurses' aides, etc.);
- physical stresses related to working in warehouses;
- biomechanical, physiological, and psychological issues in lifting techniques; and
- participatory ergonomics in red-meat packing.

Laboratory Facilities

The College has two laboratories: the Ergonomics Laboratory and the Laboratory for Prevention of Injuries to Health Care Professionals. The Ergonomics Laboratory is spacious and well equipped. All formal coursework and course projects are supported with laboratory experience. The laboratory contains two personal computers: one laptop computer; a static-strength measurement system; an isokinetic strength measurement system; Oxylog for O_2 uptake measurement; CO_2 and O_2 analyzers; an electromyographic measurement system; anthropometers; grip- and pinch-strength measuring devices; heart rate measurement and analysis systems; a VCR and camera; computer software for 2-D and 3-D biomechanical models; the NIOSH guide; energy expenditure analysis modeling, and so forth. The lab is in the process of acquiring postural-analysis systems for trunk and wrist measurements.

Educational Offerings

The objective of the Certificate in Ergonomics Program is to provide a formal program of study, training, and experience in ergonomics to those post-baccalaureate students who wish to specialize in this area. The principles learned here are applicable to a wide range of workplace settings, including industry, hospitals, nursing homes, office work, government, and academia. This novel, cooperative, 15-credit-hour program provides an avenue for a concentration in ergonomics to nondegree graduate students in various programs such as nursing, occupational therapy, and medical school. The program emphasizes theoretical principles and job analysis methods and demonstrates various techniques and case studies for implementing ergonomic concepts in practical settings. Lectures are supplemented with laboratory experience and projects as applicable.

The following degree programs, which offer concentrations in ergonomics, are also available:

- MS and PhD in engineering,
- MS and PhD in nursing,
- MS in occupational therapy, and
- MS in rehabilitation counseling.

In addition, the college also offers short nondegree courses; for example, during the month of June, a 5-day course titled "Advanced Ergonomics" is offered.

Consulting
The professional, experienced staff at the Ergonomics Laboratory provide consulting to industry on a fee-for-service basis.

Association of Occupational and Environmental Clinics

1010 Vermont Avenue, NW
Suite 513
Washington, DC 20005
202-347-4976

The Association of Occupational and Environmental Clinics (AOEC) was established in 1987 to enhance the practice of occupational and environmental medicine through information sharing, education, and research. The growing national network now includes 54 clinics and 270 individuals dedicated to research, education, and the prevention and treatment of occupational and environmental diseases. AOEC members share a strong conviction that it is not sufficient simply to respond to occupational and environmental conditions with routine diagnosis and treatment. "They believe these issues must be met with a public health response." Such a response is likely to involve the contributions of nurses, health educators, industrial hygienists, chemists, ergonomists, epidemiologists, toxicologists, and others, as well as the contribution of the primary care physician.

AOEC member clinics share the following goals:
- to aid in identifying, reporting, and preventing occupational and environmental health hazards and their effects;
- to encourage the provision of high-quality clinical services for people with work- or environmental-related health problems;

- to provide a means for member clinics to share information that will enable them to better diagnose and treat occupational and environmental diseases;
- to increase communication among member clinics concerning issues related to patient care and disease prevention;
- to facilitate liaison between clinics and agencies responsible for workplace and environmental monitoring; and
- to provide a source of data for research projects related to occupational and environmental health.

Activities

Recent activities include

- publishing the proceedings from the AOEC National Workshop on Multiple Chemical Sensitivity (MCS);
- developing curriculum materials in environmental health and sponsoring Continuing Medical Education programs for clinicians and other health professionals (subcontracts in these areas are awarded to AOEC clinic and individual members);
- cooperating with the Agency for Toxic Substances and Disease Registry (ATSDR) and the National Institute for Occupational Safety and Health (NIOSH) in various areas under ongoing agreements;
- undertaking a pilot project in which selected clinics have compiled and exchanged data on exposures through analysis of immune biomarkers;
- acting as a resource for patient referrals for ATSDR, NIOSH, and others;
- initiating joint programs with Canadian counterparts in the Great Lakes Basin to increase awareness of environmental health issues;
- designing and initiating a quality assurance program to be followed by member clinics;
- compiling and comparing different clinic views and practices at regional and national meetings; and
- promoting a climate of intellectual and productive informational exchange via the Occupational and Environmental Medicine (OEM) List and the AOEC World Wide Web home page.

All current member clinics listed in the AOEC directory offer ergonomics-related services by a trained professional; depending on the center, these services may include diagnosis and treatment, rehabilitation, educational offerings, consultations to individuals and/or companies, and research projects. For the name of an AOEC nearest to your home/ office, contact the association.

Ohio State University

Ergonomics Institute
210 Baker Systems
1971 Neil Avenue
Columbus, OH 43210-1271
614-292-4606

As mechanization and automation become increasingly common in the workplace, the demands placed on today's worker are greater than ever. Competitive markets have forced attention on improving quality, increasing productivity, and reducing costs.

A well-designed work environment considers the mental and physical capabilities of the workforce. The Ohio State University is one of the only institutions in the United States that integrates the physical and cognitive aspects of ergonomics.

The interdisciplinary approach to ergonomics at Ohio State University provides practical solutions to the complex problems in your workplace. The state-of-the-art program draws on the extensive experience of faculty, staff, and graduate students from a variety of backgrounds. The program help address ergonomics issues in the workplace through consultation, training, and research services.

Consultation

Consultation services can help
- develop and implement ergonomics processes,
- assess the risk of work-related injuries and illnesses,
- test and evaluate prototype tools and equipment,
- quantify low back disorders,

- design tasks and workstations,
- devise systems to identify and prioritize jobs for ergonomic intervention, and
- determine software usability.

Training

Ergonomics is taught through
- short courses on the fundamentals of ergonomics,
- custom-tailored ergonomics team training, and
- symposia on state-of-the-art trends in ergonomics.

Research

The Ergonomics Institute offers comprehensive research on topics such as
- developing methods to reduce occupational injury and illness,
- understanding human performance in real-world industrial and educational settings,
- developing and evaluating effective designs,
- using computers as educational tools, and
- evaluating and reducing human error.

Louisiana State University

College of Engineering
3128 CEBA
Baton Rouge, LA 70803
504-388-5367

Industrial engineering involves the synthesis and application of scientific principles to design, installation, and improvement of integrated systems of people, materials, and equipment. The goal is to provide the most efficient and effective operating and work environment. Industrial engineering combines principles of human behavior with concepts of engineering procedure and analysis.

The College of Engineering offers formal academic training in a 4-year program that includes courses such as

- human factors engineering—human performance in human-machine systems;
- safety engineering—control of hazardous physical and environmental conditions;
- fundamentals of industrial hygiene engineering—basic principles of hazards such as radiation, sound, thermal stressors, chemicals, and air contamination;
- human performance with information-processing systems—development of human-operated information systems that can be applied to practical problems in industry;
- ergonomics in work design—anthropometry, anatomy, physiology, and their application in workplace design and task assessment;
- work physiology—relationship of physiological responses and task design, worker placement, and work-rest scheduling;
- occupational biomechanics—principles of biomechanics applied to human movement and work systems; and
- human interaction with computers—ergonomics of the use of interactive computer systems.

In addition, students may take a "minor" in occupational health and safety.

Faculty

The faculty is international in scope and has research and teaching interests that include but are not limited to the following areas:

- guidelines for preventing hand-tool-related accidents and illnesses,
- back problems affecting preschool special education staff,
- relationship between posture and lifting capacity,
- psychophysical models for manual lifting tasks, and
- a biomechanical model for optimal design of manual tasks.

Marquette University

Department of Mechanical and Industrial Engineering
1515 West Wisconsin Avenue
Milwaukee, WI 53233
414-288-7259

Formal Programs

The department offers master's and doctoral programs for both full-time and part-time students. Master's students are required to take 30 semester hours of coursework and to complete either a thesis or an essay. Doctoral students must pass a qualifying exam, meet a 1-year residency requirement, and write a dissertation in addition to course work.

Students may pursue graduate studies in a variety of areas within the disciplines of mechanical engineering and industrial engineering. Programs are designed on an individual basis. Students may major in an area called "Quality Systems/Ergonomics." The department has 20 full-time faculty members, as well as adjunct and part-time faculty members.

Resources

The Industrial Ergonomics Laboratory was established to conduct quantitative research in ergonomics and implement ergonomics principles and practices in manufacturing and service industries. Emphasis is on quantifying physical risk factors in jobs and using this information to design or redesign work stations, tools, and tasks so as to reduce cost and incidence of occupational injuries, enhance productivity and quality, and improve employee morale. Injuries studied include upper-extremity cumulative trauma disorders such as carpal tunnel syndrome and low back pain.

Equipment in the laboratory includes hardware and software that measures upper-extremity (elbow, wrist, and finger) motion of factory or office workers; human vibration sensors; whole-body-strength tester; grip- and pinch-strength dynamometers and gyrometer; anthropometric measuring devices; portable data acquisition systems and computers; and advanced desktop computer systems.

Research

Current ergonomic research includes the following projects:

- evaluation and design of dental seating for dentists and hygienists,
- evaluation and design of alternative computer keyboards,
- design of biomedical instrumentation for the National Aeronautics and Space Administration,
- biomechanical modeling of the wrist joint,
- implementation of an ergonomics process in the electric power industry,
- evaluation and design of hand tools,
- monitoring of forearm and wrist motion of factory workers,
- evaluation of handle shapes and sizes for hand tools, and
- design of clinical diagnostic tools for physical therapists.

ErgoCenter

University of Connecticut Health Center
Farmington, CT 06030-6210
860-679-1285

The purpose of the Ergonomic Technology Center (ErgoCenter) is to serve as a resource for business and labor in their efforts to control the growing incidence of cumulative trauma disorders in Connecticut workplaces. The ErgoCenter will simultaneously focus on the creation of new technologies and on jobs related to the control of injuries. The makeup of the present ErgoCenter board of directors reflects a broad-based cooperative approach that will make it possible to fully address the root causes of cumulative trauma disorders. Board members are drawn from Connecticut industry, insurance, labor, medical, and academic interests with the advisory participation of Connecticut Innovations, Inc. (CII).

After 2 years of planning, the ErgoCenter is now based at the University of Connecticut Health Center and is entering its startup and development phase. As approved and funded by the Connecticut legislature, the ErgoCenter is designed to become a self-sufficient, market-driven center of ergonomic expertise and assistance. It has been charged with several interdependent goals. Most immediately, the ErgoCenter is designed as a focus for state-of-the-art identification, evaluation, treatment, and prevention of cumulative trauma disorders. ErgoCenter services will reduce workplace injuries and illnesses, while improving human performance.

The center will thus contribute to increased productivity of Connecticut business by

- reducing medical costs, lost work time, and labor recruitment and retraining costs; and
- improving work processes and work flow, as well as employee satisfaction and commitment.

Much of the funding for the ErgoCenter is earmarked for matching funds, to leverage more extensive intervention projects in companies. The center is also mandated to create jobs by identifying and developing technologies, products, and services to serve the needs of the ergonomic market. All of these activities require the ErgoCenter to perform a function now missing in the state: bridging the gap between the ongoing development of ergonomic knowledge in academic institutions and the practical needs of industry.

Services

CLINICAL SERVICES
These include

- Upper-extremity and back diagnostic and evaluation techniques/protocols such as
  1. initial injury medical exams, IMEs, complex case diagnosis;
  2. on-site diagnostic testing (lab, EMG/NCV/radiology);

   3. on-site neurology and arthritis consultation; and
   4. ongoing research and development of diagnostic methodology;
- Treatment, including
   1. conservative treatment and management modalities;
   2. specialty consultation with board-certified hand surgeon;
   3. certified occupational hand therapy and physical therapy;
   4. therapeutic exercise training and functional capacity evaluations;
   5. ongoing research and development of treatment methodology; and
   6. social work counseling, EAP, and support services;
- Fitness for duty and return-to-work evaluations.

ERGONOMIC PREVENTION SERVICES

The following injury prevention services are offered:
- work station/work process consultation, including
   1. work station simulation/videotaping/retraining,
   2. identification and evaluation of workplace risk factors for cumulative trauma injuries,
   3. cost-effective redesign/retrofit of existing workplaces and work processes to reduce risk, and
   4. design of new/proposed workplaces and processes to incorporate the most up-to-date and effective risk-reduction knowledge and equipment;
- surveillance services—high-risk job screening and recommendations;
- development of company-specific ergonomics programs, including
   1. creation or improvement of ongoing ergonomic safety committees and
   2. assistance in development of in-house capacity for continuous ergonomic improvement; and
- evaluation strategies for assessing the effectiveness of interventions.

ERGONOMIC TRAINING
Training is provided for
- management,
- employees,
- joint health and safety committees,
- company medical personnel, and
- engineers and designers.

TECHNOLOGY AND PRODUCT DEVELOPMENT
AND DEPLOYMENT
Goals include
- provision of a referral and extension service—the ErgoCenter is developing a data base of ergonomics-related products and services available in the state;
- stimulation of research on new technologies and products relevant to diagnosis, treatment, and prevention of cumulative trauma disorders; and
- provision of assistance in the development spin-off enterprises based on the new technologies and products.

Center for Industrial Ergonomics

University of Louisville
Academic Building (Room 437)
Louisville, KY 40292
502-852-7173

The Center for Industrial Ergonomics is an integral unit of the Department of Industrial Engineering. The center's research and educational activities focus on integrating people, organization, and technology at work and on improving quality and productivity through ergonomic safety and health management.

Sources of Support

The main sources of the center's support are the engineering school, research grants, and research/development projects for industry. Among the research contracts awarded to the center in the past 5 years are those funded by NIOSH, the US Public Health Service (USPHS), General Motors Company, and local industries in the Kentucky and Indiana area.

Areas of Research and Industrial Expertise

The center performs research and training in several areas of work systems design, ergonomics, and occupational health and safety management. These areas include, but are not limited to

- people-organization-technology: integrating human, organizational, and technical systems at work;
- prevention of musculoskeletal injuries at work, such as cumulative trauma disorders of the upper extremities and low back injuries: compliance with applicable labor laws;
- ergonomic workplace evaluation and engineering redesign: task analysis, methods study, and work measurement;
- human aspects of office work, human-computer interaction, ergonomics of telecommunication, and work with video display terminals;
- human factors in advanced manufacturing technology and robotics safety: implementation and design issues;
- ergonomic evaluation and design of consumer product: safety, usability, and comfort-of-use issues; and
- systems ergonomics: management of ergonomic hazards, safety, and health in the workplace.

Resources

The center is equipped with laboratory instrumentation allowing studies in workplace design, biomechanics, work physiology, engineering anthropometry, pre-employment strength testing, and environmental stress assessment. In addition, research equipment is available for studies in robotics safety, human-computer interaction, and ergonomic workplace design using SAMMIE and Human CAD software systems.

Publications and Editorial Services

Research results have been published in several international scientific journals and reports, including *Ergonomics, International Journal of Human-Computer Interaction, Applied Ergonomics,* and *Human Factors and Ergonomics in Manufacturing,* for which the center serves as editorial office.

Educational Activities

The center offers customized workshops, seminars, and short courses in applied ergonomics for industry, trade associations, labor unions, and government. The center sponsors international conferences in the areas of industrial ergonomics and safety and human aspects of advanced manufacturing systems.

Consulting Services

The center provides extensive consulting and training services in ergonomics and safety to industry and governmental agencies in Kentucky and other states.

Staff

The center's staff consists of a director, research associates/faculty members, an administrative assistant, graduate research assistants, and an instrumentation technician.

Virginia Tech

Department of Industrial and Systems Engineering
Blacksburg, VA 24061-0118
540-231-5073

The Department of Industrial and Systems Engineering is one of 12 departments in the College of Engineering. Research addresses people/process systems under four graduate option areas, one of which is human factors engineering. Human factors engineering, often called ergonomics, is concerned with designing jobs, machines, operations, and work environments so that they are compatible with human capacities and limitations. The faculty, facilities, and research program in human factors engineering at Virginia Tech are unsurpassed by those of any academic institution in the nation.

Formal Academic Program

Within the Department of Industrial and Systems Engineering, students of human factors engineering can pursue both MS and PhD degrees. Both degree programs emphasize methodology and content areas. Foundation coursework includes a detailed study of existing research, design, and evaluation methods appropriate to human factors engineering. Additionally, content courses address sensory ergonomics (which deals with sensory capabilities and human limitations), physical ergonomics (which deals with biomechanics and work physiology, cognitive ergonomics dealing with human information processing), and macroergonomics (which deals with group processes). This coursework is supplemented by research opportunities in a variety of human factors engineering application areas, including auditory, communication, computer, display, industrial, safety, sociotechnical, training, and transportation systems. The PhD curriculum builds on the MS curriculum and assumes that the graduate student has already had behavioral research experience and has completed a thesis. This degree is heavily oriented toward independent research and the development of expertise in a particular area of ergonomics. Expertise is demonstrated by in-depth interdisciplinary coursework and dissertation research.

Research, Application, and Consultation

The Human Factors Engineering Center is a consortium of research activities representing the current interests of department faculty who are involved in undergraduate and graduate programs in human factors. These faculty members are directly responsible for administering their individual research projects and for providing the necessary personnel, equipment, and facilities to conduct their research.

Seven different laboratories form the Human Factors Engineering Center: Auditory Systems, Displays and Controls, Environmental and Safety, Human-Computer Interaction, Industrial Ergonomics, Macroergonomics and Group Decision Systems, and Vehicle Analysis and Simulation. Work done in a number of these laboratories could be applied to the work environment of the dental care worker.

AUDITORY SYSTEMS

In this laboratory, methods of human factors, behavioral science and acoustics are applied to solve problems related to hearing conservation, auditory information display, driver-display interaction, communications systems, warning systems, product design, and general ergonomics. The facility supports industrial and community investigations as well as controlled laboratory experiments. An example of a research project is "assessment of industrial noise."

DISPLAYS AND CONTROLS

This laboratory is dedicated to research and development work involving visual displays and manual controls systems. The Displays and Controls Laboratory facilities include several rooms that are used for experiments in complex human-system interaction, visual psychophysics and image quality, and manual/voice control, as well as for radiometric measurements, engineering compliance evaluations, software development and device fabrication and repair. The Display and Controls Laboratory also maintains a technical library, which contains over 5000 scientific, industrial, and government documents on significant developments in displays and controls ergonomics.

ENVIRONMENT AND SAFETY

This laboratory consists of experimental rooms, a control and observation room, and an environmental chamber. A one-way mirrored window separates one experimental room from the control and observation room. Research topics in this lab have included the ergonomics of keyboard operations and the effects of blood alcohol levels on the performance of some industrial tasks.

INDUSTRIAL ERGONOMICS

This laboratory consists of one large room, sheltered from external disturbances and environmentally controlled. It can be divided into small compartments as needed for research into topics such as engineering anthropometry; biomechanics of the human body; human engineering of systems; equipment, tools, work stations, and work tasks; and ergonomic design for safety, efficiency, and high performance. Equipment and devices can be taken to outside measuring locations, such as shop floors in industry, work sites in mines, vehicles, and stationary workstations. Applications and consultations include suitability of work seats, assessment of body postures, and selection of chairs.

HUMAN-COMPUTER INTERACTION LABORATORY

This laboratory is dedicated to research on human factors problems associated with systems involving humans and computers. Some of the research topics investigated in this laboratory include training users of computer systems, designing computer systems for users with disabilities, and the design of electronic offices.

MACROERGONOMICS AND GROUP DECISION SYSTEMS

This laboratory is dedicated to the advancement of macroergonomics and sociotechnical systems theory. Macroergonomics is concerned with the research, design, development, and application of organization-machine interface technology. This discipline constitutes a third generation of ergonomics. The first generation was characterized by human-machine interface technology, and the second generation was characterized by user-interface technology. Macroergonomics or "human-organization-environment-machine interface technology," has emerged to provide an interface between organizational design and technology to optimize human-system functioning.

VEHICLE ANALYSIS AND SIMULATION

This laboratory currently has a moving-base driving simulator with supporting computational system. A variety of vehicle research projects are conducted at the laboratory with the collaboration of the Virginia Tech Center for Transportation Research.

Cornell University

College of Human Ecology
Martha Van Rensselaer Hall
Ithaca, NY 14853-4401
607-255-2168

With a student body of more than 16 000 and a faculty of more than 1400, Cornell University offers studies ranging from architecture to veterinary medicine, from art to theoretical physics. The New York State College of Human Ecology at Cornell reflects today's concerns with the quality of the human environment. The Department of Design and Environmental Analysis is one of six academic units in the College of Human Ecology.

The department's resources include design studios, photographic facilities, personal computers, a computer-aided design laboratory, a wood and materials shop, instruments for measuring human response to environments and display galleries. A major area of study within the department is the Human/Environment Relations Major.

Within the Human/Environment Relations Major four concentrations are possible: (1) applied research in human/environment relations, (2) facility planning and management, (3) housing and design, and (4) human factors and ergonomics.

Human Factors and Ergonomics

This concentration applies the knowledge base of human factors and ergonomics to environmental design concerns:

- The design of ambient conditions in the workplace may affect worker performance and well-being. Recent projects have studied the impact of lensed-indirect and

parabolic office lighting systems on the health and productivity of computer workers; the effects of alternative smoking policies on indoor air quality and sick
building syndrome symptoms; the impact of under-
floor ventilation systems on user comfort; and the effects of exposure to electrical and magnetic radiation
from computers.
- Physical design may affect user behavior, performance,
  and attitudes. Recent work includes the effects of work
  stations adjustability on user satisfaction, the ergonomic
  design of seating, and the impact of scientific visualization of computerized facilities survey information on
  diagnostic decision processes.
- User characteristics and skills, as well as task design,
  can improve physical performance. Recent projects include biomechanical analyses of tennis players, hur-
  dlers, gymnasts, as well as analysis of postural risks to
  computer users associated with carpal tunnel syndrome.

Research

The research tradition within the Human/Environment
Relations Major is based on social sciences disciplines, particularly on the discipline of environmental psychology and
human factors. The underlying premise is that systematic,
empirical research based in the social sciences—when combined with imagination—can contribute to the planning, design, and management of environments that enhance individual and organizational effectiveness. Students acquire
competence in research methods and the use of sophisticated
analytical equipment for investigating environmental design
problems. They may conduct empirical research in the Human Factors and Ergonomics Research laboratories. These facilities are well equipped with computers, state-of-the-art analytical instrumentation for measuring a variety of indoor
environmental conditions, and a video-computer motion
analysis system. Students may conduct research in
- field settings (i.e., workplaces, housing, health-care
  settings);
- issue areas (e.g., lighting, indoor air quality);

- user groups (e.g., ergonomic design for the elderly, children, or handicapped); or
- human factors tools (e.g., the development of computer programs, workplace evaluation methods, or multimedia).

Interested students may have an opportunity to work on collaborative projects with companies through the university's Industrial Extension Service.

Degrees Offered

Study in the human factors and ergonomics concentration leads to a Master of Science degree from the graduate school at Cornell University. Required coursework must be successfully completed, and an appropriate thesis based on the student's own research must be submitted.

Chapter 21

Summary

Denise C. Murphy

It is this editor's opinion that sufficient evidence now points to occupational factors as major contributors to the various musculoskeletal conditions seen in dental care workers. However, the etiology of those conditions is an issue that continues to present unanswered questions. The authors of this book have identified some of these unanswered questions and have made recommendations for future research that will help us all to better understand and therefore to prevent and/or control these hazards to our workforce.

Areas for Future Research

1. Can we collect current information about the incidence of musculoskeletal ailments among dental care workers of *all* categories (dental assistants, dental laboratory technicians, etc.)?
2. If corrective or palliative therapy is sought to resolve musculoskeletal ailments, what is the source of therapy— chiropractor, general practitioner, physical therapist, other?
3. What is the impact of ailments upon the individual's ability to work?
4. What is the profile of occupational work styles of dental care workers with musculoskeletal ailments? That is, what are (1) anatomical form and (2) usual and customary position (in the o'clocks) relative to head of patient?
5. Can we identify the physical attributes of work settings in which dental care workers perform their duties and incur musculoskeletal ailments?
6. Was "ergonomics" included in training/curricula that prepared students for their work in dentistry? That is, was the training (1) machine- or equipment-

centered training that necessitated performer adaptation or (2) human- or individual-centered training that accommodated the human performer?

7. Do conditions of work in dentistry prompt an individual to consider alternative occupations?

8. Do minor/significant adaptations allow symptomatic workers to continue working without getting worse?

9. Do small employers have the resources and ability to make ergonomic improvements without the input of professionals?

10. What are the real long-term and short-term effects of surgical-ergonomics training on the health of oral health clinicians? Are the anticipated advantages of improved surgical ergonomics reflected in lower work-related disability claims by dentists, hygienists, and dental assistants?

11. What is the real impact of the use of surgical magnification on health of oral health clinicians?

12. Are there identifiable *unavoidable* risk factors associated with providing dental care?

13. What defensible absolute guidelines can be developed for optimal layout of work site equipment and the use of that equipment in dental operatories?

14. Are all professional categories of dental care workers equally interested in the issues related to ergonomics?

15. After education and tool changes are provided, can we measure improvement via change in symptoms?

16. Can we obtain a better understanding of the relative role of the status of the individual worker and the presence of predisposing factors in the etiology of ergonomics-related disorders?

17. Can we design a nerve conduction or muscle contraction study of the hands when they are doing work with various glove materials and designs covering them? (The materials can be latex, vinyl, and nitrile, and design types can include ambidextrous, left, and right gloves.)

18. Can we modify tools to diminish upper-extremity ergonomic stress?

19. Can we identify new approaches to work methodology that incorporate ergonomic principles?
20. Can we educate dental health professionals in prevention programs that emphasize the need for early interventions?
21. Can we design instruments that will not contribute to cumulative trauma syndrome yet are effective in patient treatment?
22. Can we design an operator stool that will allow maximum support and maintenance of the neutral back?
23. Precisely what wrist movements during patient treatment are the most detrimental (flexion, extension, lateral deviation)—or does it make any real difference?
24. Can we identify practical ways to incorporate ergonomically safe postures and maintain effective patient treatment?
25. Have ergonomic interventions in the dental office reduced injuries and illness, improved the quality of care, or reduced costs?
26. Can we develop screening tools such as checklists adapted specifically to the conditions of dental care professionals? (Most checklists have been designed for industrial or office settings. Including items relevant to dental care might increase the specificity and sensitivity of these checklists.)
27. Can we conduct in-depth analysis? (There is a need to apply suites of methods to analyze the mental and physical demands of specific clinical procedures. Particular emphasis should be placed on methods that assess sensory and manipulative requirements. Such information can help improve tools design as well as scheduling of caseloads.)

Glossary

Abduction. Movement of a limb or digit away from the midline of the body.

Biomechanical factors. Grip force, loading force, arm-wrist angle, and work posture have all been assigned roles in altering surface transmission of vibratory force and in exposing susceptible tissues to greater injury. In general, acceleration and frequency have outstripped all biomechanical factors in their importance.

Body mechanics. Position and movement of the parts of the worker's body in relation to the patient and equipment.

Brachial plexus. A network of nerves that are located in the neck and that extend from the cervical spine and serve the muscles of the wrist, hand, and fingers.

Carpal tunnel. The anatomical space on the palmar side of the hand through which flexor tendons, arteries, and the median nerve enter the hand.

Carpal tunnel syndrome. The constriction of the median nerve within the carpal tunnel, which results in tingling, numbness, weakness.

Chromatic aberrations. Color deviations of a lens system.

Declination angle. The degree to which the eyes are declined (i.e., inclined downward) as a surgeon views a surgical site.

Diffractive viewing effect. A misrepresentation of the real location of the object viewed. This phenomenon can be caused by noncoaxial alignment of telescope oculars and sight lines.

Dominant hand. The hand most often used to perform work.

Extension. The movement by which two ends of a joint are moved away from each other.

Exteroceptive. Pertaining to sensory awareness based on stimuli received by the body from the external environment (e.g., smell, sound, temperature, taste, external pressure, touch).

Flexor tendons. Tendons, located on the ventral side of the arm and wrist, that travel through the carpal tunnel and flex fingers and thumbs.

Frequency range. There has been significant controversy about the extension of frequency range. The various national and international standards have cutoffs in a range of 900 to 1200 Hz. Many investigators extend through 5000 Hz. Very-high-frequency tools such as electrical dental drills have peaks at 15 000 to 20 000 Hz.

Flexion. The act of bending or the condition of being bent; the movement by which two ends of a joint are moved toward each other.

Frequency weighting. The process of down-weighting higher frequencies in the calculation of the summed acceleration. Unweighted frequencies are usually one to two orders of magnitude higher than weighted. In industry, the impact of frequencies over 1000 Hz is negligible, as most gloves and materials are effective dampers. Any evaluation of a personal hygiene item would need to take these adjustments into consideration.

Instruments. Tools, appliances, or apparatuses used to do work.

Knurled. Roughened or ridged; the gripping surface of an instrument handle may be knurled.

Micropauses. Brief interruptions (15 to 30 seconds long) in a given task that allow muscles under strain to rest.

Peak value. The maximal momentary acceleration. This value is used to characterize "impulse" for tools with large vertical displacement. While the crest value is interesting, it is not immediately relevant to the Braun product.

Proprioceptive. Pertaining to sensory awareness based on stimuli received from tissues within the body (e.g., labyrinthine balance and the sense of body and body segment position derived from internal pressure receptors in muscles and tendons).

Repetitive strain injuries. Injuries to the musculoskeletal system caused by repeated or protracted force.

Resonance frequency (RF). The natural frequency at which an object is set in free motion. RFs for the shoulder, neck, and head are all below 20 Hz. The RF for small organelles and physical and humoral receptors appears to be between 100 and 350 Hz. Ultrastructural resonances may occur at much higher frequencies.

Root mean square (rms). The effective time function value of acceleration. Vibration is commonly but not always expressed as an acceleration level. The standard unit is m/sec^2.

Sensorineural. Pertaining to afferent neurological effects.

Static loading. Excessive strain to a muscle unit caused by lack of pauses in work.

Torque. A force that causes torsion or rotation.

Vibration white fingers. A clinical condition characterized by cold-related blanching of the fingers and associated with exposure to vibratory tools.

Index